AF903284

ERECTILE DYSFUNCTION – DISEASE-ASSOCIATED MECHANISMS AND NOVEL INSIGHTS INTO THERAPY

Edited by **Kenia Pedrosa Nunes**

Erectile Dysfunction – Disease-Associated Mechanisms and Novel Insights into Therapy

Edited by Kenia Pedrosa Nunes

Published by InTech

Janeza Trdine 9, 51000 Rijeka, Croatia

Copyright © 2012 InTech

All chapters are articles distributed under the Creative Commons Non Commercial Share Alike Attribution 3.0 license, which permits to copy, distribute, transmit, and adapt the work in any medium, so long as the original work is properly cited. After this work has been published by InTech, authors have the right to republish it, in whole or part, in any publication of which they are the author, and to make other personal use of the work. Any republication, referencing or personal use of the work must explicitly identify the original source.

Statements and opinions expressed in the chapters are these of the individual contributors and not necessarily those of the editors or publisher. No responsibility is accepted for the accuracy of information contained in the published articles. The publisher assumes no responsibility for any damage or injury to persons or property arising out of the use of any materials, instructions, methods or ideas contained in the book.

Technical Editor Sonja Mujacic

Cover Designer InTech Design Team

Additional hard copies can be obtained from orders@intechopen.com

Erectile Dysfunction – Disease-Associated Mechanisms and Novel Insights into Therapy, Edited by Kenia Pedrosa Nunes
p. cm.
ISBN 978-953-51-0199-4

We are IntechOpen, the world's leading publisher of Open Access books

Built by scientists, for scientists

4,100+
Open access books available

116,000+
International authors and editors

120M+
Downloads

151
Countries delivered to

Our authors are among the
Top 1%
most cited scientists

12.2%
Contributors from top 500 universities

WEB OF SCIENCE™

Selection of our books indexed in the Book Citation Index
in Web of Science™ Core Collection (BKCI)

Interested in publishing with us?
Contact book.department@intechopen.com

Numbers displayed above are based on latest data collected.
For more information visit www.intechopen.com

For EU product safety concerns:
IN TECH d.o.o., Prolaz Marije Krucifikse Kozulić 3, 51000 Rijeka, Croatia,
info@intechopen.com or visit our website at intechopen.com.

Meet the editor

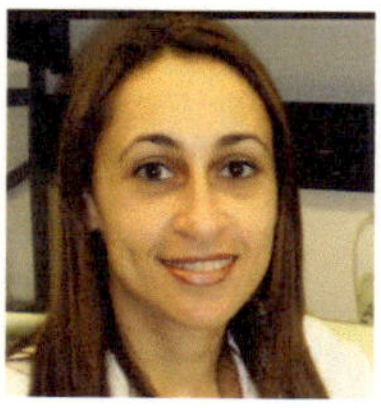

Dr Nunes has a background in physiology and pharmacology. She served as a professor of physiology in Brazil, where she started her research on erectile dysfunction (ED). She is currently a postdoctoral fellow in a laboratory specializing in vascular physiology at Georgia Health Sciences University, where her research is focused on vascular mechanisms in ED and associated diseases, such as hypertension and diabetes. Her projects involve intense collaboration with experts in the United States and Brazil. Dr Nunes' research has been supported by the American Heart Association over the last two years. She has to her credit more than 10 peer-reviewed manuscripts, book chapters and an international patent regarding pharmaceutical compositions to improve erectile function.

Contents

Preface

I am delighted to bring you the Erectile Dysfunction (ED) book. Organizing this book was an enlightening experience and an amazing adventure in science. Considering the breadth and depth of information available in the continuously expanding field of ED, this book provides information ranging from the basic mechanism of erectile function and dysfunction to updates regarding most discussed topics in ED nowadays, such as association between ED and cardiovascular diseases. Although ED disorder has been described for more than 1,000 years, the molecular basis and mechanisms of ED have yet to be completely understood. Over the last four decades, elucidation of the macroscopic structures of the erectile system ushered in a new era of therapeutic options for erectile disorders. Later, new insights into erectile neurotransmission, essentially the nitric oxide (NO) pathway, resulted in rational alternatives as a treatment. Nowadays, advances in gene discovery and intensive research regarding different mechanisms that could lead to ED have increased the working knowledge of the pathways involved in this condition. However, many questions still need to be elucidated.

This book contains chapters written by widely acknowledged experts, each of which provides a unique synthesis of information on emergent aspects of ED. All chapters take into account not only new perspectives on ED but also recent extensions of basic knowledge that presage directions for further research. The approach in this book has been to not only describe the recent popular aspects of ED, such as basic mechanism updates, etiologic factors and pharmacotherapy, but also disease-associated ED and some future perspectives in this field.

ED is a widespread problem affecting many men across all age groups and it is more than a serious quality of life problem for sexually active men. The prevalence of ED is very high and is expected to rise considerably over the next 25 years, affecting more than 300 million men by 2025. ED is a multifactorial pathology and has recently been observed as a condition that may predict cardiovascular disease, making the knowledge in this area extremely important to prevent future diseases. Finally, to you, our readers, even though this book is a small overview of ED field, I hope that it provides enough useful and updated information that you will consider joining us in studying this condition. In addition, for readers who are not physicians, I wish that basic information as well as a scientific overview about research in ED can be acquired from this work.

I would like to thank Dr R. Clinton Webb, Professor and Chairperson of the Physiology Department at Georgia Health Sciences University, for his help and advice in the preparation of this edition. Many thanks are also due to Dr Maria Elena De Lima and Dr Romulo Leite for introducing me to the scientific research world. Special thanks to my co-workers, as well as to my parents, Feliciano (*in memoriam*) and Conceição, who have always been behind the scenes supporting me. It would not be fitting for me to conclude this preface without a major acknowledgment to my beloved husband, Russell Bruhn. My husband's journalistic experience in reading and revising many parts of this book was an indispensable aid in accomplishing this work.

As it is inevitable when preparing a text, in addition to my own experience, I have called upon the help and advice of many others as I have in ten years or since I started research in this field. Thus, I'm deeply grateful to all the people who made this book possible.

Comments on this edition will be welcome.

Kenia Pedrosa Nunes
Georgia Health Sciences University, Augusta, Georgia
USA

Part 1

An Introduction of ED

1

Mechanisms in Erectile Function and Dysfunction: An Overview

Kenia Pedrosa Nunes and R. Clinton Webb
Georgia Health Sciences University, Augusta, Georgia
USA

1. Introduction

Erectile dysfunction (ED) is a widespread problem affecting many men across all age groups and it is more than a serious quality of life problem for sexually active men. Over 30 million men suffer from ED in the U.S. [1] and it is becoming a public health issue. The prevalence of ED is very high and is expected to raise considerably over the next 25 years, impacting more than 300 million men by 2025 [2]. ED is defined as the persistent inability to maintain or achieve a penile erection sufficient for satisfactory sexual performance. Its etiology is multifactorial. Various aspects affect the expression/degree of ED and risk factors include age, diabetes mellitus, neurologic diseases, smoking and cardiovascular diseases (CVD), among others [3]. Although the disorder has been described for more than 1000 years, the molecular basis and mechanisms of ED have yet to be completely understood. In the last 4 decades, elucidation of the macroscopic structures of the erectile system [4-5] ushered in a new era of therapeutic options for erectile disorders. Later, new insights into erectile neurotransmission, [6] essentially the nitric oxide (NO) pathway, [7] resulted in rational alternatives as a treatment [8]. Nowadays, advances in gene discovery and intensive research regarding different mechanisms which could lead to ED have increased the working knowledge of the pathways involved in this condition. This chapter will describe the basic penile physiology and the emergent mechanisms associated to pathophisiology of vasculogenic ED. Penile anatomy and physiology will be summarized in order to review the new insights regarding pathways and critical modifications observed in ED condition.

2. Penile anatomy

The penis is composed of three bodies of erectile tissue running in paralel; the corpus spongiosum, encompassing the urethra and terminating in the glans penis; and the two corpora cavernosa (CC) which function as blood-filled capacitors providing structure to the erect organ [9]. The penile CC are highly specialized vascular structures that are morphologically adapted to their function of becoming engorged during sexual arousal. The trabecular smooth muscle constitutes approximately 40-50% of tissue cross-sectional area, as assessed by histomorphometric analysis [10]. There are three main arteries in the penis: cavernosal, dorsal, and bulbourethral. All three arise from a shared branch of the internal pudendal artery and provide an extensive anastomotic network [11]. Nowadays, there is a tendency to perform *in vitro* experiments using the pudendal artery instead of cavernosal tissue to investigate patophysiological aspects of ED since this artery is the major resistance to penile engogerment during sexual stimulation. Novel findings suggest that the pudendal artery contributes 70% of the total penile vascular resistence [12]. The arterial blood supply in the CC is mainly fed from the deep penile cavernosal artery [9], which causes corporal enlargement during erection, whereas the deep dorsal artery causes glans enlargement. Venous drainage is not similar to arterial supply; there exists only one deep dorsal vein that runs alongside the dorsal arteries and nerves in Buck's fascia above the tunica albuginea, which is a multilayered structure where emissary veins pass. The human penile venous system is generally described as a single deep dorsal vein accompanied by a pair of dorsal arteries positioned between the tunica albuginea and Buck's fascia for the venous drainage [13]. The corpus spongiosum is erectile tissue analogous to CC, but with a thinner tunica albuginea. The urethra lies within the spongiosum. The innervations of the penis is both autonomic (sympathetic and parasympathetic) and somatic (sensory and motor). From the neurons in the spinal cord and peripheral ganglia, the sympathetic and parasympathetic nerves merge to form the cavernous nerves, which enter in the CC and corpus spongiosum to affect the neurovascular events during tumescence and detumescence [14].

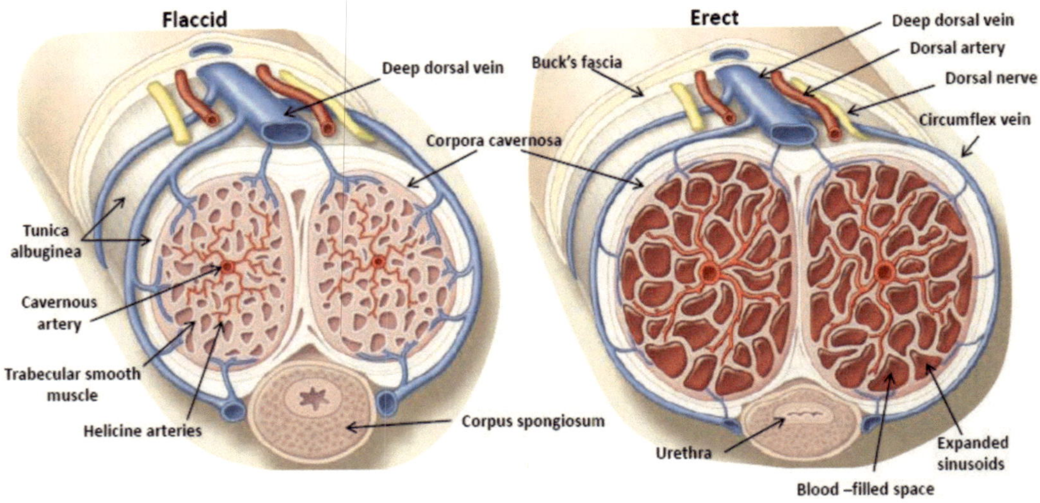

Fig. 1. Penile anatomy. Adapted from Fazio and Brock , 2004.[15]

3. Physiology of Penile Erection

Penile erection (PE) involves central and peripheral pathways. Tumescence is initiated after central processing and integration of tactile, visual, olfactory and imaginative stimuli. Upon sexual stimulation, signals are generated to the peripheral tissues involved. Thus, final response is mediated by coordinated spinal activity in the autonomic pathways to the penis, and also in the somatic pathways to the perineal striated muscles. Both central and peripheral regulation of PE involves several neurotransmitters and systems, of which details are still not completely known. Spinally, there seems to be a network consisting of primary afferents from the genitals, spinal interneurons, sympathetic, parasympathetic and somatic nuclei, which is capable of integrating all information. Peripherally, the balance between substances that control the degree of contraction of the cavernosal smooth muscle determines the functional state of the penis [16]. The dynamic interplay of vasoconstrictors and vasodilators in the penis establish the erect or flaccid state.

PE is determined by pressure changes in the cavernosal arterioles and sinuses. The vasculature of the erectile mechanism differs from most vascular beds as it is composed of arterioles and hallow blood-filled sinuses, both which are lined with smooth muscle and endothelial cells [14] as previously described. In the flaccid state, this tissue is tonically contracted, allowing only a small amount of arterial flow for nutritional purposes. The partial pressure of oxygen (PO2) in the blood is around 35mmHg [17]. On the other hand, dilation of the penile arteries is the first event in the development of erection. Its consequence is the increase of blood flow and pressure into the lacunar space. Then, the expansion of sinusoids blocks the incoming blood. Also, venous outflow is reduced by compression of venular spaces between the tunica albuginea and peripheral sinusoids. This stretches the tunica to its capacity and decreases the venous outflow to a minimum, leading to an increase in intracavernosal pressure, which is maintained at approximately 100mmHg (2). Thus, erection includes sinusoidal relaxation, arterial dilation and venous compression (3).

3.1 Mechanisms mediating erection and penile relaxation

In general, mechanisms leading to normal erectile function imply inter-connections among neurons, striated perineal muscles and androgens which are responsible for maintaining sexual behavior in adults. Locally, the stage of penile erection requires relaxation of cavernosal smooth muscle. It is triggered by release of substances from parasympathetic and non-adrenergic non-cholinergic nerves (NANC), which in turn promotes vascular and cavernosal relaxation, leading to an increase in blood flow and intracavernosal pressure resulting in erection (Figure 1). Although several vasodilators have been implicated in this process, nitric oxide (NO) still is the main vasodilator involved [18-19]. In the penis, stimulation of parasympathetic nerves inhibits noradrenalin release and evokes acetylcholine (Ach) release, which binding to muscarinic receptors in endothelial cells promoting eNOS activation and consequently NO production. Cholinergic nerves have been demonstrated within the human cavernous smooth muscle and surrounding penile arteries and ultrastructural examination has also identified terminals containing cholinergic vesicules in the same area [20]. Two decades ago, it was suggested that NO released from NANC increases the production of 3′,5′-cyclic guanosine monophosphate (cGMP), which in turn relaxes the cavernosal smooth muscle [7, 21]. Nowadays, it is well known that NO plays a critical role in erectile function. NO is formed from the precursor amino acid, L-arginine, by enzymatic action of NOS, which exists as three main isoforms: neuronal NOS (nNOS), inducible (iNOS), and endothelial NOS (eNOS). All three isoforms have been detected in the penis, although nNOS and eNOS are the main constitutively active NOS enzymes expressed in penile tissues [22], it is activated by calcium entry into the cell, binding to calmodulin associated with enzymes [23].

There are two main intracellular mechanisms for relaxing the cavernosal smooth muscle: the guanylate cyclase (GS)/cGMP and adenylate cyclase/cAMP pathways (Figure 3). NO is associated with GS/cGMP signaling, called NO/cGMP pathway. Upon its release, NO diffuses locally into adjacent smooth muscle cells of the corpus cavernosum and binds to soluble guanylyl cyclase (GC), which catalyzes the conversion of guanosine trisphosphate (GTP) to cGMP. This cyclic nucleotide then activates protein kinase G, also known as

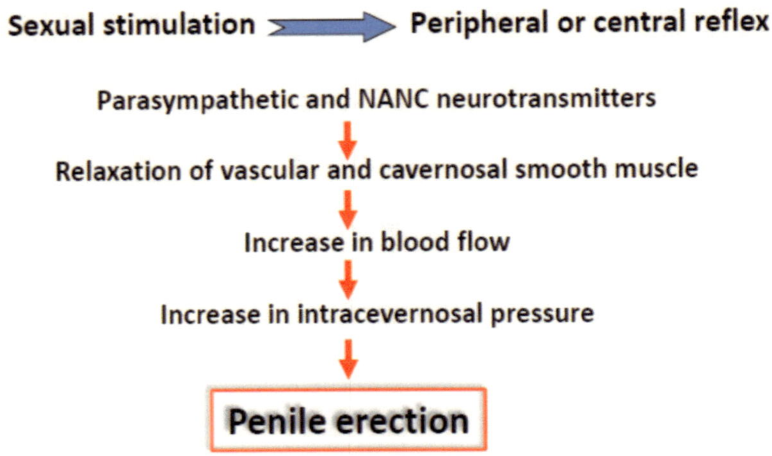

Fig. 2. Sequence of events required for penile erection. Upon sexual stimulation, substances such as Ach and NO are released from endothelial cells, parasympathetic and NANC neuronal endings evoking vascular relaxation and consequently increase in blood flow. Thus, there is an increase in intracavernosal pressure resulting in penile erection.

cGMP-dependent protein kinase I (cGKI), which decreases cytosolic Ca^{2+} by various mechanisms. cGMP also blocks RhoA migration avoiding Rho-kinase pathway activation, which is a step very important to penile relaxation. The decay in cytosolic Ca^{2+} concentration induces relaxation of the vascular and cavernosal smooth muscle cells, leading to dilation of arterial vessels, increased blood flow into the corpora cavernosa, and penile erection (Figure 3). Contributing to penile relaxation, substances such as prostaglandin E1 (PGE1) can bind to G protein coupled receptors and activate the enzyme adenylate cyclase, which catalyzes the conversion of adenosine monophosphate (AMP) to cyclic AMP (cAMP). This cyclic nucleotide activates protein kinase A (PKA), which also decreases the intracellular Ca^{2+}. PGE1, injected intracavernosally, alone or in combination, is today the second-line treatment for ED [24]. These second messengers, cGMP and cAMP activate protein kinase (PKG and PKA respectively), which in turn phosphorylate certain proteins and ion channels, resulting in opening of the potassium channels and hyperpolarization, sequestration of intracellular Ca+2 by the endoplasmatic reticulum, and inhibition of voltage-dependent Ca^{+2} channels, blocking the Ca^{+2} influx [25]. Both, cGMP and cAMP levels are modulated by phosphodiesterase (PDE) enzymes, which cleave these signaling molecules to 5′GMP and 5′AMP, respectively (Figure 3). Phosphodisterase-5 (PDE-5) is a key enzyme in the NO/cGMP signal transduction pathway and functions to restrain smooth muscle cells relaxation and erectile process [18]. Predominantly expressed in CC, PDE-5 catalyzes the hydrolysis cGMP to the inactive metabolite 5′GMP. Nowadays, the PDE5 inhibitors are the first-line treatment for ED [26].

Another mechanism which has been demonstrated to be involved in maintenance of the erectile process is the phosphatidylinositol 3-kinase (PI3-kinase) pathway that activates the serine/threonine protein kinase Akt (also known as PKB). It causes direct phosphorylation of eNOS, reducing the enzyme's calcium requirement and causing increased production of NO. It has been suggested that rapid, brief activation of nNOS initiates the erectile process, whereas PI_3-kinase/Akt-dependent phosphorylation and activation of eNOS by augmented blood flow and endothelial shear stress lead to sustained NO production and maximal erection [27].

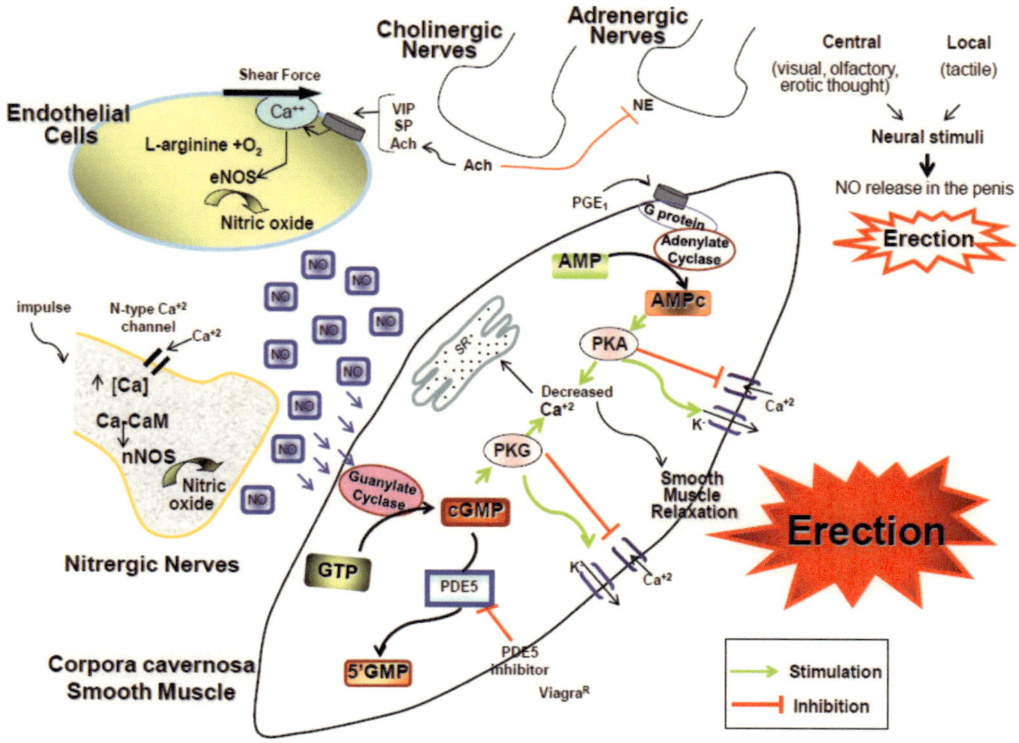

Fig. 3. Regulation of cavernosal smooth muscle relaxation by NO released from the nitrergic nerve and sinusoidal endothelium. Central and/or local excitation evoke stimulation of the endothelial cells and nitrergic nerves in the penis, causing Ca^{+2} influxes which promote eNOS and nNOS activation, increasing NO production. NO binds to soluble guanylate cyclase (GC) inside cavernous muscle smooth catalyzing the conversion of GTP in cyclic GMP (cGMP). AMPc and high levels of cGMP result in vasodilatation of arteries and sinusoidal spaces of the corpus cavernosum, by decreasing intracellular calcium concentration, which is due to activation of PKA and PKG, leading consequently to erection. In addition, PKA and PKG cause inhibition of calcium channels and activation of potassium channels. Abbreviations: CaM, calmodulin; nNOS, neuronal nitric oxide synthase; eNOS, endothelial nitric oxide synthase; GTP, guanosine triphosphate; GMP, guanosine monophosphate; cGMP, cyclic GMP; PDE5, phosphodiesterase type 5; PKG, protein kinase G; PKA, protein kinase A.

3.2 Flaccidity and detumescense

Rich adrenergic enervation found in the penis, mainly surrounding the cavernosal arteries, and norepinephrine has been suggested as the chief neurotransmitter derived from the symphatetic nervous system to control flaccidity and detumescense [8, 28]. Also, the penis is kept in the flaccid state due to endothelins. Penile smooth muscle cells not only respond to, but also synthesize, endotelin-1 (ET-1)[29]. Vasoconstriction in erectile tissue induced by ET-1 appears to be predominantly mediated by ET_A receptor. In the penis, ET-1/ET_A receptor-mediated biological effects involve activation of the inositol trisphosphate (IP_3)/calcium (Ca^{2+}) and RhoA/Rho-kinase signaling pathways [30]. However, both ET_A and ET_B receptors have been found in human CC smooth muscle membranes, and it cannot be excluded that both receptor subtypes are functional [28]. The role of ET_B receptors in the CC has not been clarified. This receptor activation is known to possibly induce a NO-mediated decrease in penile vascular tone [31].

The intracellular mechanism in the absence of arousal stimuli, initiates with activation of G proteins following ligand binding to membrane receptors in order to keep cavernosal arterioles and sinuses constricted, maintaining the penis in the non-erect state. Subsequently to G protein activation, two signaling pathways are brought into play to cause smooth muscle contraction in the arterioles and cavernosum: the well characterized Ca^{+2} dependent pathway (phopholipase C) and the recently identified RhoA/Rho-kinase pathway know as Ca^{+2} sensitization. The Rho-kinase pathway is intrinsically involved with the process of smooth muscle contraction. The Ca^{2+} sensitivity of smooth muscle reflects the ratio of activities of MLCP to myosin light-chain kinase (MLCK), resulting in contraction or relaxation. Activation of G-protein coupled receptors by several agonists such as endothelin, angiotensin II, and noradrenalin, leads to the exchange of GDP for GTP on the small monomeric GTPase RhoA. This event actives RhoA and is catalyzed by the guanine nucleotide exchange factors, which causes dissociation of RhoA from its biding partner, Rho-guanine dissociation inhibitor. As a result, RhoA translocates from the cytosol to the membrane, allowing the downstream activation of several effectors such as Rho-kinase. Phophorylation of the regulatory subunit of MLC phophatase by Rho kinase causes inhibition phosphatase activity, which increases the contractile response at a constant intracellular calcium concentration [32]. It is now widely accepted that MLCK and the RhoA/Rho-kinase pathway are two major cellular targets for regulating Ca^{2+} sensitivity of myosin light chain, and they generally operate in parallel. RhoA/Rho-kinase activity is a fundamental component to keep the penis in the non-erect state, and this pathway is upregulated in ED. Also, the essential balance between contraction and relaxation in the penis, which is maintained by the RhoA/Rho-kinase and NO/cyclicGMP pathways, is modified in this pathology [33-34]. It has been demonstrated that Rho-kinase antagonism stimulated rat penile erection independently of NO suggesting that this principle could be a potential alternative for ED treatment [35-36]. Many studies have suggested that NO inhibits RhoA/Rho-kinase activity [37-38]. Increased of RhoA/Rho-kinase activity may lead to abnormal contractility of the CC and has been suggested to be involved not only in ED, but in several diseases which are risk factors for ED such as hypertension and diabetes [39].

Another mechanism involved in penile vasoconstriction in absence of arousal stimuli, is the phospholipase C (PLC) pathway. The stimulation of PLC occurs through the binding of vasoconstrictors agonists, such as norepinephrine (NE), angiotensin II (Ang II), endothelin-1 (ET-1) and others, to their respective receptors. PLC hydrolyzes phosphatidylinositol 4,5-biphosphate (PIP_2) to release IP_3 (inositol 1,4,5-trisphosphate) and DAG (1,2-diacylglycerol). IP_3 binds to specific receptors (IP_3R) on the endoplasmatic reticulum (ER) to stimulate the release of $Ca+^2$ from the intracellular stores. DAG directly stimulates protein kinase C (PKC), which can regulate smooth muscle tone by controlling ion channels, allowing Ca^{+2} influx. PKC also phosphorylates multiple substrates to facilitate contraction (figure 4).

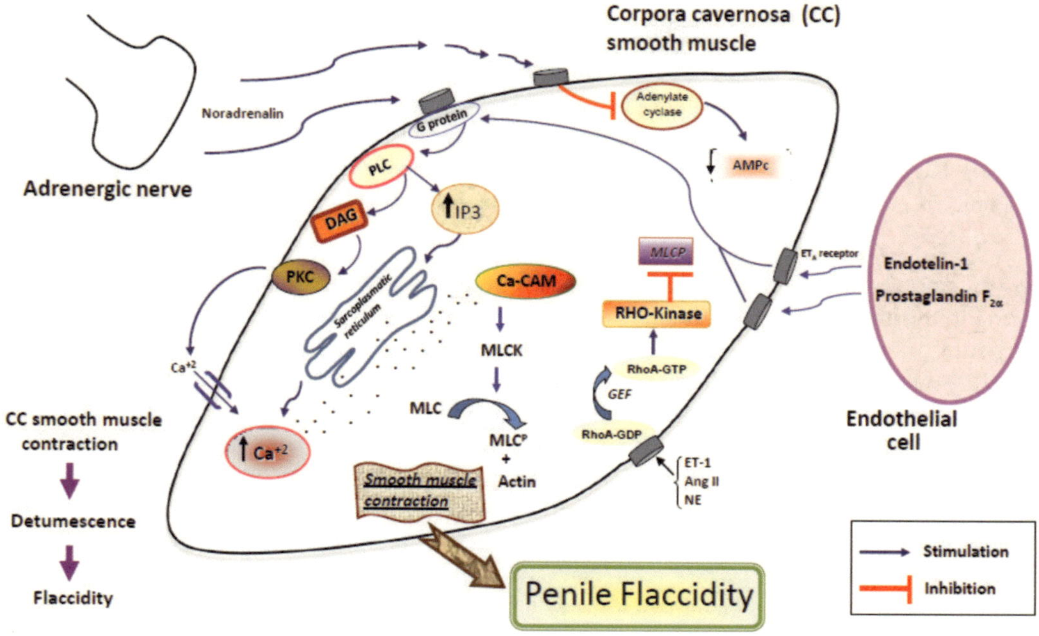

Fig. 4. Regulation of cavernosal smooth muscle contraction leading to penile flaccidity. Pathways mediating the contraction of smooth muscle in CC, which is regulated by an increase in cytosolic Ca^{+2}, are illustrated.

4. Emergent mechanisms associated with ED

Various aspects of neurotransmission, impulse propagation, and intracellular transduction of signals in penile smooth muscle remain to be elucidated. Nevertheless, the information about mechanisms involved in erection is quickly increasing and details regarding new pathways are constantly being added. The renin-angiotensin system (RAS), TNF-α, MAP Kinases and arginase II are some of the new insights in this field.

4.1 Renin-angiotensin system

In the past decade, it has become apparent that the renin-angiotesin system (RAS) is involved in the regulation of ED. There is evidence that the local RAS exists within the CC [40] and that several active peptides, particularly angiotensin II (Ang II), may be involved in the erectile mechanism. Ang II is the main effector of RAS that regulates important physiologic functions. The conventional idea of RAS as a systemic system has been extended recently. Many organs and tissues have components of RAS, working in a paracrine manner [41]. Tissue RAS synthesizes Ang II locally and is modulated independently of systemic RAS. It has been demonstrated that Ang II activates the RhoA/Rho-kinase pathway via AT_1 receptor, which is dominantly expressed in the smooth muscle and endothelial cells of the blood vessel wall, leading to the inhibition of myosin light chain phosphatase (MLCP) [42-43]. Another significant function of AT_1 is to activate nicotinamide adenine dinucleotide phosphate (NADPH) oxidase, increasing reactive oxygen species (ROS) production. ROS rapidly react with NO, reducing its bioavailability, and also stimulate RhoA/Rho-kinase activity[44-45]. Additionally, both Ang II [46] and AT_1 [47] were detected in endothelial and smooth muscle cells from CC, and comparing the different stages of penile flaccidity, tumescence, rigidity, and detumescence, Ang II levels were significantly higher during detumescence [47]. Human CC produces and secretes physiological amounts of Ang II, as much as 200-fold greater than that in plasma[46]. Furthermore, *in vivo* experiments demonstrated that injection of Ang II into the CC terminated spontaneous erections observed in anesthetized dogs[46]. Chronic infusion of exogenous Ang II for 4 weeks induced ED in Sprague-Dawley rats [48]. It seems that RAS is crucial in ED [49].

Reinforcing the association of RAS and ED, agiotensin-converting enzyme (ACE) has been found in the endothelial cells of dog CC [50], and ACE mRNA expression is up-regulated in a rat model of arteriogenic ED, although it is expressed at very low levels in the penis of control rat[51]. Results from human CC smooth muscle showed that Ang II and NO interact to modulate penile function, since an AT_1 antagonist potentiated sodium nitroprusside (a NO donor) and electrical field stimulation mediated CC relaxation. Also, the authors suggested that Ang II response involves the production of superoxide and the development of oxidative stress [52]. Taken together, evidence from many studies suggests that the main function of the RAS system is Ang II-mediated contraction, contributing to maintenance of the penis in a flaccid state. However, the RAS system consists of two major arms: a vasoconstrictor/proliferative arm in which the major mediator is Ang II acting on AT_1 receptors, and a vasodilator/antiproliferative arm in which the main effector is Ang-(1-7) acting via G protein-coupled recetors Mas [53]. The Ang-(1-7)-Mas axis may play an important role in penile erection. This receptor has been observed in rat CC, and it has been demonstrated that Ang-(1-7) acts as a mediator of penile erection by activation of Mas and subsequent NO release. Additionally, in the absence of Mas erectile function was severely compromised [54].

4.2 TNF-α

The emerging role for tumor necrosis factor-alpha (TNF-α) in ED has been discussed. It is a pro-inflammatory cytokine originally defined by its antitumoral activity and is involved in many cardiovascular diseases (CVD), including heart-failure and atherosclerosis[55-56]. In these diseases, TNF-α plasma levels are significantly increased and the vascular endothelium is the major target for the actions of TNF-α. *In vivo* administration of this cytokine induces impairment of endothelium-dependent relaxation in a diversity of vascular beds and decreases the release of NO [57]. Endothelium dysfunction is a key event in the pathophysiology of ED and, importantly, endothelium dysfunction is impaired in the presence of increased oxidative stress and inflammatory conditions[55]. A low-grade inflammatory process is associated with several CVD, and accordingly, cytokines levels, including TNF-α, are increased in response to inflammation and contribute to the changes in vascular reactivity observed in these conditions[58-59]. TNF-α has been described as an important contributor to many cardiovascular disorders[55]. Patients with ED present increased expression and elevated plasma levels of inflammatory markers and mediators among them TNF-α [60], which have been also observed in patients with hypertension. An emerging basic science and clinical data base provides a strong argument for endothelial and smooth muscle dysfunction as a central etiologic factor in systemic and peripheral vascular diseases, such as ED. It has been raising the idea of ED as an early sign of CVD [61]. Once CDV appears right after ED and after the levels of TNF-α start to increase [62-63], seems that this cytokine may represent not only a common point between ED and CVD, but its increasing levels associated with ED may be a predictor of cardiovascular events[64].

TNF-α has been associated with Rho-kinase signaling in endothelial cells. This cytokine not only induces inflammatory gene transcription, but also activation of RhoA and Rho-kinase[65]. In addition, TNF-α leads to increased Ca^{+2} sensitivity via activation of the RhoA/ROCK pathway, a mechanism that may contribute not only to TNF-α-induced airway hyperresponsiveness and hyperreactivity [66-67]. It was recently demonstrated that TNF-α KO mice shown increased number of spontaneous erections, also these animals have enhanced nNOS expression in CC tissue[68] , which suggests that TNF-α down regulates nNOS expression in this tissue [68]. In another work, the same authors showed that TNF-α-infused mice displays decreased NANC-dependent relaxation and increased symphathetic-mediated concentrations in vivo, which would contribute to penile detumecesce to occur [69]. Enhanced direct adrenergic responses were also observed in CC tissue from these animals, and it was suggested that downregulation of eNOS and nNOS may be the mechanism underlying the functional modifications in CC strips from TNF-α infused mice [69]. Endothelin-1 not only induces vasoconstriction, but it also stimulates the expression of adhesion molecules and activates transcriptional factors responsible for the coordinated increase in the expression of many cytokines and enzymes, which can in turn lead to the production of inflammatory mediators [70]. Additionally, RAS system and Ang II, the main known mediator of RAS, induces vascular injury through many mechanisms, including vasoconstriction, oxidative stress and inflammation. Both peptides have been shown to increase TNF-α levels and this pro-inflammatory cytokine also positively regulates release of these vasoactive peptides[71-72]. Finally, sexual performance has been negatively associated with circulating levels of endothelial inflammatory parameters [73]. Further studies are necessary to better clarify the role of TNF-α in ED and its mechanism in CC dysfunction. The positive point is that now we have access to target anti-TNF-α a therapy.

4.3 Arginase

The involvement of arginase in ED has been evident in recent years. Arginase catalyses the conversion of L-arginine to ornithine plus urea. Arginase exists in two isoforms, the hepatic type, arginase I and the extrahepatic type, arginase II [74]. Both isoforms are expressed in human CC tissue [75], but it seems that arginase II is the predominant isoform involved in ED mainly when this condition is associated with age and diabetes [76-77]. In mammalian cells, L-arginine is used as a substrate by both NOS and arginase. NO is derived from L-arginine by nitric oxide synthase (NOS) and both endothelial (eNOS) and neuronal (nNOS) isoforms of the CC serve as sources to generate essential levels of NO. NO production depends on NOS activity and NOS protein expression. On the other hand, NO production absolutely depends on the availability of L-arginine to NOS, since NOS shares L-arginine as a common substrate with arginase [78]. Considering this, L-arginine catabolism via the arginase pathway can act as an endogenous negative control system to regulate overall NO production. ED mechanisms involve oxidative stress and vascular inflammation [79], both of which have been associated with enhanced arginase activity and expression in the vasculature [77]. Recently, it has been demonstrated that diabetes-induced ED involves elevated arginase activity and expression [80]. Also, previous studies suggest that arginase activity in the CC is increased by hyperglycemia and aging [81].

Aging-associated ED involves abnormalities at multiple levels of the NO/cGMP signaling in the penis. These include reduced NANC nerve fibers in CC, decreased constitutive NOS activity, impaired endothelium-dependent smooth muscle relaxation and reduced NO bioavailability [82-83]. It has been observed that dietary L-arginine supplementation as well as acute infusion of L-arginine results in improved NO release and increased endothelium-dependent vasodilatation in the penis [84]. The basis by which L-arginine supplementation can improve the endothelial function and NO release is questionable. Studies have been shown that eNOS expression is upregulated with advanced age in the penis and in peripheral vasculature. However, eNOS activity is reduced such that, for any given concentration of L-arginine, vascular production of NO is reduced [85-86]. Nowadays, we have evidence of a biological role of arginase in regulating erectile function in the aged penile vascular bed at both the molecular and functional level. It has been demonstrated that penile endothelial cells isolated from the aged mouse penis overexpressed arginase and, as a result, decreased eNOS activity and impaired vascular function. Moreover, inhibition of arginase via an adeno-associated virus (AVV) gene transfer of anti-arginase in this tissue increases penile eNOS activity and cGMP levels, thus restoring endothelial-derived NO vasodilatation and erectile function [79], speculating that an antisence for arginase may represent a novel molecular therapeutic target for the treatment of age-associated vasculogenic ED. Regarding diabetes- associated ED, reduced nitrergic and endothelial dependent smooth muscle relaxation, as well as arginase activation and diminished NO production are involved [87-88]. In addition, it has been well documented that a major causative factor contributing to ED in diabetic patients is the reduction in the amount of NO synthesis in CC. Recently, it was demonstrated that arginase II deletion prevents diabetes-impairment in CC relaxation [80]. Since a specific arginase inhitor is not available, in this study they used diabetic arginase II knockout mice. These animals did not exhibit increased arginase activity and expression, as well as decreased nNOS and phospho-eNOS (at Ser-1177 and Thr-495) levels. Arginase has been involved in sexual disorders not only in men, but also in women. Administration of arginase inhibitors *in vitro* and *in vivo* enhances engorgement in male and female genitalia [89]. There is no doubt that arginase is involved in ED. However, more complete understanding about the exact mechanism leading to disruption of erectile dynamic by arginase is necessary, as well as further research.

4.4 MAP-Kinases

Mitogen-activated protein kinases (MAPK) are a group of serine/threonine protein kinases which play an important role in cellular process, such as proliferation, stress response apoptosis and immune defense [90]. The extracellular-signal-regulated kinase 1/2 (ERK1/2), p38 MAPK and the JUN N-terminal kinase (JNK) are the three most defined MAPK pathways [91]. Not long ago, evidence of involvement of ERK1/2 and p38 MAPK in the ED began. It seems that these MAPKs are indirectly associated with NOS regulation, which affects NO avaibility. It has been observed that ERK plays a key role in eNOS regulation [92]. In addition, phosphorylation of eNOS catalysed by ERK can lead to enzyme inhibition, and it was shown that *in vivo* phosphorylation of eNOS by ERK is associated with a reduction in enzyme activity. ERK inhibits eNOS by phosphorylating the enzyme in endothelial cells [92]. ERK has been involved in various pathological conditions; one major mechanism involved in the regulation of inflammatory processes is the activation of ERK [93]. Regarding cavernosal tissue, an inhibitory influence on activity of eNOS by ERK has been described in humans [94].

The first study showing a link between ERK1/2 and the CC was published in 2002 and the authors demonstrated that this kinase is present and active in human CC. Also, they found that the endothelial expression of ERK was more pronounced than muscular expression, and tissue from patients with ED showed a higher expression of the active ERK [94]. ERK can be triggered by cellular stresses such as oxidative stress and hyperglycemia, which play an important role in the development of diabetic complications [95], a disease associated with ED. Recently, it was demonstrated that ERK inhibition decreases arginase activity and improves CC relaxation in streptozotocin (STZ)-induced diabetic mice (Nunes, 2011). Hyperglycemia in STZ-induced diabetic mice stimulates adipogenic induction of lipid accumulation and

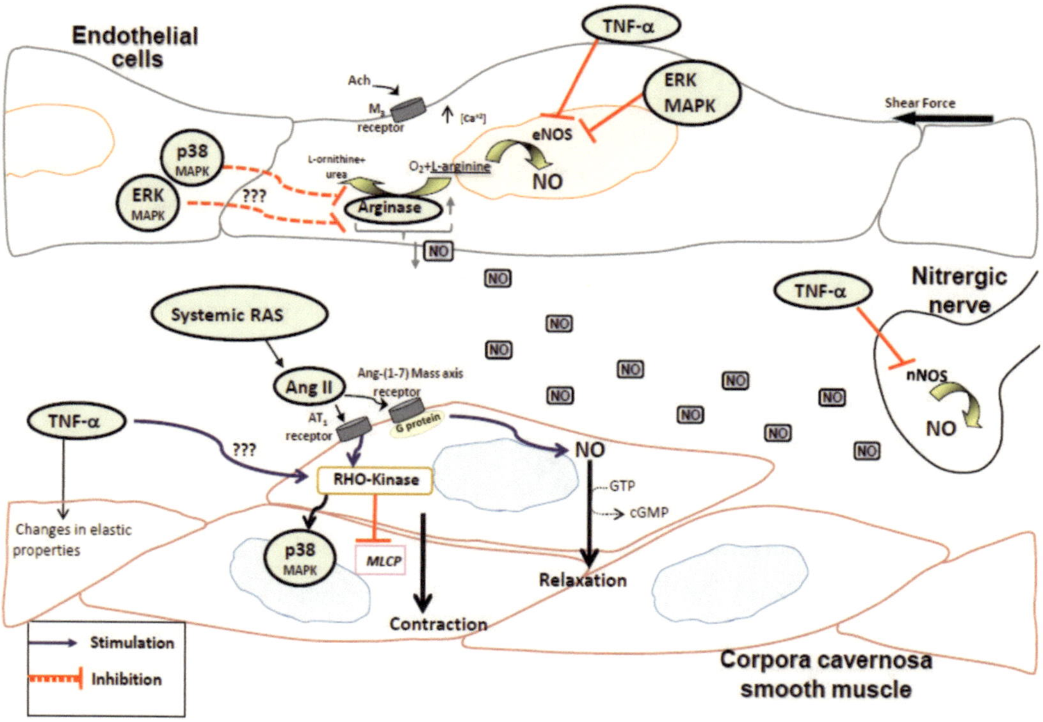

Fig. 5. Emergent pathways involved in ED. The influence of renin-angiotensin system (RAS), TNF-α, ERK and P38 MAPK, and Arginase II in ED are illustrated. Tissue RAS synthesizes Ang II locally, which acts via two different receptors: AT-1, leading to activation of RHO-kinase and consequently MLPC inhibition, contributing to penile flaccid, or Ang-1-7 Mass axis G-protein coupled receptor evoking NO release and facilitating CC relaxation. Additionally, Ang II can activates p38, which is involved in NOS regulation. TNF-α promotes downregulation of eNOS and nNOS, contributing to ED. In addition, TNF-α may lead to increased Ca^{+2} sensitivity, via activation of the RhoA/ROCK pathway, (???) in the penis. Since arginase and eNOS share L-arginine as a common substrate, increased arginase activity can limit NO availability, making the erectile function difficulty. ERK and p38 MAPKs are indirectly associated with NOS regulation, which affects NO avaibility. Inhibitors for ERK and p38 in CC tissue resulted in decreased arginase activity, suggesting an association between these kinases and arginase. However, this mechanism in ED still needs be clarified.

involves ERK signaling pathway [96]. Also, neuropathy is a common complication of long-term diabetes [97]. Accordingly, the recent study showed that diabetes increased expression of activated ERK and arginase activity in CC and this effect was blocked by acute treatment with PD98059 (an ERK inhibitor). Also, the impaired cavernosal relaxation from STZ-diabetic mice was attenuated by treatment with an ERK inhibitor, observed in nitrergic and endothelium-dependent relaxation responses. The authors suggested that ERK inhibition prevents the elevation of penile arginase activity and protects against ED caused by diabetes [98]. However, the mechanism involving ERK and arginase in ED is unclear and needs to be better understood.

There are a few studies associating ERK and P38 MAPK with ED. RhoA/Rho-kinase has been indicated as an upstream regulator of MAPK family members such as p38 MAPK [99]. Increased p38 MAPK in response to stress stimuli, including hyperglycemia, contributes to diabetic somatic neuropathy [100]. The first study connecting ED and p38 demonstrated that inhibition of p38 MAPK corrects nitrergic neurovascular function in diabetic mice CC [101]. It has been described that Ang II markedly activates p38 MAPK [102-103] and inhibition of p38 MAPK attenuates organ damage and improves vascular function in cardiovascular diseases [104-105]. Recently, it was demonstrated that p38 MAPK increases arginase activity and contributes to endothelial dysfunction in CC [106]. This study showed that acute treatment with p38 inhibitor prevents increased arginase activity and expression of phosphorylated p38 MAPK levels in CC from mice treated with Ang II. Also, decreased eNOS phosphorylation at Ser-1177 due to Ang II treatment, was prevented. [106]. Although further research is needed to better clarify the exact role of these kinases in ED, new insights pointed to these pathways as a new therapeutic target worthy of consideration for clinical trials.

5. Endothelial dysfunction in vasculogenic ED

A number of both clinical and preclinical studies on hypercholesterolemia, hypertension, diabetes, and aging have demonstrated endothelial dysfunction to be a critical factor in the development of vasculogenic ED [107]. Since the erectile function is a mechanism which requires a sensitive balance between the vasodilators and vasoconstrictors agents, any modification or impairment in endothelial function contributes to ED. Nowadays, because a systemic endothelial may functionally manifest itself early in the penile endothelium, the possibility arises that ED may be an early indicator of cardiovascular diseases [61, 108-110]. In addition, since the penis is a rich vascularized organ, penile erection is, in large part, a vascular event. The endothelium, which is a layer of epithelial cells that lines structures of the cardiovascular system, is pivotal to the regulation of vasomotor tone. Impaired vasodilatation is closely linked with endothelial dysfunction, and endothelial cells are the primary source of NO, which is a crucial vasodilatory neurotransmitter involved in the regulation of vascular wall function, specifically in the penis [19]. At the cellular level, endothelial dysfunction results in impaired release of NO. Oxidative stress, which is directly toxic to the endothelium and also interferes with NO signaling, is a strong factor responsible for the endothelial dysfunction in ED. In addition, free radical damage and impaired function, as well as NO availability, also results in increased adhesion and aggregation of platelets and neutrophils, and the release of vasoconstrictor substances [111-112]. Since the penis is a vascular organ, it may be very sensitive to changes in oxidative stress and systemic levels of NO for many reasons. The small diameter of the cavernosal arteries and the eminent amount of endothelium and smooth muscle (per gram of tissue compared to other organs) may make the penile vascular bed a sensitive indicator of systemic vascular disease [61].

Oxidative stress has been implicated in endothelial damage or destruction of NO [113] as previously mentioned. It occurs when cells are exposed to excessive levels of reactive oxygen species (ROS) as a result of an imbalance between pro-oxidants and the protective mechanisms conferred by antioxidants [114]. ROS is a superoxide (O_2^-) which interacts with NO reducing NO bioavailability and resulting peroxynitrite ($ONOO^-$) formation. It has been demonstrated that the blockade of NOS increased basal superoxide production in penile arteries, suggesting that the release of ROS is modulated by its interaction with endogenous endothelial-derived NO, probably by producing peroxynitrite that reduces the bioavailability of both radicals [115]. In addition, peroxynitrite and superoxide have been reported to increase the incidence of apoptosis in the endothelium of cavernosal smooth muscle, resulting in denudation of endothelium and further reduction of available NO [116]. NOS, enzyme responsible for NO generation, uses l-arginine as a substrate and promotes its oxidation with NADPH and O_2 consumption to yield citrulline and NO. NADPH oxidase is a big source of superoxide radicals and many authors have reported that up regulation of this enzyme is associated with an increased risk of vascular diseases [117]. Also, superoxide anions plays a role in natural aging process and the prevalence and severity of ED increase with age.

Another mechanism associated endothelial damage and ED is the recently indentified advanced glycation end products (AGEs). It is believed that when AGEs are increased, NO cannot interact with GS, resulting in decreased CGMP levels and ultimately functional ED. Recently, it has been demonstrated that inhibitors of AGE formation can prevent formation of a range of complications in experimental diabetic animals, including ED [118-119]. AGEs are elevated in diabetic human penile tissue and it has been localized to the collagen of the penile tunica and corpus cavernosum [120]. Furthermore, AGEs and their receptors have been described to elevate the activity of endothelin-1, a vasoconstrictor, in rat corpus cavernosum [121], and AGEs production is associated with increased superoxide anion. O-linked N-acetylglucosamine (O-GlcNAc) is the major AGE product implicated in cavernosal dysfunction in diabetic patients. It has been reported a significant increase in the O-GlcNAc modification of eNOS and reduced phosphorylation of eNOS at baseline and following electrical stimulation in cavernosal tissue from diabetic rats compared with the controls [122]. Finally, increased AGEs has been reported in penile tissue from aged man [123].

Although the vascular endothelium is capable of self-repairing in general, any disruption in the penile endothelium balance may affect the dynamic of erectile function since the intact endothelium is critical to normal erection. Increase production of ROS has been associated with decreased normal erectile response, mainly because the reduction in NO avaibility, which is also observed due to endothelium damage [113]. Consequently, ED can be the result of any number of structural or functional abnormalities in the penile vascular bed. Accordingly, ED may result from occlusion of the cavernosal arteries by atherosclerosis (structural vascular ED), impairment of endothelial dependent and/or independent smooth muscle relaxation (functional vascular ED), or a combination of these factors. Thus, it seems that endothelial dysfunction is sometimes a primary factor involved in ED even though reduced NO from NANC nerves has a significant contribution in ED.

6. Conclusion

The molecular and clinical understanding of ED continues to gain ground at a particularly fast rate. Significant scientific advances during the last 2 decades have increased our knowledge regarding physiology and pathophysiology of penile erection. Different parts of the pathways involving ED have been studied intensely and the investigations of new components in this mechanism are emerging. The main target in the mechanism associated with ED is still NO, and the deep understanding of NO/cGMP signaling has supported, not only the molecular understanding of the tumescence, but also added significantly in the treatment of the ED, including the possibility of stem cell use and gene therapy. Also, the new components found to be involved in ED may be a potential target for development of novel drugs. However, the erectile mechanism is not completely elucidated and despite the efficacy of current therapies, current knowledge remains insufficient to address a growing patient population who do not respond to conventional treatment.

7. References

[1] Lue TF. Erectile dysfunction. N Engl J Med. 2000;342: 1802-13.
[2] Ayta IA, McKinlay JB, Krane RJ. The likely worldwide increase in erectile dysfunction between 1995 and 2025 and some possible policy consequences. BJU Int. 1999;84: 50-6.
[3] Hafez ES, Hafez SD. Erectile dysfunction: anatomical parameters, etiology, diagnosis, and therapy. Arch Androl. 2005;51: 15-31.
[4] Lue TF, Tanagho EA. Physiology of erection and pharmacological management of impotence. J Urol. 1987;137: 829-36.
[5] Mersdorf A, Goldsmith PC, Diederichs W, et al. Ultrastructural changes in impotent penile tissue: a comparison of 65 patients. J Urol. 1991;145: 749-58.
[6] Andersson KE, Holmquist F. Regulation of tone in penile cavernous smooth muscle. Established concepts and new findings. World J Urol. 1994;12: 249-61.
[7] Ignarro LJ, Bush PA, Buga GM, Wood KS, Fukuto JM, Rajfer J. Nitric oxide and cyclic GMP formation upon electrical field stimulation cause relaxation of corpus cavernosum smooth muscle. Biochem Biophys Res Commun. 1990;170: 843-50.
[8] Andersson KE. Mechanisms of Penile Erection and Basis for Pharmacological Treatment of Erectile Dysfunction. Pharmacol Rev. 2011.
[9] Andersson KE, Wagner G. Physiology of penile erection. Physiol Rev. 1995;75: 191-236.
[10] Nehra A, Azadzoi KM, Moreland RB, et al. Cavernosal expandability is an erectile tissue mechanical property which predicts trabecular histology in an animal model of vasculogenic erectile dysfunction. J Urol. 1998;159: 2229-36.
[11] Yiee JH, Baskin LS. Penile embryology and anatomy. ScientificWorldJournal. 2010;10: 1174-9.
[12] Manabe K, Heaton JP, Morales A, Kumon H, Adams MA. Pre-penile arteries are dominant in the regulation of penile vascular resistance in the rat. Int J Impot Res. 2000;12: 183-9.
[13] Moscovici J, Galinier P, Hammoudi S, Lefebvre D, Juricic M, Vaysse P. Contribution to the study of the venous vasculature of the penis. Surg Radiol Anat. 1999;21: 193-9.
[14] Dean RC, Lue TF. Physiology of penile erection and pathophysiology of erectile dysfunction. Urol Clin North Am. 2005;32: 379-95, v.
[15] Fazio L, Brock G. Erectile dysfunction: management update. CMAJ. 2004;170: 1429-37.

[16] Gratzke C, Angulo J, Chitaley K, et al. Anatomy, physiology, and pathophysiology of erectile dysfunction. J Sex Med. 2010;7: 445-75.
[17] Sattar AA, Salpigides G, Vanderhaeghen JJ, Schulman CC, Wespes E. Cavernous oxygen tension and smooth muscle fibers: relation and function. J Urol. 1995;154: 1736-9.
[18] Leite R, Giachini FR, Carneiro FS, Nunes KP, Tostes RC, Webb RC. Targets for the treatment of erectile dysfunction: is NO/cGMP still the answer? Recent Pat Cardiovasc Drug Discov. 2007;2: 119-32.
[19] Toda N, Ayajiki K, Okamura T. Nitric oxide and penile erectile function. Pharmacol Ther. 2005;106: 233-66.
[20] Steers WD, McConnell J, Benson GS. Anatomical localization and some pharmacological effects of vasoactive intestinal polypeptide in human and monkey corpus cavernosum. J Urol. 1984;132: 1048-53.
[21] Ignarro LJ. Nitric oxide. A novel signal transduction mechanism for transcellular communication. Hypertension. 1990;16: 477-83.
[22] Burnett AL, Tillman SL, Chang TS, et al. Immunohistochemical localization of nitric oxide synthase in the autonomic innervation of the human penis. J Urol. 1993;150: 73-6.
[23] Bredt DS, Snyder SH. Isolation of nitric oxide synthetase, a calmodulin-requiring enzyme. Proc Natl Acad Sci U S A. 1990;87: 682-5.
[24] Alexandre B, Lemaire A, Desvaux P, Amar E. Intracavernous injections of prostaglandin E1 for erectile dysfunction: patient satisfaction and quality of sex life on long-term treatment. J Sex Med. 2007;4: 426-31.
[25] Saenz de Tejada I, Angulo J, Cellek S, et al. Physiology of erectile function. J Sex Med. 2004;1: 254-65.
[26] Albersen M, Mwamukonda KB, Shindel AW, Lue TF. Evaluation and treatment of erectile dysfunction. Med Clin North Am. 2011;95: 201-12.
[27] Hurt KJ, Musicki B, Palese MA, et al. Akt-dependent phosphorylation of endothelial nitric-oxide synthase mediates penile erection. Proc Natl Acad Sci U S A. 2002;99: 4061-6.
[28] Andersson KE. Pharmacology of penile erection. Pharmacol Rev. 2001;53: 417-50.
[29] Granchi S, Vannelli GB, Vignozzi L, et al. Expression and regulation of endothelin-1 and its receptors in human penile smooth muscle cells. Mol Hum Reprod. 2002;8: 1053-64.
[30] Wingard CJ, Husain S, Williams J, James S. RhoA-Rho kinase mediates synergistic ET-1 and phenylephrine contraction of rat corpus cavernosum. Am J Physiol Regul Integr Comp Physiol. 2003;285: R1145-52.
[31] Ari G, Vardi Y, Hoffman A, Finberg JP. Possible role for endothelins in penile erection. Eur J Pharmacol. 1996;307: 69-74.
[32] Hirano K. Current topics in the regulatory mechanism underlying the Ca2+ sensitization of the contractile apparatus in vascular smooth muscle. J Pharmacol Sci. 2007;104: 109-15.
[33] Andersson KE. Erectile physiological and pathophysiological pathways involved in erectile dysfunction. J Urol. 2003;170: S6-13; discussion S13-4.
[34] Jin L, Burnett AL. RhoA/Rho-kinase in erectile tissue: mechanisms of disease and therapeutic insights. Clin Sci (Lond). 2006;110: 153-65.
[35] Chitaley K, Wingard CJ, Clinton Webb R, et al. Antagonism of Rho-kinase stimulates rat penile erection via a nitric oxide-independent pathway. Nat Med. 2001;7: 119-22.

[36] Chitaley K, Webb RC, Mills TM. Rho-kinase as a potential target for the treatment of erectile dysfunction. Drug News Perspect. 2001;14: 601-6.
[37] Sawada N, Itoh H, Yamashita J, et al. cGMP-dependent protein kinase phosphorylates and inactivates RhoA. Biochem Biophys Res Commun. 2001;280: 798-805.
[38] Sauzeau V, Le Jeune H, Cario-Toumaniantz C, et al. Cyclic GMP-dependent protein kinase signaling pathway inhibits RhoA-induced Ca2+ sensitization of contraction in vascular smooth muscle. J Biol Chem. 2000;275: 21722-9.
[39] Nunes KP, Rigsby CS, Webb RC. RhoA/Rho-kinase and vascular diseases: what is the link? Cell Mol Life Sci. 2010;67: 3823-36.
[40] Becker AJ, Uckert S, Stief CG, et al. Possible role of bradykinin and angiotensin II in the regulation of penile erection and detumescence. Urology. 2001;57: 193-8.
[41] Bader M, Ganten D. Update on tissue renin-angiotensin systems. J Mol Med (Berl). 2008;86: 615-21.
[42] Ryan MJ, Didion SP, Mathur S, Faraci FM, Sigmund CD. Angiotensin II-induced vascular dysfunction is mediated by the AT1A receptor in mice. Hypertension. 2004;43: 1074-9.
[43] Ying Z, Jin L, Palmer T, Webb RC. Angiotensin II up-regulates the leukemia-associated Rho guanine nucleotide exchange factor (RhoGEF), a regulator of G protein signaling domain-containing RhoGEF, in vascular smooth muscle cells. Mol Pharmacol. 2006;69: 932-40.
[44] Jin L, Ying Z, Hilgers RH, et al. Increased RhoA/Rho-kinase signaling mediates spontaneous tone in aorta from angiotensin II-induced hypertensive rats. J Pharmacol Exp Ther. 2006;318: 288-95.
[45] Jin L, Ying Z, Webb RC. Activation of Rho/Rho kinase signaling pathway by reactive oxygen species in rat aorta. Am J Physiol Heart Circ Physiol. 2004;287: H1495-500.
[46] Kifor I, Williams GH, Vickers MA, Sullivan MP, Jodbert P, Dluhy RG. Tissue angiotensin II as a modulator of erectile function. I. Angiotensin peptide content, secretion and effects in the corpus cavernosum. J Urol. 1997;157: 1920-5.
[47] Park JK, Kim SZ, Kim SH, Park YK, Cho KW. Renin angiotensin system in rabbit corpus cavernosum: functional characterization of angiotensin II receptors. J Urol. 1997;158: 653-8.
[48] Jin L, Lagoda G, Leite R, Webb RC, Burnett AL. NADPH oxidase activation: a mechanism of hypertension-associated erectile dysfunction. J Sex Med. 2008;5: 544-51.
[49] Jin LM. Angiotensin II signaling and its implication in erectile dysfunction. J Sex Med. 2009;6 Suppl 3: 302-10.
[50] Iwamoto Y, Song K, Takai S, et al. Multiple pathways of angiotensin I conversion and their functional role in the canine penile corpus cavernosum. J Pharmacol Exp Ther. 2001;298: 43-8.
[51] Lin CS, Ho HC, Gholami S, Chen KC, Jad A, Lue TF. Gene expression profiling of an arteriogenic impotence model. Biochem Biophys Res Commun. 2001;285: 565-9.
[52] Ertemi H, Mumtaz FH, Howie AJ, Mikhailidis DP, Thompson CS. Effect of angiotensin II and its receptor antagonists on human corpus cavernous contractility and oxidative stress: modulation of nitric oxide mediated relaxation. J Urol. 2011;185: 2414-20.
[53] Santos RA, Simoes e Silva AC, Maric C, et al. Angiotensin-(1-7) is an endogenous ligand for the G protein-coupled receptor Mas. Proc Natl Acad Sci U S A. 2003;100: 8258-63.

[54] da Costa Goncalves AC, Leite R, Fraga-Silva RA, et al. Evidence that the vasodilator angiotensin-(1-7)-Mas axis plays an important role in erectile function. Am J Physiol Heart Circ Physiol. 2007;293: H2588-96.
[55] Berk BC, Abe JI, Min W, Surapisitchat J, Yan C. Endothelial atheroprotective and anti-inflammatory mechanisms. Ann N Y Acad Sci. 2001;947: 93-109; discussion 09-11.
[56] Meldrum DR, Meng X, Dinarello CA, et al. Human myocardial tissue TNFalpha expression following acute global ischemia in vivo. J Mol Cell Cardiol. 1998;30: 1683-9.
[57] Chia S, Qadan M, Newton R, Ludlam CA, Fox KA, Newby DE. Intra-arterial tumor necrosis factor-alpha impairs endothelium-dependent vasodilatation and stimulates local tissue plasminogen activator release in humans. Arterioscler Thromb Vasc Biol. 2003;23: 695-701.
[58] Zhang C. The role of inflammatory cytokines in endothelial dysfunction. Basic Res Cardiol. 2008;103: 398-406.
[59] Zhang H, Park Y, Wu J, et al. Role of TNF-alpha in vascular dysfunction. Clin Sci (Lond). 2009;116: 219-30.
[60] Giugliano F, Esposito K, Di Palo C, et al. Erectile dysfunction associates with endothelial dysfunction and raised proinflammatory cytokine levels in obese men. J Endocrinol Invest. 2004;27: 665-9.
[61] Billups KL. Erectile dysfunction as an early sign of cardiovascular disease. Int J Impot Res. 2005;17 Suppl 1: S19-24.
[62] Feldman HA, Johannes CB, Derby CA, et al. Erectile dysfunction and coronary risk factors: prospective results from the Massachusetts male aging study. Prev Med. 2000;30: 328-38.
[63] Montorsi P, Ravagnani PM, Galli S, et al. Association between erectile dysfunction and coronary artery disease: Matching the right target with the right test in the right patient. Eur Urol. 2006;50: 721-31.
[64] Carneiro FS, Webb RC, Tostes RC. Emerging role for TNF-alpha in erectile dysfunction. J Sex Med. 2010;7: 3823-34.
[65] Mong PY, Petrulio C, Kaufman HL, Wang Q. Activation of Rho kinase by TNF-alpha is required for JNK activation in human pulmonary microvascular endothelial cells. J Immunol. 2008;180: 550-8.
[66] Hunter I, Cobban HJ, Vandenabeele P, MacEwan DJ, Nixon GF. Tumor necrosis factor-alpha-induced activation of RhoA in airway smooth muscle cells: role in the Ca2+ sensitization of myosin light chain20 phosphorylation. Mol Pharmacol. 2003;63: 714-21.
[67] Morin C, Sirois M, Echave V, Gomes MM, Rousseau E. EET displays anti-inflammatory effects in TNF-alpha stimulated human bronchi: putative role of CPI-17. Am J Respir Cell Mol Biol. 2008;38: 192-201.
[68] Carneiro FS, Sturgis LC, Giachini FR, et al. TNF-alpha knockout mice have increased corpora cavernosa relaxation. J Sex Med. 2009;6: 115-25.
[69] Carneiro FS, Zemse S, Giachini FR, et al. TNF-alpha infusion impairs corpora cavernosa reactivity. J Sex Med. 2009;6 Suppl 3: 311-9.
[70] Schiffrin EL. Vascular endothelin in hypertension. Vascul Pharmacol. 2005;43: 19-29.
[71] Marsden PA, Brenner BM. Transcriptional regulation of the endothelin-1 gene by TNF-alpha. Am J Physiol. 1992;262: C854-61.

[72] Kagawa T, Takao T, Horino T, et al. Angiotensin II receptor blocker inhibits tumour necrosis factor-alpha-induced cell damage in human renal proximal tubular epithelial cells. Nephrology (Carlton). 2008;13: 309-15.
[73] Vlachopoulos C, Aznaouridis K, Ioakeimidis N, et al. Unfavourable endothelial and inflammatory state in erectile dysfunction patients with or without coronary artery disease. Eur Heart J. 2006;27: 2640-8.
[74] Mori M, Gotoh T. Regulation of nitric oxide production by arginine metabolic enzymes. Biochem Biophys Res Commun. 2000;275: 715-9.
[75] Cox JD, Kim NN, Traish AM, Christianson DW. Arginase-boronic acid complex highlights a physiological role in erectile function. Nat Struct Biol. 1999;6: 1043-7.
[76] Bivalacqua TJ, Hellstrom WJ, Kadowitz PJ, Champion HC. Increased expression of arginase II in human diabetic corpus cavernosum: in diabetic-associated erectile dysfunction. Biochem Biophys Res Commun. 2001;283: 923-7.
[77] Numao N, Masuda H, Sakai Y, Okada Y, Kihara K, Azuma H. Roles of attenuated neuronal nitric-oxide synthase protein expression and accelerated arginase activity in impairing neurogenic relaxation of corpus cavernosum in aged rabbits. BJU Int. 2007;99: 1495-9.
[78] Boucher JL, Moali C, Tenu JP. Nitric oxide biosynthesis, nitric oxide synthase inhibitors and arginase competition for L-arginine utilization. Cell Mol Life Sci. 1999;55: 1015-28.
[79] Bivalacqua TJ, Burnett AL, Hellstrom WJ, Champion HC. Overexpression of arginase in the aged mouse penis impairs erectile function and decreases eNOS activity: influence of in vivo gene therapy of anti-arginase. Am J Physiol Heart Circ Physiol. 2007;292: H1340-51.
[80] Toque HA, Tostes RC, Yao L, et al. Arginase II deletion increases corpora cavernosa relaxation in diabetic mice. J Sex Med. 2011;8: 722-33.
[81] Sakai Y, Masuda H, Kihara K, Kurosaki E, Yamauchi Y, Azuma H. Involvement of increased arginase activity in impaired cavernous relaxation with aging in the rabbit. J Urol. 2004;172: 369-73.
[82] Carrier S, Nagaraju P, Morgan DM, Baba K, Nunes L, Lue TF. Age decreases nitric oxide synthase-containing nerve fibers in the rat penis. J Urol. 1997;157: 1088-92.
[83] Cartledge JJ, Eardley I, Morrison JF. Nitric oxide-mediated corpus cavernosal smooth muscle relaxation is impaired in ageing and diabetes. BJU Int. 2001;87: 394-401.
[84] Gur S, Ozturk B, Karahan ST. Impaired endothelium-dependent and neurogenic relaxation of corpus cavernosum from diabetic rats: improvement with L-arginine. Urol Res. 2000;28: 14-9.
[85] Berkowitz DE, White R, Li D, et al. Arginase reciprocally regulates nitric oxide synthase activity and contributes to endothelial dysfunction in aging blood vessels. Circulation. 2003;108: 2000-6.
[86] Haas CA, Seftel AD, Razmjouei K, Ganz MB, Hampel N, Ferguson K. Erectile dysfunction in aging: upregulation of endothelial nitric oxide synthase. Urology. 1998;51: 516-22.
[87] Angulo J, Gonzalez-Corrochano R, Cuevas P, et al. Diabetes exacerbates the functional deficiency of NO/cGMP pathway associated with erectile dysfunction in human corpus cavernosum and penile arteries. J Sex Med. 2010;7: 758-68.
[88] Bivalacqua TJ, Champion HC, Usta MF, et al. RhoA/Rho-kinase suppresses endothelial nitric oxide synthase in the penis: a mechanism for diabetes-associated erectile dysfunction. Proc Natl Acad Sci U S A. 2004;101: 9121-6.

[89] Christianson DW. Arginase: structure, mechanism, and physiological role in male and female sexual arousal. Acc Chem Res. 2005;38: 191-201.
[90] Liu Y, Shepherd EG, Nelin LD. MAPK phosphatases--regulating the immune response. Nat Rev Immunol. 2007;7: 202-12.
[91] Johnson GL, Lapadat R. Mitogen-activated protein kinase pathways mediated by ERK, JNK, and p38 protein kinases. Science. 2002;298: 1911-2.
[92] Bernier SG, Haldar S, Michel T. Bradykinin-regulated interactions of the mitogen-activated protein kinase pathway with the endothelial nitric-oxide synthase. J Biol Chem. 2000;275: 30707-15.
[93] Kyriakis JM, Avruch J. Sounding the alarm: protein kinase cascades activated by stress and inflammation. J Biol Chem. 1996;271: 24313-6.
[94] Sommer F, Klotz T, Steinritz D, et al. MAP kinase 1/2 (Erk 1/2) and serine/threonine specific protein kinase Akt/PKB expression and activity in the human corpus cavernosum. Int J Impot Res. 2002;14: 217-25.
[95] Tomlinson DR. Mitogen-activated protein kinases as glucose transducers for diabetic complications. Diabetologia. 1999;42: 1271-81.
[96] Chuang CC, Yang RS, Tsai KS, Ho FM, Liu SH. Hyperglycemia enhances adipogenic induction of lipid accumulation: involvement of extracellular signal-regulated protein kinase 1/2, phosphoinositide 3-kinase/Akt, and peroxisome proliferator-activated receptor gamma signaling. Endocrinology. 2007;148: 4267-75.
[97] Cameron NE, Eaton SE, Cotter MA, Tesfaye S. Vascular factors and metabolic interactions in the pathogenesis of diabetic neuropathy. Diabetologia. 2001;44: 1973-88.
[98] Nunes KPT, H. A.; Caldwell, R. B.; William Caldwell, R.; Webb, R.C. Extracellular signal-regulated kinase (ERK) inhibition decreases arginase activity and improves corpora cavernosal relaxation in streptozotocin (STZ)-induced diabetic mice.. The Journal of Sexual Medicine. 2011.
[99] Marinissen MJ, Chiariello M, Tanos T, Bernard O, Narumiya S, Gutkind JS. The small GTP-binding protein RhoA regulates c-jun by a ROCK-JNK signaling axis. Mol Cell. 2004;14: 29-41.
[100] Purves T, Middlemas A, Agthong S, et al. A role for mitogen-activated protein kinases in the etiology of diabetic neuropathy. FASEB J. 2001;15: 2508-14.
[101] Nangle MR, Cotter MA, Cameron NE. Correction of nitrergic neurovascular dysfunction in diabetic mouse corpus cavernosum by p38 mitogen-activated protein kinase inhibition. Int J Impot Res. 2006;18: 258-63.
[102] Meloche S, Landry J, Huot J, Houle F, Marceau F, Giasson E. p38 MAP kinase pathway regulates angiotensin II-induced contraction of rat vascular smooth muscle. Am J Physiol Heart Circ Physiol. 2000;279: H741-51.
[103] Zhang GX, Kimura S, Nishiyama A, Shokoji T, Rahman M, Abe Y. ROS during the acute phase of Ang II hypertension participates in cardiovascular MAPK activation but not vasoconstriction. Hypertension. 2004;43: 117-24.
[104] Widder J, Behr T, Fraccarollo D, et al. Vascular endothelial dysfunction and superoxide anion production in heart failure are p38 MAP kinase-dependent. Cardiovasc Res. 2004;63: 161-7.
[105] Bao W, Behm DJ, Nerurkar SS, et al. Effects of p38 MAPK Inhibitor on angiotensin II-dependent hypertension, organ damage, and superoxide anion production. J Cardiovasc Pharmacol. 2007;49: 362-8.

[106] Toque HA, Romero MJ, Tostes RC, et al. p38 Mitogen-activated protein kinase (MAPK) increases arginase activity and contributes to endothelial dysfunction in corpora cavernosa from angiotensin-II-treated mice. J Sex Med. 2010;7: 3857-67.
[107] Watts GF, Chew KK, Stuckey BG. The erectile-endothelial dysfunction nexus: new opportunities for cardiovascular risk prevention. Nat Clin Pract Cardiovasc Med. 2007;4: 263-73.
[108] Yassin AA, Akhras F, El-Sakka AI, Saad F. Cardiovascular diseases and erectile dysfunction: the two faces of the coin of androgen deficiency. Andrologia. 2011;43: 1-8.
[109] Solomon H, Man JW, Jackson G. Erectile dysfunction and the cardiovascular patient: endothelial dysfunction is the common denominator. Heart. 2003;89: 251-3.
[110] Billups KL. Erectile dysfunction as a marker for vascular disease. Curr Urol Rep. 2005;6: 439-44.
[111] Jeremy JY, Angelini GD, Khan M, et al. Platelets, oxidant stress and erectile dysfunction: an hypothesis. Cardiovasc Res. 2000;46: 50-4.
[112] Jones RW, Rees RW, Minhas S, Ralph D, Persad RA, Jeremy JY. Oxygen free radicals and the penis. Expert Opin Pharmacother. 2002;3: 889-97.
[113] Agarwal A, Nandipati KC, Sharma RK, Zippe CD, Raina R. Role of oxidative stress in the pathophysiological mechanism of erectile dysfunction. J Androl. 2006;27: 335-47.
[114] Zalba G, Beaumont J, San Jose G, Fortuno A, Fortuno MA, Diez J. Vascular oxidant stress: molecular mechanisms and pathophysiological implications. J Physiol Biochem. 2000;56: 57-64.
[115] Prieto D, Kaminski PM, Bagi Z, Ahmad M, Wolin MS. Hypoxic relaxation of penile arteries: involvement of endothelial nitric oxide and modulation by reactive oxygen species. Am J Physiol Heart Circ Physiol. 2010;299: H915-24.
[116] Khan MA, Thompson CS, Mumtaz FH, et al. The effect of nitric oxide and peroxynitrite on rabbit cavernosal smooth muscle relaxation. World J Urol. 2001;19: 220-4.
[117] Warnholtz A, Nickenig G, Schulz E, et al. Increased NADH-oxidase-mediated superoxide production in the early stages of atherosclerosis: evidence for involvement of the renin-angiotensin system. Circulation. 1999;99: 2027-33.
[118] Usta MF, Bivalacqua TJ, Yang DY, et al. The protective effect of aminoguanidine on erectile function in streptozotocin diabetic rats. J Urol. 2003;170: 1437-42.
[119] Usta MF, Kendirci M, Gur S, et al. The breakdown of preformed advanced glycation end products reverses erectile dysfunction in streptozotocin-induced diabetic rats: preventive versus curative treatment. J Sex Med. 2006;3: 242-50; discussion 50-2.
[120] Seftel AD, Vaziri ND, Ni Z, et al. Advanced glycation end products in human penis: elevation in diabetic tissue, site of deposition, and possible effect through iNOS or eNOS. Urology. 1997;50: 1016-26.
[121] Chen D, Shan YX, Dai YT. [Advanced glycation end products and their receptors elevate the activity of endothelin-1 in rat cavernosum]. Zhonghua Nan Ke Xue. 2008;14: 110-5.
[122] Musicki B, Kramer MF, Becker RE, Burnett AL. Inactivation of phosphorylated endothelial nitric oxide synthase (Ser-1177) by O-GlcNAc in diabetes-associated erectile dysfunction. Proc Natl Acad Sci U S A. 2005;102: 11870-5.
[123] Jiaan DB, Seftel AD, Fogarty J, et al. Age-related increase in an advanced glycation end product in penile tissue. World J Urol. 1995;13: 369-75.

2

Erectile Dysfunction Etiological Factors

Rafaela Rosalba de Mendonça[1], Fernando Korkes[1]
and João Paulo Zambon[2,3]
[1]ABC School of Medicine /
[2]Albert Einstein Hospital /
[3]Federal University of São Paulo,
Brazil

1. Introduction

The prevalence of ED in men between 40 and 70 years old is approximately 50%. (Massachusetts Male Aging Study). There are many ED etiological factors, such as psychological, vascular, neurological and hormonal disorders. (Tomada, 2010; Kavoussi, 2007; Glina 2002).

In accordance with the International Society of Impotence Research, ED may be classified into three subtypes: organic (that includes iatrogenic, neurogenic, vasculogenic and hormonal), psychogenic and mixed erectile dysfunction. A thorough investigation ought to be performed by a multidisciplinary team in order to avoiding misdiagnosis. (Kavoussi, 2007)

The basic assessment is suggested by ED guidelines: detailed anamnesis and physical examination, fast serum glucose, total cholesterol and fractions, triglycerides and testosterone level. Long history of diabetes, alcohol abuse and spinal cord injuries suggest neurological ethiology. (Kavoussi; Tanagho & McAninch, 2007).

Patients without contra-indications must be recommended to use 5 phosphodiesterase (PDE5) inhibitors after first visit. Vascular integrity may be tested by PDE5 inhibitors response and good drug response usually mean vascular integrity. (Tanagho & McAninch, 2007; Glina, 2002)

Recent studies have demonstrated the association between ED and cardiovascular diseases Zambon, 2010; Bal, 2007. Ultrasensible C Reactive Protein (CRP) is an early marker of cardiovascular risk, and patients with ED have higher levels of CRP. Risk factors such as hypertension, smoking, obesity, diabetes mellitus, metabolic syndrome and sedentary lifestyle are pretty common in patients with coronary disease and ED (Zambon, 2010; Bal, 2007).

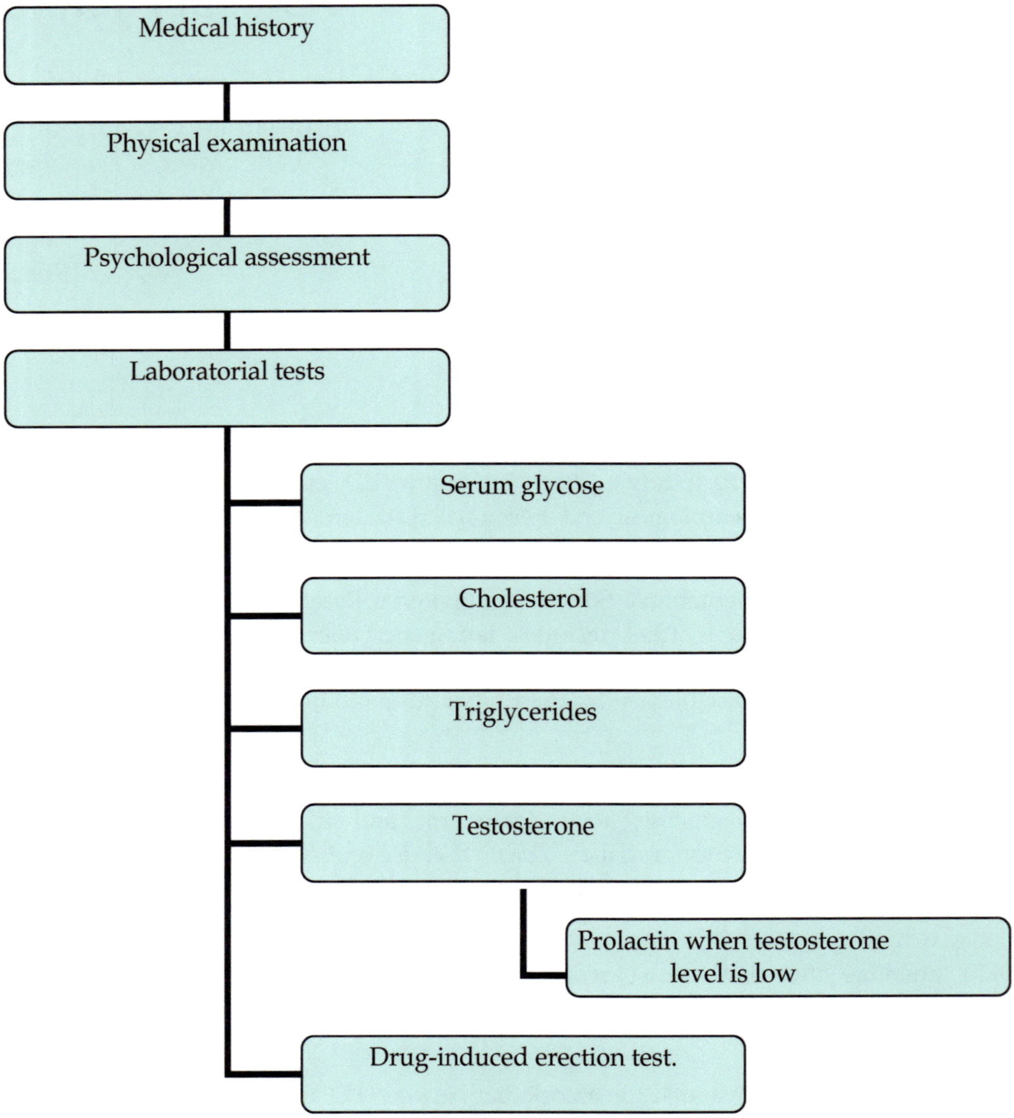

Fig. 1. Initial ED evaluation

2. Etiological factors

ORGANIC			
	Vasculogenic		
		Arteriogenic	
			Smoking
			Trauma
			Dislipidemia
			Hypertension
			Diabetes Mellitus
			Pelvic irradiation
			Pelvic surgery
		Cavernosal	
	Neurogenic		
		Central	
			Parkinson disease
			Encephalitis
			Vascular Stroke
			Brain Tumor
			Multiple Sclerosis
			Alzheimer
			Spinal cord injury
			Disc herniation
		Peripheral	
			Pelvic surgery
			Retroperitoneal surgery
			Diabetes Mellitus
			Alcohol
			Polineuropathic
	Endocrinologic		
			Hypogonadism
			Hyperprolactinemia
			Diabetes Mellitus
			Dyslipidemia
			Thyroid hormones
			Adrenal hormones
			Estradiol changes
	Anatomic		
			Peyronie disease
			Penile fracture

Table 1. ED organic causes

2.1 Anatomic factors

The most frequent physiopathology of these dysfunctions is low abnormal drainage, or severe alterations of penile geometry. Peyronie's disease, priapism and penile trauma are some examples of anatomic etiological factors. Physical examination can confirm penile shaft fibrosis, and Doppler ultrasound can identify the fibrosis with good sensitivity and specificity (Navarro, 2010; Persu, 2009).

2.2 Endocrinological factors

The endocrine disorders are directly or indirectly related with erection mechanism. Endocrine disorders can be associated or worsen the pre-existing ED. Among the etiological factors we can point out diabetes mellitus, obesity, hypogonadism, adrenals and thyroid dysfunction and Hyperprolactinemia. (Tanagho & McAninch, 2007; Kavoussi; Jabaloyas, 2010; Persu, 2009)

2.2.1 Diabetes mellitus

Diabetes Mellitus (DM) is one of the most frequent etiologies of ED. Patients with higher levels of glucose and glycated hemoglobin has higher risk of ED. The prevalence of ED in men with DM ranges from 10 to 90%. Risk factors for the emergence of ED in diabetic patients are: disease time, age, sedentary lifestyle and glycemic control. (Jabolayas, 2010)

Regarding PDE 5 inhibitors response, diabetic patients have lower response than normal patients. Furthermore, it is directly related to disease severity. Vascular and autonomic neuropathies are the main etiological alterations observed in diabetic patients. The main pathophysiological mechanisms proposed for ED in diabetic patients include the release of free radicals, increased endothelin receptor B, impaired nitric oxide synthesis and up-regulated RhoA/Rho-kinase pathway. (Jabolayas, 2010; Thorve, 2011; Moore, 2006)

2.2.2 Hypogonadism

Low testosterone level can decrease the libido, the morning erections and penile tumescence. It can also increase the risk of depression and psychiatric disorders. Furthermore, hypogonadic patients with ED have higher risk of early osteoporosis. (Tanagho & McAninch, 2007)

Studies have shown that hypogonadic men present high risk of metabolic syndrome and DM. The symptoms which are related to hypogonadism are common to many others diseases. It is advisable at least 2 consecutive dosages of total testosterone in the period between 7 and 11 a.m. The institution of compulsory treatment should be based on clinical and total dosage of testosterone. Moreover, hypogonadic patients may clinically present primary or secondary infertility. Thyroid, pituitary and adrenal disorders are less common etiologies, and in specific situations, alterations must be taken into account. (Traish, 2009)

2.2.3 Hyperprolactinemia

Hyperprolactinemia may be associated with reduced libido. The prevalence of hyperprolactinemia in men with ED varies between 2 and 13%. Prolactin above 35 ng/mL are associated with ED and decreased libido. (Jabolayas, 2010)

The mechanism by which elevated prolactin leads to ED, is not fully understood. This change is attributed to the reduction of testosterone and alterations in the pulsatile release of LH. There are several causes for elevated prolactin, for instance pituitary adenoma (most common cause), drugs (especially antipsychotics), chronic renal failure and herpes zoster. (Jabaloyas, 2010)

Guidelines recommended prolactin dosage when testosterone levels are low. The gold standard exam to evaluate pituitary adenoma is the magnetic ressonance imaging. (Tanagho & McAninch, 2007)

2.2.4 Changes in thyroid hormones

Changes in thyroid hormones are also associated with changes in libido, erectile function and ejaculation. The prevalence of thyroid diseases is variable and normalization of hormone levels can restore an adequate erection when the ethiology is the thyroid dysfunction .The hypothyroidism can decrease levels of free testosterone and SHBG, and hyperthyroidism appears to be strictly related to changes in libido. (Jabolayas, 2010; Cauni, 2009).

2.2.5 Dyslipidemia

Dyslipidemia is a risk factor for ED, and some patients are diagnosed during the ED investigation. The change in lipid metabolism is associated with endothelial dysfunction and abnormal relaxation of smooth muscle. (Vrentzos, 2007; Jabaloyas, 2010)

Hypercholesterolemia, high level of LDL and low HDL increase the risk of atherosclerosis, which may change the penile blood flow. Besides, hypercholesterolemia increases the pro-inflammatory markers and endothelial dysfunction. (Vrentzos, 2007; Bal, 2007)

Studies demonstrated a positive correlation between cardiovascular risks, hypercholesterolemia and erectile dysfunction (Zambon, 2010; Koenig, 2004) have demonstrated that men with ED had higher levels of C-reactive protein, which is an early marker of endothelial dysfunction and cardiovascular diseases. (Zambon, 2010; Koenig, 2004)

2.2.6 Changes of adrenal hormones

The role of adrenal hormones and their changes are not well established in the etiology of ED. Studies have correlated the low levels of dehydroepiandrosterone with ED. Androstenedione can be converted into testosterone and supplementation of this hormone may improve erectile function. Nevertheless, there is no justification dosage of adrenal hormones in the initial investigation of ED. In specific cases, the dosage of hormones produced in the adrenal, for example, cortisol, aldosterone, androstenedione, dehydroepiandrosterone, among others, is recommended. (Jabolayas 2010)

2.2.7 Changes in estradiol

The increased production of estradiol in men can be associated with ED. Elevated estrogen levels decrease the production of testosterone by inhibiting the LH production. The chronic liver disease may be related with the hyperestrogenism. Another uncommon etiology of hyperestrogenism is the endocrinologic neoplasms. (Jabolayas, 2010)

2.3 Vascular factors

The vascular dysfunctions are common in men with ED. Commonly, the vasoreactivity is reduced, and consequently low penile blood flow, hypoxia and fibrosis are the final results. These changes decrease the penile shaft stiffness over the time. (Tomada, 2010; Cauni, 2009; Odriozola, 2010)

ED seems to be an early marker of endothelial dysfunction, which can changes the vasoreactive substances production, such as nitric oxide and endothelin (Odriozola, 2010;

Hannan, 2010). Local growth factors seem also to be involved in the pathophysiology. Therefore, there is a reduced response to vasodilating substances and an increased sensitivity to vasoconstrictor agents. (Odriozola, 2010; Hannan, 2010)

Penile vascular abnormalities are strictly linked to cardiovascular risk factors such as hypertension, smoking, dyslipidemia, and DM among others. Diffuse and bilateral lesions in internal pudendal arteries, penile and cavernous as well are common in patients with atherosclerosis. (Odriozola, 2010, Hannan, 2010)

The evaluation of penile vascular function can be performed using Doppler ultrasound, magnetic resonance image or angiography, however, the real significance of these tests remains unclear.

2.4 Neurologic factors

The prevalence of ED as a consequence of neurological diseases ranges from 10 to 19%. In these cases, ED is moderate or severe, with poor response to oral therapy. (Cauni, 2009; Antuna, 2008)

The neurogenic etiology can be central or peripheral. Central disorders can be exemplified by Parkinson's disease, brain tumor, encephalitis, cerebral strokes, cranial trauma, epilepsy and multiple sclerosis. In the other hand, DM, spinal cord injury, and surgical trauma of the erector nerves during radical prostatectomy, polyneuropathy metabolic, toxic or congenital conditions among others, can be cited as peripheral neurogenic disorders. (Cauni, 2009; Antuna, 2008)

The basic neurological assessment must be performed in all patients with ED. Guidelines recommended the spinal cord reflexes evaluation, for example bulbocavernosum reflex, and sensitivity level. (Kavoussi, 2007)

2.4.1 Dysfunctional system

Multiple sclerosis is characterized by multiple areas of demyelization of the central nervous system. The prevalence of ED in men with multiple sclerosis is approximately 60%. Generally, multiple sclerosis is a progressive disease, with periods of acute crisis and remission. In the initial profiles, ED is mild; however, with the evolution of the disease, it becomes severe and unresponsive to conservative therapy. (Antuna, 2008)

Parkinson's disease is a neurodegenerative disease characterized by progressive decrease of gray matter's dopaminergic neurons. This process can achieve the mesolimbic and mesocortical regions and areas of the autonomic nervous system. Drug therapy with PDE-5 inhibitors can produce satisfactory results, but a careful analysis of these patients should be performed in order to improve the results and patient satisfaction. (Antuna, 2008)

In patients with epilepsy, the prevalence of ED is variable and the ethiology is multifactorial. ED secondary to cerebral strokes depends on many factors such as age, location and extent of stroke. Furthermore, co-morbidities and co-related diseases can worsen the ED prognosis. In general, traumas also can be associated with ED. Many patients develop psychogenic disorders, which may raise the ED incidence. (Antuna, 2008)

2.4.2 Spinal cord injuries

The spinal cord trauma is usually associated with automobilistic crashes. Generally, this kind of trauma affects the younger population who are economically active and the initial care of these patients should be performed by a multidisciplinary team, to avoid late sequel. (Kavoussi, 2007)

After the trauma, there is a phase of spinal shock, which has a variable duration, what occurs is a reflex abolition below the affected area. Over the time with spinal shock recovery, patients may have reflex erections. (Kavoussi, 2007)

The post spinal cord trauma depends on the level, extent and severity of trauma. In general, ED tends to be moderate to severe, and semen quality in these patients most frequently is poor. The use of medications can provide satisfactory results in some patients. A second option is the intracavernosal injections and penile prosthesis, which can be performed when other options did not have a good result. (Antuna, 2008)

In conclusion, the treatment of patients with spinal cord trauma should be individualized and carried out by a multidisciplinary team. (Antuna, 2008)

2.4.3 Peripheral dysfunction

The peripheral neuropathy may be related with many differents etiologies. The clinical manifestation is quite variable and the correct diagnosis must be made as always as possible to avoid unsuccessful treatment. ED is a symptom of this syndrome. In Brazil, in addition to DM, there is an increasing incidence of alcoholic polyneuropathy, due to the excessive consumption of alcoholic beverages. In this case, ED occurs late and is often irreversible. (Antuna, 2008; Abdo, 2006)

2.5 Pelvic surgery

Excluding skin cancer, prostate cancer is more common in men after age 60. Radical retropubic prostatectomy is the gold standard treatment of prostate cancer. The prostate-specific antigen (PSA) screening programs improve the early detection of this disease. (Zippe, 2006)

ED is a major surgical post-operative complication after pelvic surgery. The prevalence of ED after radical retropubic prostatectomy is approximately 50%, but depends on factors such as age, tumor stage, surgical technique, associated comorbidities, among others. The manipulation of the periprostatic nerve plexus can cause a transient neurological injury (neuropraxia) or permanent (neurovascular bundle injury). These lesions can induce hypoxia and collagen deposition in the corpus cavernosum. (Zippe, 2006; Gallina, 2010)

The vessel damage during surgery such as in the accessory pudendal arteries may cause a vascular insufficiency, by changing the irrigation of the erectile tissue. Furthermore, ligation of anomalous pudendal artery branches or venous plexus can induce the formation of fibrosis in the corpus cavernosum. (Zippe, 2006; Gallina, 2010)

ED can also occur after surgery to remove colon cancer, which is the most common cancers of the distal colon and at the junction between the rectum and sigmoid. Thus, the ED incidence in patients undergoing colorectal cancer surgery varies between 10-60%. This incidence increases when there is need for neoadjuvant or radiotherapy adjuvant. A permanent colostomy also increases the rate of dysfunction to leading to alteration in body image. (Zippe, 2006; Gallina, 2010)

2.6 Cardiovascular risk factors

ED may be related to cardiovascular risk and may precede a cardiovascular event in 3-5 years. Studies have shown that ED is an early marker of endothelial dysfunction and atherosclerotic disease (Bryan, 2011; Blumentals, 2004).

The prevalence of ED in men with cardiovascular disease varies between 44 and 75%. (Muller & Mulhall, 2006). There is a strong correlation between cardiovascular disease and ED, since the risk factors are the same, such as hypertension, dyslipidemia, obesity, smoking, DM and sedentary lifestyle (Kupelian, 2006; Bal, 2007; Feldman, 2000; Derby, 2000)

The endothelium and the cavernous nerves are two sources of nitric oxide. Nitric oxide acts on smooth muscle relaxation during erection. The production and release of this substance depends on the integrity of endothelium. A nitric oxide response in men with ED is lower than in men with a preserved erection (Muller & Mulhall, 2006; Giugliano, 2004). Endothelial dysfunction is an early stage of vascular damage. Cardiovascular risk factors can cause endothelial damage leading to an impaired nitric oxide release, atherosclerosis and vascular stenosis. Endothelial dysfunction seems to play an important role in the development of both ED and cardiovascular diseases. Organic erectile dysfunction in a majority of men is due to the vascular diseases. (Muller & Mulhall, 2006).

Obesity is a multifactorial disease with high prevalence worldwide. Genetic, environmental and behavioral factors were identified as etiological factors. The incidence of obesity in men with ED is 30% higher than men without ED, (Muller & Mulhall, 2006). It is usually associated with other diseases such as, dyslipidemia, diabetes mellitus and hypertension.. In obese ones there is a peripheral resistance to insulin and a consequent hyperinsulinemia. Patients with higher body mass index are at greater risk of ED, even at the prospect of weight loss. Clinical factors like waist-hip ratio, body mass index and resting heart rate are significantly higher in patients with ED (Muller & Mulhall, 2006; Zambon, 2010).

Regarding hypertension, it has been demonstrated that the chronic changes in blood pressure, altering the flow of small vessels and penile vessels, which are associated with the development of the atherosclerotic disease can cause severe ED. A number of anti-hypertensive medications, such as beta-blocking drugs may have ED as a side effect (Muller & Mulhall, 2006).

Smoking as above mentioned is a risk factor for ED. It changes the mechanism of penile erection because it affects the smooth muscle relaxation. The prevalence among men with ED is 27.3% vs. 12.5% among men without ED. Not only the smoker, but passive exposure to cigarette smoke has a higher incidence of erectile dysfunction.Therefore, smoking increase the ED grade. (Feldman, 2000; Zambon, 2010; Muller & Mulhall, 2006).

Metabolic syndrome is also a significant risk factor in patients aged 40 to 49. In elderly men, this effect of metabolic syndrome on erectile function was not prominent, probably because aging itself is a risk factor for erectile dysfunction. (Bal, 2007) ED may provide a warning sign and an opportunity for early intervention among men who had previously been considered to have lower risk of metabolic syndrome and cardiovascular disease (Kupelian, 2006; Muller & Mulhall, 2006; Zambon, 2010).

Preventive actions such as regular diet, physical activity, and hypertension and diabetes controls can decrease these risks and improve erectile function (Kratsky, 2009; Derby, 2000).

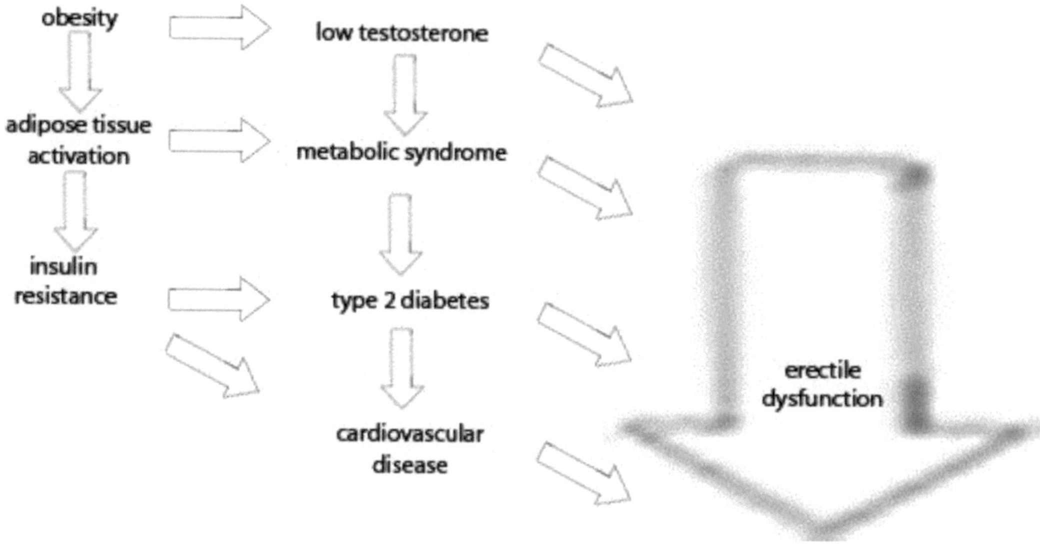

Fig. 2. Metabolic syndrome

2.7 Chronic renal failure

ED has a high incidence in patients with chronic renal failure (20-50%) and those underwent to renal transplantation. There is a positive relationship between the severities of both diseases. The cause of ED in these patients is multifactorial, including endothelial dysfunction, comorbidities, chronic hyperuricemia and psychogenic factors. Kidney transplantation can improve erectile function, due to the improvement of uremic neuropathy and anemia. (Phé 2008; Cauni, 2009).

2.8 Drug induced ED

Drug use may be responsible for up to 25% of all cases of ED. Among the medications that can induce it, we can highlight the drugs which affect the cardiovascular and autonomic nervous systems. Cauni, 2009).

Several studies have shown that intravitreal drugs such as bevacizumab (antivascular endothelial growth factor) can lead to a transient ED. The mechanism is not well established, but it is postulated that the systemic drug absorption may lead to an interaction with nitric oxide in the corpus cavernosum (Yohendran & Chauhan, 2010). . Moreover, injection trauma can be associated with psychological effect, leading to temporary loss of erection. (Yohendran & Chauhan, 2010).

Anthyhipertensive agents			
	Diuretics	Thiazide	
	B adrenergic blockers		
	A adrenergic blockers		
Antiandrogens (mechanism)			
		Estrogenes	
		Cyproterone acetate	
		Ketoconazole	
Psycotropics			
	Antipsycotics		
	Antidepressants		
		Monoamine oxidade inhibitors	
		Selective serotonin reuptake inhibitors	
		Tricyclics	
	Anxiolitics		
Digoxin			
Opiates			
Statin			
Alcohol			
Retroviral and chemothrapeutic agents			
Histamine H2 receptor antagonist			
Fenitoin			
Antimuscarinic			

Table 2. Drugs induced **ED**

2.9 Psychogenic

In the past, psychogenic cause was considered the most important etiologic factor of ED, however, currently organic factors account for 60-90% of this condition. (Cauni 2009)

The pathogenesis of psychogenic ED is not well established. Many etiological factors have been studied, such as: neurotransmitters imbalance, autonomic dysfunction, etc. (Kavoussi 2007)

Psycogenic		
	Generalized	
		Generalized unresponsible
		Generalized inhibition
	Situational	
		Partner related
		Performance related
		Adjustment related

Table 3. Psycogenic ED causes

Performance anxiety related to several different causes ends up being the most common cause. Other causes are: an inappropriate sex education, traumatic childhood sexual experiences, a troubled marriage or relationship, stressful situations or psychiatric disorders. (Monseny, 2010)

Usually, psychogenic ED has short duration. Most commonly, patients have satisfactory erection in specific situations. (Abdo, 2006) Socioeconomic factors such as low income and poor educational background also have been associated withED. (Abdo, 2006).

3. Conclusions

ED has a high prevalence in men over than 50 years. The incidence increase with aging and its ethiology appears to be multifactorial. The anamnesis and detailed physical evaluation ought to be performed in order to detect the main etiological factors. The best approach to obtain better results is to identify the main etiology. A multidisciplinary evaluation should be recommended for all patients.

4. References

Abdo, CHN.; Oliveira Jr, WM.; Scanavino, MT. & Martins, FG. (2006). Erectile dysfunction: results of the Brazilian sexual life study. *Rev Assoc Med Bras.* Vol. 52, No 6 (Nov-Dec 2006),pp.424-9, ISSN 0104-4230.

Bal, K.; Oder, M. & Sahin, AS. et al. (2007). Prevalence of metabolic syndrome and its association with erectile dysfunction among urologic patients: metabolic backgrounds of erectile dysfunction. *Urology,* Vol. 69, No 2, pp.3356-60, ISSN 0090-4295.

Blumentals, WA.; Gomez-Caminero, A.; Joo, S. & Vannappagari, V. (2004) Should erectile dysfunction be considered as a marker for acute myocardial infarction? Results from a retrospective cohort study. *Int J Impot Res.* Vol 16, No 4, pp. 350-3, ISSN 0955-9930.

Bryan, G.; Schwartz, Robert A. Kloner.(2011). Physician Update: Erectile Dysfunction and Cardiovascular Disease. *Circulation.* Vol. 123, pp.98- 101, ISSN 0009-7322.

Derby, C.; Mohr, BA.; Goldstein, I.; et al. (2000). Modifiable risk factors and erectile dysfunction: can lifestyle changes modify risk? *Urology.* Vol. 56, No 2, pp.302-6, ISSN 0090-4295.

Feldman, HA.; Johannes, CB.; Derby, CA.; et al. (2000). Erectile dysfunction and coronary risk factors: prospective results from the Massachusetts male aging study. *Prev Med.* Vol 30, No 4,pp.328-38, ISSN: 0091-7435.

Gallina, A.; Briganti, A.; Suardi, N.; Capitanio, U.; Abdollah, F.; Zanni, G.; Salonia,A.; Rigatti, P. & Montorsi F. (2010). Surgery and erectile dysfunction.*Arch Esp Urol.* Vol. 63, No 8 (OUT 2010),pp.640-8, ISSN 0004-0614.

Giugliano, F.; Espósito, K.; Di Palo, C.; et al. (2004). Erectile dysfunction associates with endothelial dysfunction and raised proinflammatory cytokine levels in obese men. *J Endocrinol Invest.* Vol, 27, No 7, 2004,pp.665-9, ISSN 1720-8386.

Glina, S.; Puech-Leao, P.; Reis, JMSM. & Pagani, E. (2002). *Difunção sexual masculina: conceitos básicos: diagnóstico e tratamento* (1ª edition), Instituto H. Ellis, ISBN 858-94-1301-2 , São Paulo.

Hannan, JL.; Blaser, MC.; Oldfield, L.; Pang, JJ.; Adams, SM.; Pang, SC. & Adams, MA. (2010) Morphological and functional evidence for the contribution of the pudendal artery in aging-induced erectile dysfunction.*J Sex Med.* Vol 7, No 10 (oct 2010), pp.3373-84, ISSN: 1743 6095.

Jabaloyas, JM. Hormonal etiology in erectile dysfunction. (2010) *Arch Esp Urol..* Vol. 63, No 8 (Out 2010), pp.621-7, ISSN 0004-0614

Kavoussi, L.; Novick, A.; Partin, A.; Peters, C.; Wein, A.(Ed(s)). (2007). *Campbell-Walsh Urology.* Saunders-Elsevier, ISBN 13-978-8089-2353-4, Philadelphia.

Koenig, W.; Lowel, H.; Baumert, J. & Meisinger, C. (2004). C-reactive protein modulates risk prediction based on the Framingham Score: implications for future risk assessment: results from a large cohort study in Southern Germany. *Circulation.* Vol 23. (2004),pp.1349-53, ISSN 0009-7322.

Kratzik, CW.; Lackner, JE.; Märk, I.; et al. (2009). How much physical activity is needed to maintain erectile function? Results of the Androx Vienna Municipality Study. *Eur Urol.* Vol. 55, No 2 (2009),pp. 509-16, ISSN: 0302-2838.

Kupelian, V.; Shabsigh, R.; Araujo, AB.; O'Donnell, AB. & McKinlay, JB. (2006). Erectile dysfunction as a predictor of the metabolic syndrome in aging men: results from the Massachusetts Male Aging Study. *J Urol.* Vol. 176, No 1(2006), pp.222-6, ISSN:0022-5347.

Monseny, JM. (2010) Psicogenic erectile dysfunction. *Arch Esp Urol.* Vol 63, No 8 (oct 2010), pp.599-602, ISSN 0004-0614 .

Moore, CR. & Wang,R. (2006). Pathophysiology and treatment of diabetic dysfunction. *Asian J Androl.* Vol. 8, No 6 (2006),pp.675-84, ISSN: 0105-6263 .

Muller, A. & Mulhall JP. (2006). Cardiovascular disease, metabolic syndrome and erectile dysfunction. *Curr Opin Urol.* Vol. 16, No 6 (2006),pp.435-43, ISSN: 0963-0643.

Navarro, NC. (2010) Penile structural erectile dysfunction. *Arch Esp Urol.* Vol. 63, No 8 (Oct 2010), pp.628-36, ISSN 0004-0614.

Odriozola, AA.; Quintanilla, MG.; Arias JGP.; Tamayo, AL. & Gonzalez, GI. (2010). Disfuncion erétil de origen vascular. *Arch Esp* Urol. Vol. 63, No 8 (2010),pp.611-20, ISSN 0004-0614.

Persu, C.; Cauni, V.; Gutue, S.; Albu, ES.; Jinga, V. & Geavlete P. (2009). Diagnosis and treatment os erectile dysfunction-a pratical update. *Journal of Medicine and Life.* Vol. 2, No 4 (Oct-dec 2009),pp.394-400, ISSN: 1844122X.

Phé, V.;Roupret, M.;Ferhi, K.;Barrou, B.; Cussenot, O. ;Traxer, O.; Haab, F.& Beley, S. (2008). Erectile dysfunction and renal chronic insufficiency: etiology and management. *Progres en urologie.*Vol. 19, No 1 (Jan 2009),pp.1-7, ISSN:1166-7087.

Tanagho, EA. & McAninch, JW. (Ed(s).). (2007). *Smiths General Urology,* Editora Manole, ISBN 978-85-204-2224-3, Barueri, SP.

Thorve, VS.; Kshirsagar, AD.; Vyawahare, NS.; Joshi, VS.; Ingale, KG. & Mohite, RJ. (2011). Diabetes-induced erectile dysfunction: epidemiology, pathophysiology and management. *J. Diabetes Complications.* Vol. 25, No 2(Mar-Apr 2011),pp.129-36, ISSN: 1056-8727.

Tomada, I.; Tomada, N. & Neves, D. Disfunção Eréctil:Doença (Cardio)Vascular. (2010) *Acta Urológica* .Vol 27. No 1 (2010), pp.27-3

Traish, AM.; Guay, A.; Feeley, RJ.& Saad, F.(2009). The dark side of testosterone deficiency: I. Metabolic Syndrome and erectile dysfunction. *J Androl.* Vol, 30, No 1 (Jan-Feb 2009),pp.10-22, ISSN: 1365-2605 .

Vrentzos, GE.; Paraskevas, KI. & Mikhailidis, DP. (2007). Dyslipidemia as a risk factor for erectile dysfunction. *Curr Med Chem.* Vol. 14, No 16 (2007),pp.1765-70, ISSN 1875-533X.

Yohendran, J. & Chauhan, D. (2010). Erectile dysfunction following intravitreal bevacizumab. *MiddleEast Afr J Ophthalmol.* Vol. 17 (Jul 2010),pp.281-4, ISSN: 0974-9233.

Zambon, JP.; Mendonça, RR.; Wroclawski, ML.; Karam Junior, A.; Santos, RD.; Carvalho, JA. & Wroclawski, ER.(2010). Cardiovascular and metabolic syndrome risk among men with and without erectile dysfunction: case-control study. *Sao Paulo Med J.* Vol. 128, No 3 (2010),pp.137-40, ISSN 1516-3180.

Zippe, C.; Nandipati, K.; Agarwal, A. & Raina, R. (2006). Sexual dysfunction after pelvic surgery. *Int J Impot Res.* Vol. 18, No 1(Jan-Feb 2006), pp.1-18, ISSN: 0955-9930.

3

Erectile Dysfunction and Quality of Life

Quek Kia Fatt
School of Medicine & Health Sciences
Monash University Sunway Campus,
Selangor Darul Ehsan,
Malaysia

1. Introduction

Erectile dysfunction (ED) affects the quality of life (QoL) of millions of people worldwide (Rosen et al., 2004; Aytac et al., 1999; National Institutes of Health Consensus Development Panel on Impotence, 1993). Nowadays, QoL measurements have become an important health status indicator in determining the general health of a person. ED affects a man's self-esteem, relationships with sexual partners, family, friends and colleagues and overall QoL.

The impact of ED on QoL has been becoming very important in the management of ED. QoL is used to assess the overall well-being of a person. Most of the medical treatments for ED now are focussing on improving QoL of patients (Althof, 2002).

2. What is quality of life/ health-related quality of life

2.1 Quality of life

QoL is defined as the perception of a person's life in the cultural and value systems in which he or she lives in regards to his or her goals, expectations and standards. QoL is affected by a person physical health, psychological state, level of independence, social relationships, environment and spiritual/religion/personal beliefs (WHOQOL, 1997).

QoL is a construct that encompasses physical function, psychological function, somatic sensation, social interaction, occupational and financial (Schipper et al., 1996). QoL is a good indicator of functional status and well-being of a person who undergone treatment for medical conditions (Stewart et al., 1989). QoL is becoming important in the evaluation of treatment and assessment of medical conditions (Wagner et al., 2000).

The overall QoL encompasses disease free, physical, emotional and social well-being (Tsai et al., 2008). QoL is one's ability to enjoy normal life activities. Some medical treatments can impair one's QoL while there are treatments can improve it.

The main goal of health care is to maintain or improve the QoL of people. Apart from health status, factors such as religion, environment, financial etc are important determinants of a person's QoL (Chen et al., 2005; WHOQOL, 1997).

2.2 Health-Related Quality of Life

Health-Related Quality of Life (HRQoL) is widely used among health care/medical professionals and is an important measure to assess a person's well-being (Wilson and Cleary, 1995). HRQoL includes the physical, functional, psychological, emotional, social function, mental and overall well-being of an individual (Fallowfield, 2009).

ED can affect both men and women, as they may suffer due to ED. Men will also suffer if their female partners have sexual dysfunction. These problems need to be look into as an overall health issue (Wagner et al., 2000).

3. ED and QOL

ED is associated with many psychosocial problems such as decreased QoL, low self-esteem, depression, anxiety, relationship problems, and marital tension (Althof, 2002; Litwin et al., 1998; Shabsigh et al., 1998). According to many studies, it is undeniable that ED has a strong impact on QoL (Tsai, 2008; Althof, 2002; Litwin et al., 1998).

There are many studies showing ED has an effect on QoL of men with this condition (Rosen et al., 2004; Althof 2002). Satisfaction in sexual life has been shown to affect overall satisfaction in life (Fugl-Meyer et al., 1997). Studies have shown that QoL parameters, especially social relationship and psychological well-being is affected by ED (Tsai et al., 2008; Litwin et al., 1998). Men with ED suffer deterioration in emotional well-being as noted in some studies (Litwin et al., 1998; Rosen, 1998).

One HRQOL study showed that ED is associated with physical function and emotional function (Litwin et al., 1998). This study also found that emotional domains are more affected than physical domains in patients with ED.

The majority of studies showed that men who suffer ED will have poor QoL especially in physical, mental and social domains (Sanchez-Cruz et al., 2003). Laumann et al. 1999 found there is an association between ED with health status and emotional function /problems / satisfaction, stress, deterioration of general health and physical satisfaction.

3.1 Young and old men

Younger males show lower social function as compared to older men and significant differences were observed between non-ED and ED subjects in young age group (Sanchez-Cruz et al., 2003). For example, it was found that men with ED tend to have lower QoL especially among young men compared to men without ED. One of the reasons is probably older men reported more sexual satisfaction than younger men as reported in one study (Gralla et al., 2008).

3.2 Sexual activity and QoL

Satisfaction in sexual activity is important in achieving good QoL. Sexual activity has been found to contribute to the overall QoL (Robinson & Molzahn, 2007). The psychological and social well-being of a man will be affected if he lacks sexual activity. However, there are some men who consider ED as a part of the aging process (Martin-Diaz et al., 2006).

3.3 ED with co-morbid condition and QoL

It is difficult to assess the real effect of ED on QoL because ED could be due to psychological or other medical conditions. It was also found that men with ED with co-morbid medical condition such as hypertension or diabetes mellitus have lower QoL (Rosen et al., 2004). Men with both comorbid medical condition and ED were found to have poorer QoL as they are more distress and less satisfied with their sexual life (Berardis et al., 2002). It is noted that a man's age is associated with QoL as suggested by Guest & Gupta, (2002). The QoL of men with ED who are younger than 65 years was found to be poorer (Guest & Gupta, 2002) compared to men of similar age who do not suffer ED (Kind, 1999). Those men younger than 45 years old were found to have poorer QoL compared to those aged 74 years or older. The deterioration of QoL in the younger age group was noted due to deterioration of erectile function (Feldman et al., 1994). The QoL in the older group was much better because they focus less attention or less emphasize on sexual activity (Guest & Gupta, 2002). Men from all age groups who had co-morbid illnesses were found to have poorer QoL as compared to those without co-morbid illnesses. ED has been shown to have contributed to the deterioration of emotional well being and relationship but improved after treatment (Paige et al., 2001). Some men with ED tend to worry about their sexual performance thus this may lead to premature ejaculation (Williams et al., 1984).

3.4 ED and relationship with partner

ED can lead to the breakdown of relationships due to conflicts with their partners and this affects their general health and QoL (Guest & Gupta, 2002). Study has shown that approximately 12%-28% of men with ED believed ED is one of the main causes that affect their relationships (Guest & Gupta, 2002).

Men with ED who are single were found to be unable to develop a new relationship, thus, this affects their QoL (Guest & Gupta, 2002). This suggests ED may hinder them from forming a new relationship or may deteriorate their current relationship which may lead to separation.

However, sometimes relationships can be improved through other ways other than having sexual intercourse such as focusing family activities or having relaxation. Pharmacological intervention has shown to improve men's QoL e.g sildenafil citrate and transurethral alprostadil (Quirk et al., 1998; William et al., 1998; Kaiser et al., 1997).

3.5 Quality of life following treatment of ED

Several studies showed sexual function improves the QoL in both men and their partners following treatment (Rosen et al., 2004; Shabsigh et al., 2001). It has been shown that the mood, overall sexual function, satisfaction in relationships and their overall QoL improves after treatment of ED (Rosen at al., 2004).

The level of sexual life satisfaction which was noted to be low prior to treatment for ED, were significantly improved after treatment (Fugl-Meyer et al., 1997). Men with ED and depression, their QoL were also improved after undergoing treatment for depression (Muller & Benkert, 2001).

4. Anxiety

Anxiety is a feeling of worry, fear, nervousness and apprehension exhibited by psychological, and physiological state such as emotional, cognitive and behavioral symptoms. Anxiety due to daily activities may lead to distress and deterioration of normal activity (Corretti & Baldi, 2007).

Anxiety disorders include panic disorder (PD), specific and social phobia, obsessive-compulsive disorder (OCD), post-traumatic stress disorder (PTSD), acute stress disorder (ASD), and generalized anxiety disorder (GAD) (Corretti and Baldi, 2007).

The relationship between anxiety and sexual function is complex. However, anxiety and ED can have a two-way or bilateral relationship. Anxiety can cause sexual dysfunction and sexual dysfunction can cause anxiety. Sexual dysfunction and anxiety are not causally related. They may express differently but the symptoms may derive from one common source (Corretti and Baldi, 2007).

Anxiety contributes to the development of problems associated with ED. Psychological impact from ED can lead to uneasiness, distance and conflicts (Hedon, 2003). This will lead to low sexual contact, less time together and lack of communication between partners which can lead to deterioration of relationship (Hedon, 2003).

The prevalence of anxiety disorder were noted to be varies from 1.7% - 37% in men with ED (Mallis et al., 2005; Farre et al., 2004; Lee et al., 2000). Some studies showed there were some relationships or association between anxiety and ED (Corona et al., 2006; Sugimori et al., 2005).

4.1 ED and performance anxiety

If a man suffers some degree of ED, he may feel worried of the condition and this may lead to performance anxiety. Performance anxiety will affect men such as embarrassment if they are unable to perform, achieve erection or unable to satisfy their partners. They will feel disappointed and guilty, thus, this will affect their QoL.

When a person suffers from anxiety disorder, it is important to investigate his/her sexual life and vice-versa. Studies have shown that anxiety plays a major role in the development of ED.

There are many factors which can lead to anxiety and to ED. For example, job related stress and family problems (divorce, conflicts) which can increase anxiety thus leading to ED (Hedon, 2003).

Anxiety can impair sexual arousal/desire via increased sympathetic tone which leads to weak erection (Graziottin, 2000; Maggi et al., 2000; Kaplan, 1988). Anxiety can also impact orgasm where it can lead to premature ejaculation (PE) (Dunn et al., 1999; Zilbergeld, 1999; Hawton & Catalan, 1986). Anxiety can affect the ejaculation control through sympathetic hyperactivity (Williams, 1984; Wolpe, 1982).

Men who are anxious during sexual intercourse are found to be worried about their sexual performance and this affects their sexual satisfaction (Kaplan, 1989; Kaplan, 1974). There are other studies which support these findings (Corona at al., 2006; Corretti et al., 2006; Tignol et al., 2006).

5. Depression

Depression can lead to feelings of fatigue, worthlessness, suicidal thoughts, agitation, weight loss or weight gain. It can caused by grief, family and social isolation, physical, genetics, biological, psychological factors. All these contribute to the deterioration of QoL. The person may not sleep well and/or eating well and may resort to smoking, alcohol or drugs to overcome the depression.

Many studies have showed an association between ED and depression regardless of sociodemographic or co-morbidities (Shabsigh et al, 2006; Moreira et al., 2001; Araujo et al., 1998; Feldman et al., 1994). In a study by Araujo et al., 1999, subjects who were depressed were found to have a 1.82 times higher chance of getting ED compared with patients without depression. Another study showed men with ED were 2.6 times more likely to have depressive symptoms as compared to men suffering from benign prostatic hyperplasia (BPH) alone (Shabsigh et al., 1998).

Depression most of the time are due to the loss of mood/interest in daily activities. ED can affect the mood, family or partner relationships thus affecting QoL (Rosen et al., 2004).

Depression and ED is a two-way or bilateral relationship (Shabsigh et al., 2001; Araujo et al., 1998; Smith, 1998). ED has aetiology in affective components which were described in many studies (Smith, 1998; Barlow, 1986; Hengeveld, 1983; Jacobs et al., 1983). It was noted that depression may cause or exacerbate ED and that ED may cause depression. Until today, no one knows which one comes first. Patients presenting with ED should be screened for depression while patients with depression will need to be screeened for ED (Araujo et al., 1998). One study by Nicolosi et al., 2004, found a relationship between ED, depression, sexual activity and sexual satisfaction.

ED associated with depression has been observed in many studies (Araujo et al., 1998). Men with ED tend to feel embarrassed, frustrated and sad. This will affect his self-esteem thus lead to depression. Men often associate their ability to perform sex with their manhood and self-esteem. When they are unable to perform, they will feel disappointed and this will lead to depression. If the condition is not treated, ED may affect his relationship with his partners, friends and family. If the men treated for depression, it may become worse as medication may have side effects on erection (Bartlik et al., 1999).

Depression is found to affect sexual performance as indicated in the Massachusetts Male Aging Study (MMAS)(Araujo et al., 1998). The findings of this study showed that those who are depressed are more likely to suffer moderate and severe ED (Araujo et al., 1998). This study also shows that the cognitive and behavioral factors may also contribute to sexual performance. Another study showed patients who were depressed are twice likely as the general population to have sexual dysfunctions (Angst, 1998).

Depressed men can be too critical of themselves. This will lead to performance anxiety and thus will hinder their ability to achieve an erection. Depression also can affect sexual drive (Heiman & Rowland, 1983; Bartlik et al., 1999) and sexual drive is important for helping men to achieve an erection. Men with low sexual drive (libido) tend to have difficulties in achieving erection.

Depression is found to be associated with neurophysiological disturbances which can affect the autonomic nervous system. Due to this, the parasympathetic nervous system unable to assist the relaxation of the penile smooth muscle tissue which require for erection (Saenz de Tejada I, 1985). Men with severe depression can develop a reversible loss of nocturnal penile tumescence (Roose et al., 1982). Studies have shown depression can deteriorate the erectile function but improved following treatment with antidepressants (Nofzinger et al., 1993).

It was found that men with the severe depression had higher chance of getting moderate and severe ED (Melman & Gingell, 1999). The relationship between depression and ED is affected by the low frequency of sexual intercourse and poor sex life.

ED is one of the symptoms of depressive disorder which associated with deterioration or loss of sexual drive, erectile function, and sexual activity (Seidman et al., 2001). This condition will get worse if the person is on medications such as antidepressants which can cause ejaculation, erection, orgasm and libido problems (Nurnberg et al., 2001; Seidman & Roose, 2000; Rosen et al., 1999).

5.1 Depression, ED and treatment

Depression with ED or vice versa is treatable. With proper counseling, men will be able to overcome the depression and cope with ED as there are many treatment options available for ED.

The inability to achieve and maintain sexual performance often causes other problems apart from problems related to sexual activity. It is important for a man to seek help if he is experiencing depression or ED or both.

Studies have shown that treatment is successful in improving the QoL in men with ED co-morbid with depression.

6. Marital problem

Many men with ED will stay silent and not like to talk about their problems to others. Men with ED tend to think they are failures and thinking their partner is not happy. These men will find excuses to avoid having sex or having intimate relationships.

Some will find excuses or changing their topics of conversation to avoid talking about sex. When men start to withdraw themselves from their partners and others, they will be thinking of their ED problem. Thus, this may affect their daily activities and general health.

When a man is unable to perform sexual intercourse or unable to satisfy his partner's sexual needs, he may feel useless, embarrassed and guilty. Thus, he may find difficult to communicate with his partner about ED. ED affects a man's life and marriage and it was noted that ED contributed to one in five failed marriages (Wespes et al., 2002).

ED affects men psychologically. Because of miscommunication and misunderstanding, the partner may abandon him. Men tend to blame their partner for leaving them due to ED.

Men are found to be sensitive in their relationships. Any withdrawals from the relationship due to ED may affect their overall general health and well-being (National Institutes of Health Consensus Development Panel on Impotence, 1993). The relationship between sexual and marital problems was more obvious in men compared to women as shown in one study (Rust et al., 1988).

From the partner point of view, the partner will feel unattractive, lonely, depressed and unwanted. The partner may think that their partner is having an affair. This becomes worse when men do not communicate with their partner regarding their ED. Many men refuse to seek medical advice due to apprehension. Apart from that there are also misunderstanding and poor communications which may lead to the relationship breakdown with their partners.

The prevalence of sexual dysfunction was noted higher in women especially when their partner suffering from ED. Women who have been sexually active before will suffer some sexual dysfunction. The severity of ED can influence their partners' sexual satisfaction and frequency of orgasm (Fisher et al., 2005). Women suffer deterioration of sexual desire, unable to achieve orgasm and dissatisfied with their sexual life when their partner suffering from ED. However, this improved after their partners' undergone treatment. One study has shown women whose partners who were on pharmacological therapy (e.g. PDE5 inhibitors) had more satisfying sexual satisfaction than those whose partners did not use pharmacological therapy (Fisher et al., 2005).

7. Summary

Although ED is not a life-threatening condition, it has an effect on not only the QoL of men but that of their sexual partners as well. The effect of ED on QoL is hard to determine because the dysfunction can be due to the psychological problem. However, ED can cause anxiety, sadness, depression, low self-confidence, low self-esteem, marital tension, deteriorating relationships, guilt, anger, frustration etc. All these will lead to deterioration of QoL.

It is important for men to discuss their anxiety regarding their ED with their partners. It will help them to reduce their fears while their partner will be able to help them to cope. Men should realize that they are not alone in ED. There are many avenues where they can seek help where they are many qualified ED medical professionals who can provide counseling and also there are treatments and guidelines available in the management of male sexual dysfunction (Wespes et al., 2009). Men should communicate with their partners because they need moral support to overcome their ED problem. When it comes to HRQoL for men, it is vital to assess their erectile function.

8. References

Althof SE. Quality of life and erectile dysfunction. Urology 2002; 59(6): 803–810.

Angst J. Sexual Problem in Healthy and Depressed Persons. International Clinical Psychopharmacology. 1998; 13(6):S1-S4.

Araujo AB, Durante R, Feldman HA, Goldstein I, McKinlay JB. The Relationship Between Depressive Symptoms and Male Erectile Dysfunction: Cross-Sectional Result From the Massachusetts Male Aging Study. Psychosomatic Medicine. 1998; 60(4): 458-465

Aytac IA, McKinlay JB, Krane RJ. The likely worldwide increase in erectile dysfunction between 1995 and 2025 and some possible policy consequences British Journal Urology International. 1999; 84(1): 50–6.

Barlow DH. Causes of sexual dysfunction: The role of anxiety and cognitive interference. Journal of Consulting and Clinical Psychology. 1986; 54(2):140-148

Bartlik B, Kocsis JH, Legere R, Villaluz J, Kossoy A, Gelenberg AJ. Sexual dysfunction secondary to depressive disorder. Journal Gender Specific Medicine. 1999; 2(2): 52-60.

Berardis GD, Franciosi M, Belfiglio M, Di Nardo B, Greenfield S, Kaplan SH, Pellegrini F, Sacco M, Tognoni G, Valentini M, Nicolucci A; for the Quality of Care and Outcomes in Type 2 Diabetes (QuED) Study Group. Erectile Dysfunction and Quality of Life in Type 2 Diabetic Patients. A serious problem too often overlooked. Diabetes Care. 2002; 25(2):284–291.

Chen TH, Li L, Kochen MM. A systematic review: How to choose appropriate health-related quality of life (HRQOL) measures in routine general practice? Journal of Zhejiang University Science. 2005; 6B(9): 936–940.

Corretti G, Baldi I. The Relationship Between Anxiety Disorders and Sexual Dysfunction. Psychiatric Times. 2007; 24(9).

Corretti G, Pierucci S, De Scisciolo M, Nisita C. Comorbidity between social phobia and premature ejaculation: study on 242 males affected by sexual disorders. Journal of Sexual and Marital Therapy. 2006;32(2):183-187.

Corona G, Mannucci E, Petrone L, Ricca V, Balercia G, Giommi R, Forti G, Maggi M. Psychobiological correlates of free-floating anxiety symptoms in male patients with sexual dysfunctions. Journal of Androlology. 2006; 27(1):86-93.

Dunn KM, Croft PR, Hackett GI. Association of sexual problem with social, psychological, and physical problems in men and women: a cross sectional population survey. Journal of Epidemiology and Community Health. 1999;53(3):144-148.

Fallowfield L. What is quality of life? Health Economics 2nd ed., Hayward Medical Communications, pp1-7.

Farre JM, Fora F, Lasheras MG. Specific aspects of erectile dysfunction in psychiatry. International Journal of Impotence Research. 2004; 16(suppl 2):S46-S49.

Feldman HA, Goldstein I, Hatzichristou DG, Krane RJ, McKinlay JB. Impotence and its medical and psychosocial correlates: results of the Massachusetts Male Aging Study. Journal of Urology. 1994; 151(1): 54–61.

Fisher WA, Rosen RC, Eardley I, Sand M, Goldstein I. Sexual experience of female partners of men with erectile dysfunction: the Female Experience of Men's Attitudes to Life Events and Sexuality (FEMALES) study. Journal of Sexual Medicine. 2005;2(5):675–684.

Fugl-Meyer AR, Lodnert G, Branholm I-B, Fugl-Meyer KS. On life satisfaction in male erectile dysfunction. Internationl Journal of Impotence Research. 1997;9(3): 141–148.

Gralla O, Knoll N, Fenske S, Spivak I, Hoffmann M, Ronnebeck C, Lenk S, Hoschke B, May M. Worry, desire, and sexual satisfaction and their association with severity of ED and age. Journal of Sexual Medicine. 2008; 5(11):2646-2655.

Graziottin A. Libido: The biologic scenario. Maturitas. 2000;34:S9-S16.

Guest JF, Das Gupta R. Health-related quality of life in a UK-based population of men with erectile dysfunction. Pharmacoeconomics. 2002; 20(2): 109–117.

Hawton K, Catalan J. Prognostic factors in sex therapy. Behaviour Research and Therapy. 1986; 24(4):377-385.

Hedon F. Anxiety and erectile dysfunction: a global approach to ED enhances results and quality of life. International Journal of Impotence Research. 2003; 15(2): S16–S19.

Heiman JR, Rowland DL. Affective and physiological sexual response patterns: The effects of instructions on sexually functional and dysfunctional men. Journal of Psychosomatic Research. 1983; 27(2):105-116.

Hengeveld MW. Erectile dysfunction: A sexological and psychiatric review. World Journal of Urology. 1983; 1(4): 227-232.

Jacobs JA, Fishkin R, Cohen S, Goldman A, Mulholland SG. A multidisciplinary approach to the evaluation and management of male sexual dysfunction. Journal of Urology. 1983; 129(1):35-38.

Kaiser FE, Weldon K, Gesundheit N, MUSE Study Group. Treatment of erectile dysfunction with transurethral alprostadil: effects on quality of life. Journal of the American Geriatric Society. 1997; 45: A33.

Kaplan HS. The New Sex Therapy. New York: Brunner-Mazel; 1974.

Kaplan HS. Anxiety and sexual dysfunction. Journal of Clinicial Psychiatry. 1988;49(Suppl 21-5): 21-25.

Kaplan HS. PE: How to Overcome Premature Ejaculation. New York: Brunner-Mazel; 1989.

Kind P, Hardmann G, Macran S. UK population norms for EQ-5D. Discussion paper 172, 1999. York: University of York.

Laumann EO, Paik A, Rosen RC. Sexual dysfunction in the United States. Prevalence and predictors. Journal of the American Medical Association. 1999; 281(6):537–544.

Lee JC, Surridge D, Morales A, Heaton JPW. The prevalence and influence of significant psychiatric abnormalities in men undergoing comprehensive management of organic erectile dysfunction. International Journal of Impotence Research. 2000; 12(1): 47-51.

Litwin MS, Nied RJ, Dhanani N. Health-related quality of life in men with erectile dysfunction. Journal of General Internal Medicine. 1998; 13(3):159–166.

Maggi M, Filippi S, Ledda F, Magini A, Forti G. Erectile dysfunction: from biochemical pharmacology to advances in medical therapy. European Journal of Endocrinology. 2000;143(1):143-154.

Mallis D, Moysidis K, Nakopoulou E, Papaharitou S, Hatzimouratidis K, Hatzichristou D. Psychiatric morbidity is frequently undetected in patientswith erectile dysfunction. Journal of Urology. 2005;174(5):1913-1916.

Martin-Diaz F, Reig-Ferrer A, Ferrer-Cascales R. Sexual function and quality of life in hemodialysis male patients. Nefrologia. 2006;26(4):452-460.

Melman A, Gingell JC. The epidemiology and pathophysiology of erectile dysfunction. Journal of Urology. 1999;161(1):5–11.

Muller MJ, Benkert O. Lower self-reported depression in patients with erectile dysfunction after treatment with sildenafil. Journal of Affective Disorders. 2001; 66(2-3): 255–261.

Moreira EDJr, Najjar Abdo CH, Torres EB, Lisboa Lobo CF, Saraiva Fittipaldi JA. Prevalence and correlates of erectile dysfunction: results of the Brazilian study of sexual behavior. Urology. 2001; 58(4): 583–588.

Nicolosi A, Moreira ED Jr, Villa M, Glasser DB. A population study of association between sexual satisfaction and depressive symptoms in men. Journal of Affective Disorder. 2004; 82(2):235-243.

National Institutes of Health Consensus Development Panel on Impotence. NIH Consensus Conference: Impotence. Journal of the American Medical Association. 1993; 270(1): 83-90.

Nofzinger EA, Thase ME, Reynolds CF 3rd, Frank E, Jennings JR, Garamoni GL, Fasiczka AL, Kupfer DJ. Sexual function in depressed men. Assessment by self-report, behavioral, and nocturnal penile tumescence measures before and after treatment with cognitive behavior therapy. Archives of General Psychiatry. 1993; 50(1): 24–30.

Nurnberg HG, Gelenberg A, Hargreave TB, Harrison WM, Siegel RL, Smith MD. Efficacy of sildenafil citrate for the treatment of erectile dysfunction in men taking serotonin reuptake inhibitors. American Journal of Psychiatry. 2001; 158(11): 1926–1928.

Paige NM, Hays RD, Litwin MS, Rajfer J, Shapiro MF. Improvement in emotional well-being and relationships of users of sildenafil. Journal of Urology. 2001; 166(5): 1774–1778.

Quirk F, Giuliano F, Pena B, Mishra A, Smith MD, Hockey H. Effect of sildenafil (Viagra) on quality of life parameters in men with broad-spectrum erectile dysfunction. Journal of Urology. 1998; 159 (Suppl. 260): A 998

Robinson JG, Molzahn AE. Sexuality and quality of life. Journal of Gerontology Nursing. 2007;33(3):19-27.

Roose SP, Glassman AH, Walsh BT, Cullen K. Reversible loss of nocturnal penile tumescence during depression: a preliminary report. Neuropsychobiology. 1982; 8(6): 284–288

Rosen RC. Quality of life assessment in sexual dysfunction trials. International Journal of Impotence Research. 1998;10(Suppl 2):S21-3; discussion S24-6.

Rosen RC, Lane RM, Menza M. Effects of SSRIs on sexual function: a critical review. Journal of Clinical Psychopharmacology. 1999; 19(1): 67- 85.

Rosen RC, Fisher WA, Eardley I, Niederberger C, Nadel A, Sand M. The multinational men's attitudes to life events and sexuality (MALES) study: I. Prevalence of erectile dysfunction and related health concerns in the general population. Current Medical Research and Opinions. 2004; 20(5): 607-617.

Rosen RC, Seidman SN, Menza MA, Shabsigh R, Roose SP, Tseng LJ, Orazem J, Siegel RL. Quality of life, mood, and sexual function: a path analytic model of treatment effects in men with erectile dysfunction and depressive symptoms. International Journal of Impotence Research. 2004; 16(4): 334–340.

Rust J, Golombok S, Collier J. Marital problems and sexual dysfunction: how are they related? British Journal of Psychiatry. 1988; 152:629-631.

Sanchez-Cruz JJ, Cabrera-Leon A, Martın-Morales A, Fernandez A, Burgos R, Rejas J. Male Erectile Dysfunction and Health-Related Quality of Life. European Urology. 2003; 44(2): 245–253.

Saenz de Tejada I, Goldstein I, Blanco R, Cohen RA, Krane RJ. Smooth muscle of the corpora cavernosae: Role in penile erection. Surgical Forum. 1985;36:623-624.

Schipper H, Clinch JJ, Olweny CLM. Quality of life studies: definitions and conceptual issues. In: Spilker B, ed. Quality of life and pharmacoeconomics in clinical trials. 2nd ed. Philadelphia, PA: Lippincott-Raven; 1996: 11-23

Seidman SN, Roose SP, Menza MA, Shabsigh R, Rosen RC. Treatment of erectile dysfunction in men with depressive symptoms: Results of a placebo-controlled trial with sildenafil citrate. American Journal of Psychiatry. 2001; 158(10): 1623–1630.

Seidman SN, Roose SP. The relationship between depression and erectile dysfunction. Current Psychiatry Reports. 2000; 2:201–205.

Shabsigh R, Klein LT, Seidman S, Kaplan SA, Lehrhoff BJ, Ritter JS. Increased incidence of depressive symptoms in men with erectile dysfunction. Urology. 1998; 52(5): 848–852.

Shabsigh R, Zakaria L, Anastasiadis AG, Seidman AS. Sexual Dysfunction and Depression: Etiology, Prevalence, and Treatment. Current Urology Reports. 2001; 2(6): 463-467.

Shabsigh R, Perelman MA. Men With Both Premature Ejaculation (PE) and Erectile Dysfunction (ED) Experience Lower Quality of Life Than Men With Either PE or ED Alone. In: Selected abstracts of presentations during the XVII World Congress of Sexology. Journal of Sex Research. 2006. 43(1): 2-37.

Smith, AD. Psychologic factors in the multidisciplinary evaluation and treatment of erectile dysfunction. Urologic Clinics of North America. 1998; 15(1):41-51

Stewart AL, Greenfield S, Hays RD, Wells K, Rogers WH, Berry SD, McGlynn EA, Ware JE Jr. Functional status and well-being of patients with chronic conditions. Results from the medical outcomes study. Journal of the American Medical Association. 1989; 262(7):907-913.

Sugimori H, Yoshida K, Tanaka T, Baba K, Nishida T, Nakazawa R, Iwamoto T. Relationships between erectile dysfunction, depression, and anxiety in Japanese subjects. Journal of Sexual Medicine. 2005; 2(3):390-396.

Tignol J, Martin-Guehl C, Aouizerate B, Grabot D, Auriacombe M. Social phobia and premature ejaculation: a case-control study. Depression and Anxiety. 2006; 23(3):153-157.

Tsai TF, Chang LC, Hwang TIS. Effect of Erectile Dysfunction on the Health-Related Quality of Life of Elderly People. Journal of Taiwan Urological Association. 2008; 19(4): 216-221

Wagner G, Fugl-Meyer KS and Fugl-Meyer AR. Impact of erectile dysfunction on quality of life: patient and partner perspectives. International Journal of Impotence Research. 2000; 12(Suppl 4): S144-S146.

Wespes E, Amar E, Hatzichristou D, Montorsi F, Pryor J, Vardi Y; European Association of Urology. Guidelines on erectile dysfunction. European Urology. 2002; 41(1):1-5.

Wespes E, Amar E, Eardley I, Giuliano F, Hatzichristou D, Hatzimouratidis K, Montorsi F, Vardi Y. Guidelines on Male Sexual Dysfunction: Erectile dysfunction and premature ejaculation. European Association of Urology. 2005.

WHOQOL. Measuring Quality of life. The World Health Quality of Life Instrument (The WHOQOL-100 and The WHOQOL-BREF), World Health Organization, Geneva, 1997.

Williams G, Abbou CC, Amar ET, Desvaux P, Flam TA, Lycklama a Nijeholt GA, Lynch SF, Morgan RJ, Muller SC, Porst H, Pryor JP, Ryan P, Witzsch UK, Hall MM, Place VA, Spivack AP, Todd LK, Gesundheit N. The effect of transurethral alprostadil on the

quality of life of men with erectile dysfunction, and their partners. MUSE Study Group. British Journal of Urology International. 1998; 82(6): 847–854.
Williams W. Secondary premature ejaculation. Australian and New Zealand Journal of Psychiatry. 1984;18(4):333-340.
Wilson IB, Cleary PD. Linking clinical variables with health related quality of life. Journal of the American Medical Association. 1995:273(1):59-65.
Wolpe J. The practice of behaviour therapy. Toronto: Pergamon; 1982.
Zilbergeld B. The New Male Sexuality. New York: Bantam Books; 1999.

Part 2

Diseases-Associated ED

4

The Role Erectile Dysfunction Plays in Cardiovascular Diseases

Sandra Crestani[1,2], Kenia Pedrosa Nunes[2], Maria Consuelo Andrade Marques[1], José Eduardo Da Silva Santos[3] and R. Clinton Webb[2]
[1]*Federal University of Parana*
[2]*Georgia Health Sciences University, Augusta, Georgia*
[3]*Federal University of Santa Catarina*
[1,3]*Brazil*
[2]*USA*

1. Introduction

Erectile dysfunction (ED) is defined as the persistent inability to maintain or achieve a penile erection sufficient for satisfactory sexual performance (1-2). ED is a very common condition in middle-aged men (3). According to the National Institute of Health (NIH) this physiological disorder affects 30 million men in the United States (US) (2). The outlook for 2025 is scary because this number is expected to grow to approximately 322 million (4). Although ED is directly associated with aging (5), its etiology is considered multifactorial. Both conditions, ED and aging, share a variety of risk factors such as atherosclerosis, sedentary lifestyle, abnormal lipids, diabetes, smoking, metabolic syndrome and hypertension (2, 6-7). In addition, ED is considered an important marker of cardiovascular disease (CVD) (8). Studies over the last decade suggest vascular changes as a common factor between ED and CVD (1, 7, 9). Also, the most important vascular alteration mentioned in these pathologies cited above is endothelial dysfunction. According to several authors, endothelial and smooth muscle dysfunction are crucial factors involved in systemic and peripheral vascular diseases, especially ED (10). In this chapter we will discuss the association between the main CVD and ED.

2. ED and atherosclerosis

Atherosclerosis begins with oxidation of Low Density Lipoproteins (LDL) particles in the arterial wall (11). Oxidatively modified LDL (oxLDL) damages the endothelial layer in the artery (8, 11), and then the elasticity of the arteries deteriorates. Impaired arterial elasticity and increased levels of circulating oxLDL, as well as elevated fibrinogen and resting heart rate associated with subclinical atherosclerosis have increased CVD risk (12-17). The decrease and/or loss of elasticity impair the blood flow because the cholesterol builds up in the blood vessel walls and forms plaque. When plaque becomes very advanced, it can completely stop blood from passing through the wall, characterizing a heart attack (18).

Diseases due to atherosclerosis are common and are becoming a growing health problem in industrialized and developing countries, evoking a huge impact on quality of life and life expectancy (2, 19). Atherosclerosis affects not only the blood vessels supplying the heart (coronary arteries), but also blood vessels throughout the entire body. In addition, various alterations disturbing normal body function can occur when atherosclerosis develops leading to more complex pathologies such as angina, heart attacks, strokes, and ED (18).

The artery size hypothesis is a pathophysiologic mechanism proposed in recent years to explain the relationship between ED and coronary artery diseases (CAD) (20). It is based on the fact that atherosclerosis, a systemic disorder, should theoretically affect all major vascular beds at the same time and extent. However, symptoms at different points in the system rarely become evident at the same time. This is probably the result of larger vessels being able to better tolerate equivalent amount of plaque compared with smaller ones. The diameter of these vessels confirms this idea: penile artery has an arterial diameter of 1-2 millimeters (mm), coronary artery is 3-4 mm, internal carotid artery is 5-7 mm and femoral artery is 6-8 mm. Results from patients with 50% obstruction in the penile artery with no coronary circulation critically affected could be explained because larger systemic arteries would be impacted later than the smaller penile artery. Thus, it suggests a mechanism for the absence of concomitant CAD in early stage ED (20-21).

The initial step in the development of atherosclerosis is endothelial dysfunction. Since the normal penile erection requires an intact endothelium, it has been proposed that patients with ED show a higher probability of developing atherosclerosis (2, 19). Regarding penile erection, nitric oxide (NO) plays an important role in physiological conditions. The sexual stimulus makes the parasympathetic nerves in the penis produce NO, triggering a cascade of events that culminate with increased dilatation of the corpora cavernosum sinusoids to induce penile erection. Many other agents are involved in this process that requires a perfect balance between vasodilators and vasoconstrictors. Thus, the physiological complexity makes it difficult to identify the etiology of ED. As a result, this condition is considered multifactorial and includes arterial, neurogenic, hormonal, cavernosal, iatrogenic, and psychogenic causes. However, it is now accepted that organic ED, in a substantial majority of men, is due to underlying vascular causes (22-23). Endothelial dysfunction is thought to be the main etiologic factor in systemic and peripheral vascular diseases, including ED (24). It has been associated with impaired vasodilatation, preceding the development of atherosclerotic lesions through the impaired release of NO, which is modulated by parasympathetic nonadrenergic, noncholinergic nerves (NANC) and by vascular endothelial cells (7). Moreover NO production is also influenced by oxidative stress, which is deleterious to the endothelium.

Reactive oxygen species (ROS) are very important in the pathophysiology of vascular disease, especially atherosclerosis. Under normal physiological conditions, ROS destruction by antioxidant enzymes is sufficient to maintain a controlled activation of signaling cascades. In contrast, in vascular diseases, the production of ROS in excess of endogenous antioxidant capacity leads to oxidative stress, which in turn results in abnormal physiological responses. Interaction between ROS and NO is implicated in many vascular diseases such as atherogenesis and play an important role in ED (25). One of the most detrimental ROS is superoxide ($O_2^{-\cdot}$), which interacts with NO decreasing NO bioavailability and resulting in formation of peroxynitrite ($ONOO^-$). All types of vascular cells produce O_2^-

and H_2O_2, two of the most significant ROS in the vessel wall. H_2O_2 can also be metabolized by myeloperoxidase, a heme enzyme produced by macrophages that converts H_2O_2 into reactive nitrogen and reactive chlorine. These reactive species can attack both LDL and HDL, enhancing cholesterol intake, reducing cholesterol efflux and contributing to plaque formation (26). In pathological situations homeostasis disruption by oxidative stress contributes to activation of proinflamatory, profibrotic and mitogenic signaling pathways leading to oxidative damage in the vasculature which in turn results in increased vasoreactivity, endothelial dysfunction, vascular remodeling, reduced vascular compliance and elevated blood pressure (BP)(26-28). All these factors also contribute to an increased adhesion and aggregation of platelets and neutrophils, and release of vasoconstrictor substances (29-30).

3. Stroke and ED

Stroke is a neuroendovascular event resulting in death of brain cells due to an ischemic lesion. According to the World Health Organization (WHO), stroke can be classified based on the size and site of lesion and its clinical consequences. Most cases of subarachnoid hemorrhage, intracranial hemorrhage and cerebral infarction are examples of stroke (31-33). Cerebrovascular diseases are the third leading cause of death in the United States, affecting 5.5 million people a year. When analyzing diseases that cause long-term consequences , the frequency of stroke is largest compared with others (34). Stroke has been responsible for 50 million deaths worldwide. In adults, cerebrovascular disease is the most frequent pathology that induces severe damage (35). It is predicted that over the next 20 years, stroke will rise from 7th in the DALY league table to 4th, principally influenced by the aging of populations especially in less economically developed countries (31, 36).

It has been hypothesized that ED represents "the tip of the iceberg" of a systemic vascular disorder. Thus, ED would potentially precede larger damage in the body, working as a sentinel event (5). Additionally, ED could be an indicator of potentially life-threatening coronary heart disease (CHD), hypertension, hyperlipidemia and stroke (37-42), which are diseases that have been the cause of morbidity and mortality among adults in industrialized societies (43).

In most studies about stroke, only the cognitive and emotional ability of the patient after the stroke has been discussed. (34) . However, the sexual function of these men has recently been investigated deeper. Since 1998 Koperlainen et al, showed that stroke patients and their wives have some level of dissatisfaction with sexual function (44). Also, ED in stroke patients has been linked with psychological causes (45). In this case, it has been speculated that impairment of cerebral erectile control functions, physical limitations after the stroke, and emotional changes, generate psychogenic and neurogenic ED (34, 46). Studies compared unilateral stroke patients compared with those showing stroke lesions in the right cerebral hemisphere. The results reported that both patients experienced ejaculation disorders besides a significant decrease in sexual desire and intercourse frequency (34, 47).

Until recently, it was believed that ED was a health problem in patients after stroke. However, increasing evidence supports an idea that men with ED have more comorbidities than men who do not. More importantly, men with ED were more likely to have strokes than those without. In the others words, ED has been cited as a strong indicator of stroke, as well as a clinical marker for cerebrovascular diseases (22, 48-49). Ponholzer et al , reported that 2,561 men with moderate to severe ED had an increased risk of stroke over 10 years (24.7% and 43.6%) (50). Furthermore, it has been suggested that ED is an independent risk factor for stroke. In this study, 1,209 men from the Massachusetts Male Aging Study were evaluated over a 15 year period and it was reported that those men who have had ED were approximately three times more likely to have a stroke if compared to those without ED (5).

The penile arteries have a smaller diameter than internal carotid, coronary and others major arteries. Thus lumen obstruction may lead to the development of ED prior to cardiac signs or stroke (22). Corroborating with this idea Lojanapiwat et al performed studies showing that patients who developed ED had endothelial dysfunction prior to the clinical symptoms. Also laboratory results for this patients indicated cardiovascular risks (51). In addition, Vicenzini et al suggested that cerebrovascular reactivity was reduced in patients with ED without other signs of clinical atherosclerosis (52). Finally Chung et al, suggested that men with ED have a significant increased risk for stroke 5 years after ED symptoms first began (22).

4. Hypertension and ED

Arterial hypertension is a systemic disorder characterized by altered regulation of cardiovascular hemodynamic, including arterial vascular resistance and cardiac index, leading to an increase in arterial blood pressure (53). It is accompanied by proliferation, migration of VSMCs, and varying levels of inflammation of the arterial wall, processes that together constitute vascular remodeling (54). Hypertension is associated with increased vasoconstrictor and reduced vasodilator responses (55-57). The pathological changes resulting from altered vascular function include injury to the brain, kidney and heart (55). Several studies have established a clinical correlation between incidence of hypertension and ED (58). According to Buccchardt et al, 30% of hypertensive patients have ED and the severity of this sexual disorder is directly proportional to the severity of hypertension. Nowadays, this fact has been well accepted because both pathologies are an unbalance between endogenous contractile and relaxing substances. In addition, since both are pathological vascular disorders, it is supposed that ED in hypertensive patients is highly prevalent and more severe than in the other people (3).

Deficiency of NO has been hypothesized to be a major cause of ED in patients with hypertension. Another substance that is important in hypertension and ED is endothelin (ET-1). ET-1 is considered a physiological antagonist of NO. ET-1 induces vasoconstriction and activates transcriptional factors that coordinate an increase of cytokines and enzymes, thus enhancing inflammation, oxidative stress and tissue damage. All these factors are very important in hypertension associated vascular dysfunction (59). Several studies have underlined the potential importance of ET-1 in the modulation of corpus cavernosum (CC) smooth muscle tone (60), since these cells can synthesize ET-1. The fetal human and adult penile cells, and several animal species, also express endothelin converting enzyme 1, the endothelin recepotors A (ETA) and B (ETB) subtypes (61-63). Furthermore, Melegy et al showed that ET-1 levels were significantly greater in patients with ED than the normal group (64).

Even though NO is well known as the major vasodilator involved in ED, other mediators are also involved. Activation of B1 or B2 kinin receptors by bradykinin (BK) induce NO and/or prostacyclin release from endothelial cells (65-66). Teixeira et al reported the existence of functional B2 kinin receptors in human erectile tissues and demonstrated that activation of it resulted in NO release. These findings were supported by results from Becker et al. They demonstrated that BK is able to promote relaxation in CC. This effect appear to involve more cAMP than cGMP (67). However, both cGMP and cAMP are associated with relaxation in systemic or penile vessel circulation.

O-GlcNAcylation is an important regulatory mechanism that also modulates stress responses in the cardiovascular system and may have significant influence on vascular blood pressure (68). Glucosamine (GlcN) is an amino sugar that can stimulate *O*-linked-*N*-acetylglucosamine (*O*-GlcNAc) modification of proteins by increasing flux through the hexosamine biosynthesis pathway, thus increasing production of UDP-GlcNAc. UDP-GlcNAc is a substrate for *O*-GlcNAc transferase (OGT), which catalyzes the *O*-linked addition of GlcNAc to serine and threonine residues of nucleocytoplasmic proteins in higher eukaryotes (68). GlcN has anti-inflammatory effects in a variety of inflammatory models and cell types. Recently, it has been demonstrated that systemic treatment with glucosamine and PUGNAc, which increases *O*-GlcNAc modification of proteins by inhibiting *O*-GlcNAcase, can inhibit acute inflammatory and neointimal responses to endoluminal arterial injury in rat's carotid artery (69). ET-1-induced changes in vascular contractile responses are mediated by O-GlcNAc modification of proteins. Aortas from Doca-salt rats, which exhibit ET-1 augment, displayed increased contractions to phenylephrine and enhanced levels of O-GlcNAC proteins. Treatment of Doca-salt rats with an endothelin A antagonist abrogated augmented vascular levels of O-GlcNAc and prevented the increase in phenylephrine vasoconstriction, suggesting that ET-1 indeed augments O-GlcNAc levels and this modification contributes to the vascular changes induced by this peptide (70). On the other hand, *O*-GlcNAcylation is also involved in ED. A new line of investigation has pointed to the significance of hyperglycemia-induced *O*-GlcNAc associated with modification of eNOS, as well as inactivation of the enzyme. It has been demonstrated that O-GlcNAc inactives eNOS in diabetes-associated ED (71). However, the exact mechanism through *O*-GlcNAcylation is correlated with hypertension or ED is still not well understood. In the last decade, another mechanism involved in the regulation of ED has been the renin-angiotensin system (RAS). Evidence has shown that there is a RAS inside of the corpus cavenosum. According Becker et al human CC is able to produce and secrete physiologically relevant amounts of angiotensin II (Ang II) (67). Ang II is the main active metabolite of the renin-angiotensin cascade. The most important physiologic effect of Angio II is induction of vascular smooth muscle contraction. This action contributes to the maintenance of systemic blood pressure through various mechanisms in the cardiovascular and renal systems. Ang II is also an important modulator of erectile function (72). Reinforcing the association of RAS and ED, angiotensin-converting enzyme (ACE) has been found in the endothelial cells of dog CC (73), and ACE mRNA expression is up-regulated in a rat model of arteriogenic ED, although it is expressed at very low levels in the penis of control rats (74).

Arginase pathway has been cited as another mechanism that may be involved in both, hypertension and ED. Growing evidence suggests that arginage misregulation plays a key role in the pathophysiology of essential hypertension and that the involvement of arginase in ED has been apparent in recent years. Arginase exists in two isoforms, the hepatic type, arginase I and the extrahepatic type, arginase II (75). Both isoforms are expressed in human CC tissue (76). Surprisingly, the role of arginase in hypertension is poorly documented. Augmented arginase activity (AA)/expression were reported in different vascular beds in models of essential or secondary hypertension (77-78). Recent studies reported that arginase inhibitor improved aortic endothelial function via a NO-dependent mechanism in pre-hypertensive or young adult SHR, and also prevented the development of hypertension (79-80).

During hypertension or ED, elevated levels of arginase can compete with NOS for available L-arginine, reducing NO and increasing superoxide production via NOS uncoupling (81). Considering this, arginase pathway can regulate overall NO production. Additionally, elevated superoxide combines with NO to form peroxynitrite further reducing NO, and also oxidative species increase arginase activity (82). ED mechanisms involve oxidative stress and vascular inflammation (83), both of which have been associated with enhanced arginase activity and expression in the vasculature (84). Furthermore, up-regulated arginase is mechanistically linked to the pathogenesis of vascular dysfunction with hypertension through increases in the polyamine and proline precursor L-ornithine, which contributes to VSM cell proliferation and intimal thickening (81, 85). There is evidence of a biological role of arginase in regulating erectile function in the aged penile vascular bed, at both the molecular and functional level (83). Also, endothelial arginase II has been proposed as a novel target for the treatment of atherosclerosis (80). Taking into account that in pathological conditions arginase can influence NO avaibility and consequently disrupt the perfect balance necessary to keep the VSM tone, arginase can be considered involved in both hypertension and ED. However, a more complete understanding about the exact mechanism leading to disruption of vascular dynamics by arginase in ED and hypertension is needed.

Regarding hypertension and ED, another important factor is the unwanted side effects from anti-hypertensive drugs. The treatment for hypertension can be associated with ED because some medicines affect erectile function, for example, diuretics. Several studies suggest that about 10% to 20% of patients taking thiazide can have ED (86), as well as patients that use an aldosterone antagonist (87). Fortunately, the effect of diuretics on ED is completely reversible after cessation of administration. β-adrenergic receptor blockers have also been suggested by several studies to be associated with ED, specially propranolol (88). However, the new generation of β-blockers appears to have less effect on erectile function, such as nebivolol. This drug enhances erectile response and reverses ED in diabetic rats, as well as potentiates NO/cGMP-mediated relaxation of human penile tissues (89). Interestingly, angiotensin-converting enzyme inhibitors (ACEI) and angiotensin receptor blockers (ARB) appear to favorably affect sexual function (90). Patients treated with captopril showed improved sexual function by 40% to 80% compared to non-treated patients (91). The same has been observed for hypertensive patients treated with valsartan; reduced ED and improved orgasmic function and sexual satisfaction (92). Also, it was found that losartan helps preserve erectile function in male rats after bilateral cavernous nerve injury by counter-acting fibrotic activator factors (93). However, recent study showed no change in ED progression in humans with ACEI or angioten-receptor blocker (ARB) therapy (94).

Regarding the α-adrenoceptor agents to treat hypertension, has been showed that direct cavernosal injection of α1-antagonists cause erection in both, experimental and humans, although this effect is not observed with α2-selective drugs. Notably, it has been observed that patients treated with α1-blockers of the adrenergic receptors exhibited improvement of their sexual activity. On the other hand, especial attention is necessary for hypertensive patients treated with vasodilators such as α-blockers because if those patients have ED, they should not take PDE5 inhibitors, otherwise, combining these drugs will result in hypotension. The treatment with calcium channel blockers, which dilate arteries by reducing calcium influx into cells also efectively lower blood pressure. The currently available ones inhibit L-type channels in humans and seem to have a neutral effect on erection (95). Possibly this is because this channel is linked with nNOS activation from cholinergic nerve endings into the penis, which is important for NO release and consequently erection. However, although this channel is inhibited, nNOS from nitrergic nerves will be activated, allowing the erectile process to begin. Finally, direct vasodilators such as hydralazine and minoxidil have rarely been reported to cause ED.

5. Heart failure and ED

Heart failure (HF) is a syndrome manifesting as the inability of the heart to fill with or eject blood due to structural or functional cardiac conditions (96). Some authors believe that HF can be considered as the last stage of heart disease and a significant cause of mortality and morbidity worldwide (97). According to the American Heart Association (AHA), HF is a condition that affects nearly 5.7 million Americans of all ages (98). Nevertheless, in the last decade improvement in survival of myocardial infarction and HF has been observed, concurrent with consequences from these diseases. It is believed that the prevalence of these diseases will continue to increase in the population, with an estimated number of more than 10 million patients by the year 2037. Coronary artery disease, with or without myocardial infarctions, with a subsequent development of ischemic cardiomyopathy or loss of contractile proteins, remains the major cause of chronic HF progression, especially among the elderly population (99). Looking at chronic heart failure (CHF) the numbers are equally alarming. The AHA has estimated more than 4.9 million people in the US have CHF (98). As this pathophysiology progresses, patients experience an increase in fatigue, shortness of breath, palpitations, or angina, decreasing their quality of life and potentially interfering with their sexual performance (90).

While HF per se can have many effects on a patient's lifestyle, ED can further aggravate these effects and contribute to poor quality of life and depression. Studies showed the prevalence of ED is around 67% in men 65 or older, and 68% in men older than 79 (100). The prevalence of ED in patients with HF appears to be significantly higher. Baraghoush et al, found a prevalence of 84% general sexual dysfunction in the male population with an average of 59 years of age and chronic compensated HF (99, 101).

It is common sense that the physiology behind an erection is a primarily vascular phenomenon. In patients with HF, several factors that come into play at the microvascular level, such as reduced arterial compliance, endothelial dysfunction, and generalized focal atherosclerosis (99). There are few theories that explain the mechanism of endothelial dysfunction in patients with HF. Impaired relaxation mediated by L-arginine-NO was found in smooth muscle cells (SMC) and in the penis from animals and humans with atherosclerotic coronary arteries (102). However, systemic endothelium-dependent vasodilatation has been shown to decrease ED in men with and without clinical CVD (103). In addition, decreased NO production via downregulation of endothelial NO synthase (eNOS) and cyclooxygenase (COX) was observed after the onset of pacing-induced HF in dogs (104). Rho-kinase signaling is very important in erectile function because in the absence of arousal, the penis remains in the non-erect state by cavernosal vasoconstriction induced mainly by norepinephrine and endothelin 1 (ET-1), which are Rho-kinase mediated responses. Thus, its upregulation leads to

ED (105). Also, this pathway is involved in the regulation of myofibrillar Ca^{+2} sensitivity in cardiac muscle and contributes to irreversible myocardial damage. Rho-kinase is involved also in the pathogenesis of cardiovascular remodeling and its inhibition plays a significant role in treatment of the failing heart by limiting infarct size, which is the major contributor to the development of heart failure. The cardioprotective effect of Rho-kinase inhibition involves PI3K/AKT and NOS activation. However, Rho-kinase inhibitor compounds need to be evaluated for their efficacy during varying index ischemia periods, a wide dose range, and *in vivo* animal models mimicking the clinical setting more closely (105).

Becker et al reported that patients with HF have vasomodulators, systemic levels unbalanced and this change can lead to increased SMC tone and vasoconstriction in the penile vessels through a variety of mechanisms (106). According to Pedersen et al, the ET-1, RhoA/Rho-kinase and ROS are not the only mechanism that can be modified, vasopressin also is elevated in patients with HF (107). Compared to patients with CHF, the situation is very similar. In 2005 Rastogi et al suggested that multiple factors may be involved in the onset of ED in patients with CHF. These patients have arterial compliance abnormalities and often atherosclerosis, which reduce blood flow into the CC (108). In addition, endothelial dysfunction decreased the production or increases the breakdown of NO. Other vasoconstrictors are also increased in patients with CHF and can be interfering with their ability to achieve and maintain an erection (109). Finally, several medicines commonly used to treat HF have been shown to either cause or worsen ED (99). Digoxin for example, is a drug that can cause ED even though the mechanism by which this happen is not really clear, but it has been speculated that this drug creates a sexual hormonal unbalance (110) and the inhibition of cavernosal sodium/ potassium-adenosine triphosphate activity, consequently impairing NO relaxation (111).

	No. of Events			
End Points	***Total***	***No ED During Study***	***ED prior to Cardiovascular event***	***ED after to Cardiovascular event***
Angina	297	12	241	44
Miocardial infarction	571	57	57	50
Miocardial infarction or angina	801	68	649	84
Stroke	181	16	157	8
Congestive Heart failure	33	7	25	1
Transient ischemic attack	113	7	96	10
Arrhythmia	193	21	149	23
First cardiovascular event	1186	113	955	118
Death due to any cause	457	75	382	0

Table 1. **Relationship between the first report of ED and subsequent cardiovascular disease.** Incident ED was statistically significant associated with subsequent angina, myocardial infarction and stroke (red circles). Also, number of patients who showed ED prior the cardiovascular event was extremely higher compared to those who shoed ED after cardiovascular event (red circle). Men with incident ED had a significantly increased risk of myocardial infarctation or angina relative to men without a report of ED. Adapted from Thompson et al, 2005 (112).

6. The link between ED and CVD

An emerging basic science and clinical database provides a strong argument for endothelial and smooth muscle dysfunction as a central etiologic factor in systemic and peripheral diseases, including ED (113). The endothelium is the single layer of cells that line the luminal surface of blood vessels. It is far more than just a structural lining; it has a range of important physiological functions. It acts as a direct interface between the components of circulating blood and local tissue, and regulates numerous local blood vessel functions, including vascular tone, cell adhesiveness, coagulation, inflammation and permeability. The endothelium produces and responds to several potent, locally and active mediators. The most important of these is NO, which is a nonadrenergic-noncholinergic (NANC) vasodilator neurotransmitter involved in the regulation of vascular wall function (113). This highly reactive gas presents potent anti-atherogenic properties, in addition to inhibiting platelet aggregation and regulating vascular tone (114). Moreover, in the atherosclerosis installation process there are leucocytes adhesion and inflammatory agents that contribute to plaque instability and rupture, and this event can be inhibited by NO.

The vasodilatation induced by NO is initiated with the synthesis from L-arginine by nitric oxide synthases (NOS) (115). Physiological amounts of NO can be produced by endothelium (eNOS) or neuronal (nNOS) enzymes and both are involved in penile erection. Down regulation of eNOS in pathological conditions results in reduced bioavailability of NO and consequently endothelial dysfunction (8). Inhibition of nNOs attenuated erectile responses (116). Erectile function was also found to be preserved in mice lacking eNOS. However, incracavernosal pressure during erection was significantly decrease in eNOS-deficient mice and over all, NOS activity was only 60% of the activity observed in wild type mice. Thus, physiologic penile erection is mediated by both nNOS and eNOS (7, 117).

NO activates a soluble guanylyl cyclase that forms cyclic guanosine monophosphate (cGMP) (118) in vascular smooth muscle cells, resulting in penile relaxation (8, 23). Reports of ED in cGMP-dependent kinase-I (cGKI)-deficient mice suggest that cGMP is indeed the main second messenger in ED (119). These findings are supported by clinical data showing that phosphodiesterase type 5 inhibitor (PDE5, e.g. sildenafil) prevents the degradation of cGMP (120). In cGKI-deficient mice cAMP-mediated pathway cannot compensate deficient cGMP-dependent signaling *in vivo* (119). However, in humans prostaglandin E1 and its derivative alprostadil, which induce relaxation predominantly via cAMP pathway, were found to be highly effective in the treatment of ED (121-122).

Dysfunction of the endothelium may be interpreted as homeostasis disturbance due to breakdown. Also, endothelial dysfunction can be caused by vascular insults, such as diabetes, smoking, hyperlipidemia and hypertension (123). At the cellular level, endothelial dysfunction outcomes in impaired release of NO, which may be considered a key pathomechanism in both endothelial (124-125) and erectile dysfunction (115, 126). Oxidative stress, which is directly toxic to the endothelium and also interferes with the NO pathway, is a causal factor in clinically evident occlusive CVD and vascular damage associated with preclinical disease. Free radical damage, impaired function and availability of NO can also result in increased adhesion, aggregation of platelets and neutrophils, besides the release of vasoconstrictor substances (29-30, 113). In addition NOS depends on tetrahydrobiopterin as a co-factor. Endothelial dysfunction associated with tetrahydrobiopterin depletion could be reversed by supplementation of this substance (127-129). Indeed the treatment with tetrahydrobiopterin increased NOS activity by 30% in rabbit CC (130).

Over the past years studies have showed that many men will realize the onset of ED occurs before they are diagnosed with CVD. The anatomic structure of the penis and the physiology of getting and maintaining an erection provide clues as to the reason the penile vascular bed has some unique properties that facilitate early detection of systemic vascular disease (113). Nowadays, it is well known that ED can result from any number of structural or functional abnormalities in the penile vascular bed. For instance, ED may be a consequence of the cavernosal arteries oclusion by atherosclerosis, impairment of endothelial-dependent and/or independent smooth muscle relaxation, or a combination of these two factors. It is believed that ED caused by functional vascular factors occurs early and is likely associated with oxidative stress and decreased NO availability. Initially these factors result in poor relaxation of penile endothelium and in smooth muscle that presents clinically as ED, with difficulty to maintain a firm erection. This early clinical symptom probably occurs before the development of structural, occlusive penile arterial disease and may be among the earliest signs of systemic CVD. Thus, it has been accepted that endothelial dysfunction is the etiologic connection between ED and systemic cardiovascular diseases (9, 30).

Corroborating this idea, Lojanapiwat et al examined 41 ED patients and 30 age-matched normal control, subjects were investigated for cardiovascular risks and endothelial function. Changes in brachial arterial diameter after its occlusion were compared between the groups. Results did not show differences in baseline characteristics for cardiovascular risks and lipid levels. However, a significant difference regarding endothelial dysfunction in ED patients without clinical cardiovascular risks versus control patients was observed. They concluded that patients who developed ED showed endothelial dysfunction and cardiovascular risk markers prior to the clinical symptoms. In addition, a study evaluating systemic vascular structure and function in 30 patients with ED and 27 age-matched normal controls, investigated whether patients with vascular ED and no other clinical CVD have structural and functional abnormalities of other vascular beds. Systemic endothelial function using flow mediated brachial artery vasodilatation showed that men with ED exhibited significantly lower brachial artery flow-mediated, vascular defect in endothelium-dependent and independent vasodilatation, which happen before the development of structural or functional systemic vascular disease, when compared to controls. According to the authors these data suggest the presence of peripheral vascular abnormality in the NO pathway (131). In another study, biochemical markers of endothelial cell activation were used to compare 45 men with ED and no clinical CVD with 25 age-matched healthy. The results showed that the carotid intima-media thickness (IMT) was similar between the groups. However, soluble P-selectin (intracellular adhesion molecule-1) and endothelin-1 levels were significantly higher in men with ED and no CVD (132).

Alterations in the several signalling pathways, mainly in Rho-kinase signaling, are common in ED as well as CDV, contributing to a further increase in endothelial dysfunction. Rho-kinase, is involved in the sequence of events that stimulates vascular smooth muscle contraction, stress fiber formation, cell migration, and, indirectly, blood pressure regulation. In this way, RhoA/Rho-kinase activation has significant effects on various cardiovascular diseases, such as arterial hypertension (133), atherosclerosis (134), heart attack (135), stroke

(136), coronary vasospasm (137), myocardial hypertrophy (138), myocardial ischemia-reperfusion injury (139), vascular remodeling (140) and ED. Since the main function of Rho-kinase is the regulation of smooth muscle tone (141), the upregulation of the Rho-kinase pathway increases cavernosal smooth muscle contraction, leading to ED (142-143). Furthermore, studies indicate that Rho-kinase isoforms are activated in patients with a cardiovascular disorder or associated risk factors (144-145). Also, RhoA mRNA expression and activity is increased in aortas from aged rats, suggesting a role of RhoA in the development of age-related cardiovascular disease (146).

7. Conclusion

Although the link between ED and CVD has been previously documented, convincing evidence of the direction and magnitude of the effect has not been available. However, several studies support the idea that ED precedes overt structural occlusion of larger blood vessels, and ED is often an early manifestation of systemic vascular disease. The evaluation of ED in the medical history as an early symptom of endothelial dysfunction and atherosclerosis may be a predictor of future cardiovascular events, including death. This might be relevant to identifying patients with a particularly high risk of experiencing cardiovascular events even though is not clear yet what kind evaluation or parameters should be prompted in ED condition.

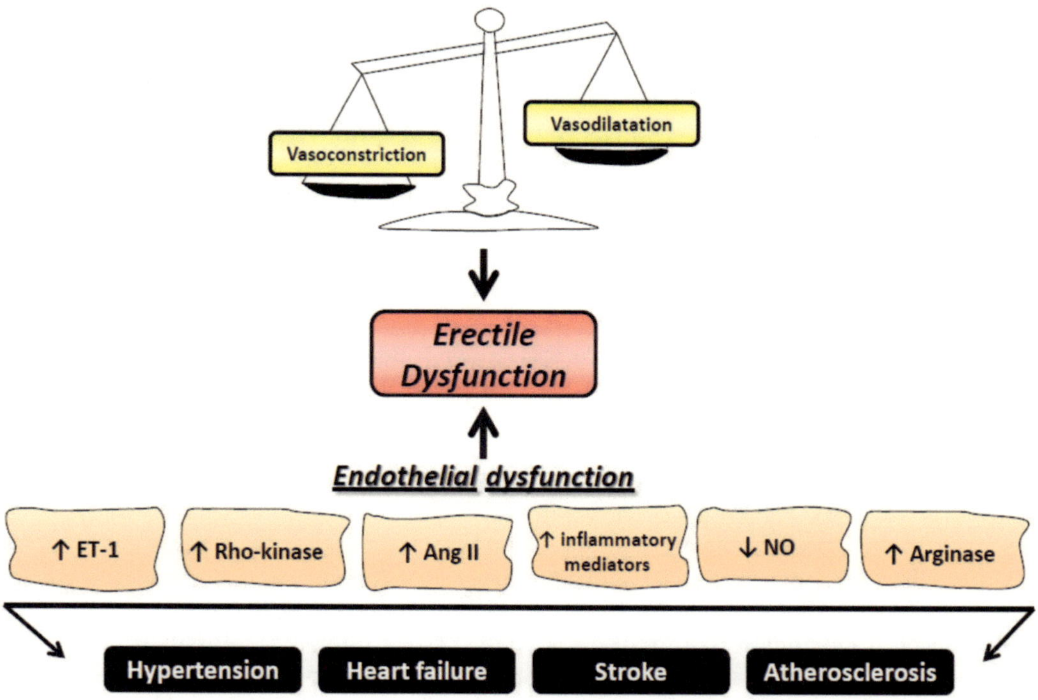

Fig. 1. **Endothelial dysfunction is a common situation in both CVD and ED.** Generally ED is caused by unbalance between vasoconstrictors (Ang II, ET-1, Rho-kinase, arginase) and vasodilators (NO) endogenous agents. Endothelial dysfunction leads to ED development and later to onset of CVD.

8. References

[1] Fung MM, Bettencourt R, Barrett-Connor E. Heart disease risk factors predict erectile dysfunction 25 years later: the Rancho Bernardo Study. J Am Coll Cardiol. 2004 Apr 21;43(8):1405-11.

[2] NIH Consensus Conference. Impotence. NIH Consensus Development Panel on Impotence. JAMA. 1993 Jul 7;270(1):83-90.

[3] Burchardt M, Burchardt T, Baer L, Kiss AJ, Pawar RV, Shabsigh A, et al. Hypertension is associated with severe erectile dysfunction. J Urol. 2000 Oct;164(4):1188-91.

[4] Ayta IA, McKinlay JB, Krane RJ. The likely worldwide increase in erectile dysfunction between 1995 and 2025 and some possible policy consequences. BJU Int. 1999 Jul;84(1):50-6.

[5] Feldman HA, Goldstein I, Hatzichristou DG, Krane RJ, McKinlay JB. Impotence and its medical and psychosocial correlates: results of the Massachusetts Male Aging Study. J Urol. 1994 Jan;151(1):54-61.

[6] Derby CA, Mohr BA, Goldstein I, Feldman HA, Johannes CB, McKinlay JB. Modifiable risk factors and erectile dysfunction: can lifestyle changes modify risk? Urology. 2000 Aug 1;56(2):302-6.

[7] Maas R, Schwedhelm E, Albsmeier J, Boger RH. The pathophysiology of erectile dysfunction related to endothelial dysfunction and mediators of vascular function. Vasc Med. 2002 Aug;7(3):213-25.

[8] Kirby M, Jackson G, Simonsen U. Endothelial dysfunction links erectile dysfunction to heart disease. Int J Clin Pract. 2005 Feb;59(2):225-9.

[9] Solomon H, Man JW, Jackson G. Erectile dysfunction and the cardiovascular patient: endothelial dysfunction is the common denominator. Heart. 2003 Mar;89(3):251-3.

[10] Billups KL. Erectile dysfunction as an early sign of cardiovascular disease. Int J Impot Res. 2005 Dec;17 Suppl 1:S19-24.

[11] Stocker R, Keaney JF, Jr. Role of oxidative modifications in atherosclerosis. Physiol Rev. 2004 Oct;84(4):1381-478.

[12] Cohn JN, Finkelstein S, McVeigh G, Morgan D, LeMay L, Robinson J, et al. Noninvasive pulse wave analysis for the early detection of vascular disease. Hypertension. 1995 Sep;26(3):503-8.

[13] Boutouyrie P, Tropeano AI, Asmar R, Gautier I, Benetos A, Lacolley P, et al. Aortic stiffness is an independent predictor of primary coronary events in hypertensive patients: a longitudinal study. Hypertension. 2002 Jan;39(1):10-5.

[14] van Popele NM, Grobbee DE, Bots ML, Asmar R, Topouchian J, Reneman RS, et al. Association between arterial stiffness and atherosclerosis: the Rotterdam Study. Stroke. 2001 Feb;32(2):454-60.

[15] Holvoet P, Mertens A, Verhamme P, Bogaerts K, Beyens G, Verhaeghe R, et al. Circulating oxidized LDL is a useful marker for identifying patients with coronary artery disease. Arterioscler Thromb Vasc Biol. 2001 May;21(5):844-8.

[16] Danesh J, Lewington S, Thompson SG, Lowe GD, Collins R, Kostis JB, et al. Plasma fibrinogen level and the risk of major cardiovascular diseases and nonvascular mortality: an individual participant meta-analysis. JAMA. 2005 Oct 12;294(14):1799-809.

[17] Cooney MT, Vartiainen E, Laatikainen T, Juolevi A, Dudina A, Graham IM. Elevated resting heart rate is an independent risk factor for cardiovascular disease in healthy men and women. Am Heart J. 2010 Apr;159(4):612-9 e3.

[18] Schwartz BG, Kloner RA. Cardiology patient page: cardiovascular implications of erectile dysfunction. Circulation. 2011 May 31;123(21):e609-11.
[19] Vlachopoulos C, Aznaouridis K, Ioakeimidis N, Rokkas K, Vasiliadou C, Alexopoulos N, et al. Unfavourable endothelial and inflammatory state in erectile dysfunction patients with or without coronary artery disease. Eur Heart J. 2006 Nov;27(22):2640-8.
[20] Montorsi P, Montorsi F, Schulman CC. Is erectile dysfunction the "tip of the iceberg" of a systemic vascular disorder? Eur Urol. 2003 Sep;44(3):352-4.
[21] Montorsi P, Ravagnani PM, Galli S, Rotatori F, Briganti A, Salonia A, et al. The artery size hypothesis: a macrovascular link between erectile dysfunction and coronary artery disease. Am J Cardiol. 2005 Dec 26;96(12B):19M-23M.
[22] Chung SD, Chen YK, Lin HC. Increased risk of stroke among men with erectile dysfunction: a nationwide population-based study. J Sex Med. 2011 Jan;8(1):240-6.
[23] Lue TF. Erectile dysfunction. N Engl J Med. 2000 Jun 15;342(24):1802-13.
[24] Costa C, Virag R. The endothelial-erectile dysfunction connection: an essential update. J Sex Med. 2009 Sep;6(9):2390-404.
[25] Agarwal A, Nandipati KC, Sharma RK, Zippe CD, Raina R. Role of oxidative stress in the pathophysiological mechanism of erectile dysfunction. J Androl. 2006 May-Jun;27(3):335-47.
[26] Lyle AN, Griendling KK. Modulation of vascular smooth muscle signaling by reactive oxygen species. Physiology (Bethesda). 2006 Aug;21:269-80.
[27] Berk BC. Redox signals that regulate the vascular response to injury. Thromb Haemost. 1999 Aug;82(2):810-7.
[28] Cave AC, Brewer AC, Narayanapanicker A, Ray R, Grieve DJ, Walker S, et al. NADPH oxidases in cardiovascular health and disease. Antioxid Redox Signal. 2006 May-Jun;8(5-6):691-728.
[29] Jeremy JY, Angelini GD, Khan M, Mikhailidis DP, Morgan RJ, Thompson CS, et al. Platelets, oxidant stress and erectile dysfunction: an hypothesis. Cardiovasc Res. 2000 Apr;46(1):50-4.
[30] Jones RW, Rees RW, Minhas S, Ralph D, Persad RA, Jeremy JY. Oxygen free radicals and the penis. Expert Opin Pharmacother. 2002 Jul;3(7):889-97.
[31] Bener A, Al-Ansari A, Al-Hamaq AO, Elbagi IE, Afifi M. Prevalence of erectile dysfunction among hypertensive and nonhypertensive Qatari men. Medicina (Kaunas). 2007;43(11):870-8.
[32] Aho K, Harmsen P, Hatano S, Marquardsen J, Smirnov VE, Strasser T. Cerebrovascular disease in the community: results of a WHO collaborative study. Bull World Health Organ. 1980;58(1):113-30.
[33] Asplund K, Bonita R, Kuulasmaa K, Rajakangas AM, Schaedlich H, Suzuki K, et al. Multinational comparisons of stroke epidemiology. Evaluation of case ascertainment in the WHO MONICA Stroke Study. World Health Organization Monitoring Trends and Determinants in Cardiovascular Disease. Stroke. 1995 Mar;26(3):355-60.
[34] Jung JH, Kam SC, Choi SM, Jae SU, Lee SH, Hyun JS. Sexual dysfunction in male stroke patients: correlation between brain lesions and sexual function. Urology. 2008 Jan;71(1):99-103.
[35] Werner RA, Kessler S. Effectiveness of an intensive outpatient rehabilitation program for postacute stroke patients. Am J Phys Med Rehabil. 1996 Mar-Apr;75(2):114-20.

[36] Ebrahim S. Conference report. World Stroke Congress, 25-29 November 2000, Melbourne, Australia. Int J Epidemiol. 2001 Feb;30(1):189.
[37] Ma RC, So WY, Yang X, Yu LW, Kong AP, Ko GT, et al. Erectile dysfunction predicts coronary heart disease in type 2 diabetes. J Am Coll Cardiol. 2008 May 27;51(21):2045-50.
[38] Chew KK, Finn J, Stuckey B, Gibson N, Sanfilippo F, Bremner A, et al. Erectile dysfunction as a predictor for subsequent atherosclerotic cardiovascular events: findings from a linked-data study. J Sex Med. 2010 Jan;7(1 Pt 1):192-202.
[39] Miner MM. Erectile dysfunction and the "window of curability": a harbinger of cardiovascular events. Mayo Clin Proc. 2009 Feb;84(2):102-4.
[40] Chew KK, Bremner A, Jamrozik K, Earle C, Stuckey B. Male erectile dysfunction and cardiovascular disease: is there an intimate nexus? J Sex Med. 2008 Apr;5(4):928-34.
[41] Salem S, Abdi S, Mehrsai A, Saboury B, Saraji A, Shokohideh V, et al. Erectile dysfunction severity as a risk predictor for coronary artery disease. J Sex Med. 2009 Dec;6(12):3425-32.
[42] Araujo AB, Travison TG, Ganz P, Chiu GR, Kupelian V, Rosen RC, et al. Erectile dysfunction and mortality. J Sex Med. 2009 Sep;6(9):2445-54.
[43] Seftel AD, Sun P, Swindle R. The prevalence of hypertension, hyperlipidemia, diabetes mellitus and depression in men with erectile dysfunction. J Urol. 2004 Jun;171(6 Pt 1):2341-5.
[44] Korpelainen JT, Kauhanen ML, Kemola H, Malinen U, Myllyla VV. Sexual dysfunction in stroke patients. Acta Neurol Scand. 1998 Dec;98(6):400-5.
[45] Monga TN, Lawson JS, Inglis J. Sexual dysfunction in stroke patients. Arch Phys Med Rehabil. 1986 Jan;67(1):19-22.
[46] Pistoia F, Govoni S, Boselli C. Sex after stroke: a CNS only dysfunction? Pharmacol Res. 2006 Jul;54(1):11-8.
[47] Coslett HB, Heilman KM. Male sexual function. Impairment after right hemisphere stroke. Arch Neurol. 1986 Oct;43(10):1036-9.
[48] Schouten BW, Bohnen AM, Bosch JL, Bernsen RM, Deckers JW, Dohle GR, et al. Erectile dysfunction prospectively associated with cardiovascular disease in the Dutch general population: results from the Krimpen Study. Int J Impot Res. 2008 Jan-Feb;20(1):92-9.
[49] Araujo AB, Hall SA, Ganz P, Chiu GR, Rosen RC, Kupelian V, et al. Does erectile dysfunction contribute to cardiovascular disease risk prediction beyond the Framingham risk score? J Am Coll Cardiol. 2010 Jan 26;55(4):350-6.
[50] Ponholzer A, Temml C, Obermayr R, Wehrberger C, Madersbacher S. Is erectile dysfunction an indicator for increased risk of coronary heart disease and stroke? Eur Urol. 2005 Sep;48(3):512-8; discussion 7-8.
[51] Lojanapiwat B, Weerusawin T, Kuanprasert S. Erectile dysfunction as a sentinel marker of endothelial dysfunction disease. Singapore Med J. 2009 Jul;50(7):698-701.
[52] Vicenzini E, Altieri M, Michetti PM, Ricciardi MC, Ciccariello M, Shahabadi H, et al. Cerebral vasomotor reactivity is reduced in patients with erectile dysfunction. Eur Neurol. 2008;60(2):85-8.
[53] Reffelmann T, Kloner RA. Sexual function in hypertensive patients receiving treatment. Vasc Health Risk Manag. 2006;2(4):447-55.

[54] Kai H, Kudo H, Takayama N, Yasuoka S, Kajimoto H, Imaizumi T. Large blood pressure variability and hypertensive cardiac remodeling--role of cardiac inflammation. Circ J. 2009 Dec;73(12):2198-203.
[55] Chitaley K, Weber D, Webb RC. RhoA/Rho-kinase, vascular changes, and hypertension. Curr Hypertens Rep. 2001 Apr;3(2):139-44.
[56] Mombouli JV, Vanhoutte PM. Endothelial dysfunction: from physiology to therapy. J Mol Cell Cardiol. 1999 Jan;31(1):61-74.
[57] Rudic RD, Sessa WC. Nitric oxide in endothelial dysfunction and vascular remodeling: clinical correlates and experimental links. Am J Hum Genet. 1999 Mar;64(3):673-7.
[58] Chitaley K, Webb RC, Dorrance AM, Mills TM. Decreased penile erection in DOCA-salt and stroke prone-spontaneously hypertensive rats. Int J Impot Res. 2001 Dec;13 Suppl 5:S16-20.
[59] Lima VV, Giachini FR, Hardy DM, Webb RC, Tostes RC. O-GlcNAcylation: a novel pathway contributing to the effects of endothelin in the vasculature. Am J Physiol Regul Integr Comp Physiol. 2011 Feb;300(2):R236-50.
[60] Sullivan ME, Thompson CS, Dashwood MR, Khan MA, Jeremy JY, Morgan RJ, et al. Nitric oxide and penile erection: is erectile dysfunction another manifestation of vascular disease? Cardiovasc Res. 1999 Aug 15;43(3):658-65.
[61] Granchi S, Vannelli GB, Vignozzi L, Crescioli C, Ferruzzi P, Mancina R, et al. Expression and regulation of endothelin-1 and its receptors in human penile smooth muscle cells. Mol Hum Reprod. 2002 Dec;8(12):1053-64.
[62] Dai Y, Pollock DM, Lewis RL, Wingard CJ, Stopper VS, Mills TM. Receptor-specific influence of endothelin-1 in the erectile response of the rat. Am J Physiol Regul Integr Comp Physiol. 2000 Jul;279(1):R25-30.
[63] Carneiro FS, Nunes KP, Giachini FR, Lima VV, Carneiro ZN, Nogueira EF, et al. Activation of the ET-1/ETA pathway contributes to erectile dysfunction associated with mineralocorticoid hypertension. J Sex Med. 2008 Dec;5(12):2793-807.
[64] El Melegy NT, Ali ME, Awad EM. Plasma levels of endothelin-1, angiotensin II, nitric oxide and prostaglandin E in the venous and cavernosal blood of patients with erectile dysfunction. BJU Int. 2005 Nov;96(7):1079-86.
[65] de Nucci G, Gryglewski RJ, Warner TD, Vane JR. Receptor-mediated release of endothelium-derived relaxing factor and prostacyclin from bovine aortic endothelial cells is coupled. Proc Natl Acad Sci U S A. 1988 Apr;85(7):2334-8.
[66] de Nucci G, Warner T, Vane JR. Effect of captopril on the bradykinin-induced release of prostacyclin from guinea-pig lungs and bovine aortic endothelial cells. Br J Pharmacol. 1988 Nov;95(3):783-8.
[67] Becker AJ, Uckert S, Stief CG, Truss MC, Machtens S, Scheller F, et al. Possible role of bradykinin and angiotensin II in the regulation of penile erection and detumescence. Urology. 2001 Jan;57(1):193-8.
[68] Lima VV, Rigsby CS, Hardy DM, Webb RC, Tostes RC. O-GlcNAcylation: a novel post-translational mechanism to alter vascular cellular signaling in health and disease: focus on hypertension. J Am Soc Hypertens. 2009 Nov-Dec;3(6):374-87.
[69] Xing D, Feng W, Not LG, Miller AP, Zhang Y, Chen YF, et al. Increased protein O-GlcNAc modification inhibits inflammatory and neointimal responses to acute endoluminal arterial injury. Am J Physiol Heart Circ Physiol. 2008 Jul;295(1):H335-42.

[70] Lima VV, Giachini FR, Choi H, Carneiro FS, Carneiro ZN, Fortes ZB, et al. Impaired vasodilator activity in deoxycorticosterone acetate-salt hypertension is associated with increased protein O-GlcNAcylation. Hypertension. 2009 Feb;53(2):166-74.
[71] Musicki B, Kramer MF, Becker RE, Burnett AL. Inactivation of phosphorylated endothelial nitric oxide synthase (Ser-1177) by O-GlcNAc in diabetes-associated erectile dysfunction. Proc Natl Acad Sci U S A. 2005 Aug 16;102(33):11870-5.
[72] Kifor I, Williams GH, Vickers MA, Sullivan MP, Jodbert P, Dluhy RG. Tissue angiotensin II as a modulator of erectile function. I. Angiotensin peptide content, secretion and effects in the corpus cavernosum. J Urol. 1997 May;157(5):1920-5.
[73] Iwamoto Y, Song K, Takai S, Yamada M, Jin D, Sakaguchi M, et al. Multiple pathways of angiotensin I conversion and their functional role in the canine penile corpus cavernosum. J Pharmacol Exp Ther. 2001 Jul;298(1):43-8.
[74] Lin CS, Ho HC, Gholami S, Chen KC, Jad A, Lue TF. Gene expression profiling of an arteriogenic impotence model. Biochem Biophys Res Commun. 2001 Jul 13;285(2):565-9.
[75] Mori M, Gotoh T. Regulation of nitric oxide production by arginine metabolic enzymes. Biochem Biophys Res Commun. 2000 Sep 7;275(3):715-9.
[76] Cox JD, Kim NN, Traish AM, Christianson DW. Arginase-boronic acid complex highlights a physiological role in erectile function. Nat Struct Biol. 1999 Nov;6(11):1043-7.
[77] Rodriguez S, Richert L, Berthelot A. Increased arginase activity in aorta of mineralocorticoid-salt hypertensive rats. Clin Exp Hypertens. 2000 Jan;22(1):75-85.
[78] Demougeot C, Prigent-Tessier A, Bagnost T, Andre C, Guillaume Y, Bouhaddi M, et al. Time course of vascular arginase expression and activity in spontaneously hypertensive rats. Life Sci. 2007 Feb 27;80(12):1128-34.
[79] Demougeot C, Prigent-Tessier A, Marie C, Berthelot A. Arginase inhibition reduces endothelial dysfunction and blood pressure rising in spontaneously hypertensive rats. J Hypertens. 2005 May;23(5):971-8.
[80] Ryoo S, Gupta G, Benjo A, Lim HK, Camara A, Sikka G, et al. Endothelial arginase II: a novel target for the treatment of atherosclerosis. Circ Res. 2008 Apr 25;102(8):923-32.
[81] Michell DL, Andrews KL, Chin-Dusting JP. Endothelial dysfunction in hypertension: the role of arginase. Front Biosci (Schol Ed). 2011;3:946-60.
[82] Durante W, Johnson FK, Johnson RA. Arginase: a critical regulator of nitric oxide synthesis and vascular function. Clin Exp Pharmacol Physiol. 2007 Sep;34(9):906-11.
[83] Bivalacqua TJ, Burnett AL, Hellstrom WJ, Champion HC. Overexpression of arginase in the aged mouse penis impairs erectile function and decreases eNOS activity: influence of in vivo gene therapy of anti-arginase. Am J Physiol Heart Circ Physiol. 2007 Mar;292(3):H1340-51.
[84] Numao N, Masuda H, Sakai Y, Okada Y, Kihara K, Azuma H. Roles of attenuated neuronal nitric-oxide synthase protein expression and accelerated arginase activity in impairing neurogenic relaxation of corpus cavernosum in aged rabbits. BJU Int. 2007 Jun;99(6):1495-9.
[85] Peyton KJ, Ensenat D, Azam MA, Keswani AN, Kannan S, Liu XM, et al. Arginase promotes neointima formation in rat injured carotid arteries. Arterioscler Thromb Vasc Biol. 2009 Apr;29(4):488-94.

[86] Wassertheil-Smoller S, Blaufox MD, Oberman A, Davis BR, Swencionis C, Knerr MO, et al. Effect of antihypertensives on sexual function and quality of life: the TAIM Study. Ann Intern Med. 1991 Apr 15;114(8):613-20.
[87] Menard J. The 45-year story of the development of an anti-aldosterone more specific than spironolactone. Mol Cell Endocrinol. 2004 Mar 31;217(1-2):45-52.
[88] Fogari R, Zoppi A, Poletti L, Marasi G, Mugellini A, Corradi L. Sexual activity in hypertensive men treated with valsartan or carvedilol: a crossover study. Am J Hypertens. 2001 Jan;14(1):27-31.
[89] Angulo J, Wright HM, Cuevas P, Gonzalez-Corrochano R, Fernandez A, Cuevas B, et al. Nebivolol dilates human penile arteries and reverses erectile dysfunction in diabetic rats through enhancement of nitric oxide signaling. J Sex Med. 2010 Aug;7(8):2681-97.
[90] Mandras SA, Uber PA, Mehra MR. Sexual activity and chronic heart failure. Mayo Clin Proc. 2007 Oct;82(10):1203-10.
[91] DiBianco R. A large-scale trial of captopril for mild to moderate heart failure in the primary care setting. Clin Cardiol. 1991 Aug;14(8):676-82.
[92] Dusing R. Effect of the angiotensin II antagonist valsartan on sexual function in hypertensive men. Blood Press Suppl. 2003 Dec;2:29-34.
[93] Canguven O, Lagoda G, Sezen SF, Burnett AL. Losartan preserves erectile function after bilateral cavernous nerve injury via antifibrotic mechanisms in male rats. J Urol. 2009 Jun;181(6):2816-22.
[94] Bohm M, Baumhakel M, Teo K, Sleight P, Probstfield J, Gao P, et al. Erectile dysfunction predicts cardiovascular events in high-risk patients receiving telmisartan, ramipril, or both: The ONgoing Telmisartan Alone and in combination with Ramipril Global Endpoint Trial/Telmisartan Randomized AssessmeNt Study in ACE iNtolerant subjects with cardiovascular Disease (ONTARGET/TRANSCEND) Trials. Circulation. 2010 Mar 30;121(12):1439-46.
[95] Papatsoris AG, Korantzopoulos PG. Hypertension, antihypertensive therapy, and erectile dysfunction. Angiology. 2006 Jan-Feb;57(1):47-52.
[96] Hunt SA, Abraham WT, Chin MH, Feldman AM, Francis GS, Ganiats TG, et al. ACC/AHA 2005 Guideline Update for the Diagnosis and Management of Chronic Heart Failure in the Adult: a report of the American College of Cardiology/American Heart Association Task Force on Practice Guidelines (Writing Committee to Update the 2001 Guidelines for the Evaluation and Management of Heart Failure): developed in collaboration with the American College of Chest Physicians and the International Society for Heart and Lung Transplantation: endorsed by the Heart Rhythm Society. Circulation. 2005 Sep 20;112(12):e154-235.
[97] Bocchi EA, Vilas-Boas F, Perrone S, Caamano AG, Clausell N, Moreira Mda C, et al. I Latin American Guidelines for the Assessment and Management of Decompensated Heart Failure. Arq Bras Cardiol. 2005 Sep;85 Suppl 3:49-94; 1-48.
[98] Lloyd-Jones D, Adams RJ, Brown TM, Carnethon M, Dai S, De Simone G, et al. Heart disease and stroke statistics--2010 update: a report from the American Heart Association. Circulation. 2010 Feb 23;121(7):e46-e215.
[99] Baraghoush A, Phan A, Willix RD, Jr., Schwarz ER. Erectile dysfunction as a complication of heart failure. Curr Heart Fail Rep. 2010 Dec;7(4):194-201.

[100] Chew KK, Bremner A, Stuckey B, Earle C, Jamrozik K. Sex life after 65: how does erectile dysfunction affect ageing and elderly men? Aging Male. 2009 Jun-Sep;12(2-3):41-6.
[101] Schwarz ER, Rastogi S, Kapur V, Sulemanjee N, Rodriguez JJ. Erectile dysfunction in heart failure patients. J Am Coll Cardiol. 2006 Sep 19;48(6):1111-9.
[102] Boger RH, Bode-Boger SM, Frolich JC. The L-arginine-nitric oxide pathway: role in atherosclerosis and therapeutic implications. Atherosclerosis. 1996 Nov 15;127(1):1-11.
[103] Yavuzgil O, Altay B, Zoghi M, Gurgun C, Kayikcioglu M, Kultursay H. Endothelial function in patients with vasculogenic erectile dysfunction. Int J Cardiol. 2005 Aug 3;103(1):19-26.
[104] Smith CJ, Sun D, Hoegler C, Roth BS, Zhang X, Zhao G, et al. Reduced gene expression of vascular endothelial NO synthase and cyclooxygenase-1 in heart failure. Circ Res. 1996 Jan;78(1):58-64.
[105] Nunes KP, Rigsby CS, Webb RC. RhoA/Rho-kinase and vascular diseases: what is the link? Cell Mol Life Sci. 2010 Nov;67(22):3823-36.
[106] Becker AJ, Uckert S, Stief CG, Truss MC, Hartmann U, Jonas U. Systemic and cavernous plasma levels of endothelin (1-21) during different penile conditions in healthy males and patients with erectile dysfunction. World J Urol. 2001 Aug;19(4):267-71.
[107] Pedersen CA, Boccia ML. Vasopressin interactions with oxytocin in the control of female sexual behavior. Neuroscience. 2006;139(3):843-51.
[108] Rastogi S, Rodriguez JJ, Kapur V, Schwarz ER. Why do patients with heart failure suffer from erectile dysfunction? A critical review and suggestions on how to approach this problem. Int J Impot Res. 2005 Dec;17 Suppl 1:S25-36.
[109] Schwarz ER, Rodriguez J. Sex and the heart. Int J Impot Res. 2005 Dec;17 Suppl 1:S4-6.
[110] Neri A, Zukerman Z, Aygen M, Lidor Y, Kaufman H. The effect of long-term administration of digoxin on plasma androgens and sexual dysfunction. J Sex Marital Ther. 1987 Spring;13(1):58-63.
[111] Gupta S, Salimpour P, Saenz de Tejada I, Daley J, Gholami S, Daller M, et al. A possible mechanism for alteration of human erectile function by digoxin: inhibition of corpus cavernosum sodium/potassium adenosine triphosphatase activity. J Urol. 1998 May;159(5):1529-36.
[112] Thompson IM, Tangen CM, Goodman PJ, Probstfield JL, Moinpour CM, Coltman CA. Erectile dysfunction and subsequent cardiovascular disease. JAMA. 2005 Dec 21;294(23):2996-3002.
[113] Billups KL. Sexual dysfunction and cardiovascular disease: integrative concepts and strategies. Am J Cardiol. 2005 Dec 26;96(12B):57M-61M.
[114] Vane JR, Anggard EE, Botting RM. Regulatory functions of the vascular endothelium. N Engl J Med. 1990 Jul 5;323(1):27-36.
[115] Rajfer J, Aronson WJ, Bush PA, Dorey FJ, Ignarro LJ. Nitric oxide as a mediator of relaxation of the corpus cavernosum in response to nonadrenergic, noncholinergic neurotransmission. N Engl J Med. 1992 Jan 9;326(2):90-4.
[116] Ignarro LJ, Bush PA, Buga GM, Wood KS, Fukuto JM, Rajfer J. Nitric oxide and cyclic GMP formation upon electrical field stimulation cause relaxation of corpus cavernosum smooth muscle. Biochem Biophys Res Commun. 1990 Jul 31;170(2):843-50.

[117] Escrig A, Marin R, Abreu P, Gonzalez-Mora JL, Mas M. Changes in mating behavior, erectile function, and nitric oxide levels in penile corpora cavernosa in streptozotocin-diabetic rats. Biol Reprod. 2002 Jan;66(1):185-9.
[118] Arnold WP, Mittal CK, Katsuki S, Murad F. Nitric oxide activates guanylate cyclase and increases guanosine 3':5'-cyclic monophosphate levels in various tissue preparations. Proc Natl Acad Sci U S A. 1977 Aug;74(8):3203-7.
[119] Hedlund P, Aszodi A, Pfeifer A, Alm P, Hofmann F, Ahmad M, et al. Erectile dysfunction in cyclic GMP-dependent kinase I-deficient mice. Proc Natl Acad Sci U S A. 2000 Feb 29;97(5):2349-54.
[120] Goldstein I, Lue TF, Padma-Nathan H, Rosen RC, Steers WD, Wicker PA. Oral sildenafil in the treatment of erectile dysfunction. Sildenafil Study Group. N Engl J Med. 1998 May 14;338(20):1397-404.
[121] Padma-Nathan H, Hellstrom WJ, Kaiser FE, Labasky RF, Lue TF, Nolten WE, et al. Treatment of men with erectile dysfunction with transurethral alprostadil. Medicated Urethral System for Erection (MUSE) Study Group. N Engl J Med. 1997 Jan 2;336(1):1-7.
[122] Porst H. The rationale for prostaglandin E1 in erectile failure: a survey of worldwide experience. J Urol. 1996 Mar;155(3):802-15.
[123] Kirby M, Jackson G, Betteridge J, Friedli K. Is erectile dysfunction a marker for cardiovascular disease? Int J Clin Pract. 2001 Nov;55(9):614-8.
[124] Moncada S, Higgs A. The L-arginine-nitric oxide pathway. N Engl J Med. 1993 Dec 30;329(27):2002-12.
[125] Kelm M, Rath J. Endothelial dysfunction in human coronary circulation: relevance of the L-arginine-NO pathway. Basic Res Cardiol. 2001 Apr;96(2):107-27.
[126] Kim N, Azadzoi KM, Goldstein I, Saenz de Tejada I. A nitric oxide-like factor mediates nonadrenergic-noncholinergic neurogenic relaxation of penile corpus cavernosum smooth muscle. J Clin Invest. 1991 Jul;88(1):112-8.
[127] Stroes E, Kastelein J, Cosentino F, Erkelens W, Wever R, Koomans H, et al. Tetrahydrobiopterin restores endothelial function in hypercholesterolemia. J Clin Invest. 1997 Jan 1;99(1):41-6.
[128] Heitzer T, Brockhoff C, Mayer B, Warnholtz A, Mollnau H, Henne S, et al. Tetrahydrobiopterin improves endothelium-dependent vasodilation in chronic smokers : evidence for a dysfunctional nitric oxide synthase. Circ Res. 2000 Feb 4;86(2):E36-41.
[129] Tiefenbacher CP, Bleeke T, Vahl C, Amann K, Vogt A, Kubler W. Endothelial dysfunction of coronary resistance arteries is improved by tetrahydrobiopterin in atherosclerosis. Circulation. 2000 Oct 31;102(18):2172-9.
[130] Bush PA, Gonzalez NE, Ignarro LJ. Biosynthesis of nitric oxide and citrulline from L-arginine by constitutive nitric oxide synthase present in rabbit corpus cavernosum. Biochem Biophys Res Commun. 1992 Jul 15;186(1):308-14.
[131] Kaiser DR, Billups K, Mason C, Wetterling R, Lundberg JL, Bank AJ. Impaired brachial artery endothelium-dependent and -independent vasodilation in men with erectile dysfunction and no other clinical cardiovascular disease. J Am Coll Cardiol. 2004 Jan 21;43(2):179-84.
[132] Bocchio M, Desideri G, Scarpelli P, Necozione S, Properzi G, Spartera C, et al. Endothelial cell activation in men with erectile dysfunction without cardiovascular risk factors and overt vascular damage. J Urol. 2004 Apr;171(4):1601-4.

[133] Jin L, Ying Z, Hilgers RH, Yin J, Zhao X, Imig JD, et al. Increased RhoA/Rho-kinase signaling mediates spontaneous tone in aorta from angiotensin II-induced hypertensive rats. J Pharmacol Exp Ther. 2006 Jul;318(1):288-95.
[134] Zhou Q, Liao JK. Rho kinase: an important mediator of atherosclerosis and vascular disease. Curr Pharm Des. 2009;15(27):3108-15.
[135] Hamid SA, Bower HS, Baxter GF. Rho kinase activation plays a major role as a mediator of irreversible injury in reperfused myocardium. Am J Physiol Heart Circ Physiol. 2007 Jun;292(6):H2598-606.
[136] Rikitake Y, Kim HH, Huang Z, Seto M, Yano K, Asano T, et al. Inhibition of Rho kinase (ROCK) leads to increased cerebral blood flow and stroke protection. Stroke. 2005 Oct;36(10):2251-7.
[137] Sato M, Tani E, Fujikawa H, Kaibuchi K. Involvement of Rho-kinase-mediated phosphorylation of myosin light chain in enhancement of cerebral vasospasm. Circ Res. 2000 Aug 4;87(3):195-200.
[138] Higashi M, Shimokawa H, Hattori T, Hiroki J, Mukai Y, Morikawa K, et al. Long-term inhibition of Rho-kinase suppresses angiotensin II-induced cardiovascular hypertrophy in rats in vivo: effect on endothelial NAD(P)H oxidase system. Circ Res. 2003 Oct 17;93(8):767-75.
[139] Bao W, Hu E, Tao L, Boyce R, Mirabile R, Thudium DT, et al. Inhibition of Rho-kinase protects the heart against ischemia/reperfusion injury. Cardiovasc Res. 2004 Feb 15;61(3):548-58.
[140] Miyata K, Shimokawa H, Kandabashi T, Higo T, Morishige K, Eto Y, et al. Rho-kinase is involved in macrophage-mediated formation of coronary vascular lesions in pigs in vivo. Arterioscler Thromb Vasc Biol. 2000 Nov;20(11):2351-8.
[141] Puetz S, Lubomirov LT, Pfitzer G. Regulation of smooth muscle contraction by small GTPases. Physiology (Bethesda). 2009 Dec;24:342-56.
[142] Mills TM, Lewis RW, Wingard CJ, Linder AE, Jin L, Webb RC. Vasoconstriction, RhoA/Rho-kinase and the erectile response. Int J Impot Res. 2003 Oct;15 Suppl 5:S20-4.
[143] Jin L, Burnett AL. RhoA/Rho-kinase in erectile tissue: mechanisms of disease and therapeutic insights. Clin Sci (Lond). 2006 Feb;110(2):153-65.
[144] Kishi T, Hirooka Y, Masumoto A, Ito K, Kimura Y, Inokuchi K, et al. Rho-kinase inhibitor improves increased vascular resistance and impaired vasodilation of the forearm in patients with heart failure. Circulation. 2005 May 31;111(21):2741-7.
[145] Shimokawa H, Hiramori K, Iinuma H, Hosoda S, Kishida H, Osada H, et al. Anti-anginal effect of fasudil, a Rho-kinase inhibitor, in patients with stable effort angina: a multicenter study. J Cardiovasc Pharmacol. 2002 Nov;40(5):751-61.
[146] Miao L, Calvert JW, Tang J, Parent AD, Zhang JH. Age-related RhoA expression in blood vessels of rats. Mech Ageing Dev. 2001 Oct;122(15):1757-70.

5

Erectile Dysfunction: A Chronic Complication of the Diabetes Mellitus

Eulises Díaz-Díaz[1], Mario Cárdenas León[1], Nesty Olivares Arzuaga[2], Carlos M. Timossi[3], Rita Angélica Gómez Díaz[4], Carlos Aguilar Salinas[5] and Fernando Larrea[1]

[1]Department of Reproductive Biology,
[2]Department of Experimental Pathology,
[5]Department of Endocrinology and Metabolism,
Instituto Nacional de Ciencias Médicas y Nutrición: "Salvador Zubirán"
[3]Duplicarte, Medical Editorial
[4] Medical Unit of Investigation in Clinical Epidemiology. Hospital de Especialidades, Centro Médico Nacional "Siglo XXI", Instituto Mexicano del Seguro Social
México

1. Introduction

Erectile dysfunction (ED) is defined as the persistent or repeated inability to achieve and/or maintain an adequate erection to accomplish a complete and satisfactory sexual activity. The term ED defines more accurately the nature of such dysfunction than the term impotence (National Institutes of Health (NIH) Consensus Conference, 1993; World Health Organization (WHO), 2000). ED manifests itself in the general population of adult males and increases with age. But it is more pronounced in individuals who suffer from diabetes, cardiovascular and metabolic problems. ED is one of the chronic complications of diabetes mellitus (DM), so the prevalence rate is very high in this group of men, and is one of the medical affectations with greatest impact on the quality of life of these patients. Because of the characteristic physiopathological alterations of DM, the damage caused mainly to the nervous and circulatory system favors the increased prevalence of ED (Kadioglu et al., 1994; Romero et al., 1997). In this chapter we discuss some aspects related to the epidemiology of ED and its prevalence in DM subjects, as well as the physiopathological mechanisms involved in this condition.

2. Epidemiology of ED

2.1 Epidemiology of ED in the general population

It has been estimated that ED affects around 100-150 million men worldwide and it is expected an increase of 322 million by 2025 (Bloomgarden et al., 1998; Laumann et al., 1999); being DM one of the main causes. It is important to note that ED is also reflected in conditions that frequently coexist with DM, such as hypertension and cardiovascular disease (Benet & Melman, 1995). Epidemiological studies clearly show the high prevalence of this pathology. According with a number of studies, variables such as and the methodology employed, the estimated prevalence of ED varies from 19% to 75%. The data also showed that in addition to age, as an important factor, others such as lifestyle, food and tobacco consumption are highly associated to ED. It is estimated that the prevalence of ED varies according to the age of the population from 39% at the age of 40 years to 75% in men aged 80 years (Morley, 1986). In the Massachusetts Male Aging Study (MMAS), it was noted that the prevalence rate of ED of any grade was 52% (17% classified as a minimum, 25% moderate, and 10% severe) (Feldman et al., 1994). In another study performed in Spain known as EDEM [by its Spanish acronym: Epidemiología de la Disfunción Eréctil Masculina, (The Epidemiology of Male ED)], it was noted that the 19% of men between 25 and 70 years old have some degree of ED (16% classified as minimum, 2% moderate, 1% severe). This prevalence increases with age (8.6% in males aged from 25 to 39 years, 13.7% aged 40-49 years, 24.5% between 50 and 59 years, and 49% in people aged from 60 to 70 years) (Martin-Morales et al., 2001). Further information can be found in the work carried out by Kubin et al., in which they describe other several studies about the incidence of ED made around the world (Kubin et al., 2003).

2.2 Prevalence of ED in the diabetic population

Prevalence of ED is significantly higher in DM when compared to that found in the general population. The ED is associated with an increase in age (Fedele et al., 2001; McCulloch et al, 1980; Roth et al., 2003), poor metabolic control (Roth et al., 2003), time of evolution of DM (Klein, 1996; Roth, 2003), smoking (Bortolotti et al, 2001), consumption of alcoholic beverages, neurological damage (Lundberg et al., 2001), depression (Fedele et al., 2000), use of some drugs (Kleinman et al., 2000) and microvascular complications (Romeo et al., 2000) among other factors. Diabetic patients, with an inadequate control of their glycemic status, chronically suffer from neurological and vascular damages of penile smooth muscle, disruptions of endothelial function, a sustained increase in oxidative stress, formation of advanced glycation end-products, among others, all closely related to the physiology of erection. All these aspects are reviewed in detail in later sections of this chapter.

Epidemiological data show that the population of men with DM is more likely to develop ED. Data reported about ED in this population show a prevalence rate ranging from 35% to 78% depending on the age and general metabolic state of patients analyzed. In a study performed in 541 DM men aged 20-59 years, a prevalence rate of 35% of ED, and mainly attributed to microangiopathy; however, as mentioned before other factors such as age, type of treatment: oral hypoglycemic agents or insulin, the presence of retinopathy, symptomatic peripheral neuropathy, and symptomatic autonomic neuropathy (McCulloch et al., 1980) are also highly associated. Other studies report higher prevalence rates of 78%, of which 6% are mild, 36% moderate, and 36% severe. In this same study, it was found that the patients with non-insulin dependent diabetes that suffered of ED, had associated higher cardiovascular risks compared with the diabetic patients who did not have ED. Likewise, it was observed that the increase in cardiovascular risk factors is closely related to the severity of ED in diabetic patients (Meena et al., 2009). These elements suggest that ED is a common problem in diabetic patients and is a direct consequence of an inadequate control of metabolic state in general and particularly of the glycemic state. ED has a multifactorial etiology but an appropriate diabetic patient's metabolic control is the best way to prevent this chronic complication of DM.

2.3 Prevalence of ED among patients with type-1 and type-2 DM

It is unclear whether erectile disorder is more common among men with non-insulin dependent diabetes (type-2, T2DM, late onset) or those with insulin-dependent diabetes (type-1, T1DM, early onset). Only a few studies include a prevalence of erectile disorder by diabetic type. In this regarding, one study reported that men with elevated body mass index (BMI) and T1DM showed a significantly higher risk of ED than men with elevated BMI and T2DM. The same study also showed that the age-adjusted prevalence of ED was higher in men with T1DM (51%) than with T2DM (37%) (Fedele et al., 2000). But Miccoli et al., found that 40% and 52% of insulin-dependent and non-insulin dependent DM participants respectively had impotence (Miccoli et al., 1987). Fedele et al., in 2001 also reported that the incidence of ED in Italian men with diabetes was higher in T2DM than in T1DM (74 *versus* 45 cases per 1,000 person-years) (Fedele et al., 2001).

3. Basic mechanism of penile erection

Stimuli that can lead to penile erection include tactile stimuli to the penis and genitalia which will produce a reflex erection, while erotic stimuli, whether visual, auditory, olfactory or imaginative also produce penile erection by a mechanism which involves the paraventricular nucleus and medial preoptic area of the hypothalamus. A third mechanism is involved in the production of nocturnal erections that occur in all men during REM sleep (Eardley, 2002). The degree of contraction of the corpus cavernosum smooth muscle and the functional state of the penis is determined by the balance between proerectile and antierectile mechanisms that operate physiologically in the penis. Vasoconstriction maintains the penis in the flaccid state. Erectile function is dependent on relaxation of the cavernous smooth muscle, and its mechanism of action is mediated by Nitric Oxide (NO). NO synthesized from L-arginine is the key mediator of endothelium-dependent smooth muscle relaxation, and likewise it is the key mediator of penile erection. After any stimulation, NO is released from non-adrenergic non-cholinergic (NANC) nerves through activation of neuronal nitric oxide synthase (nNOS). Binding of NO to soluble guanylate cyclase increases cyclic guanosine monophosphate (cGMP) levels and cGMP-dependent protein kinase-1 (PKG-1) activity, leading to smooth muscle cell relaxation and cavernosal dilation. Subsequent hemodynamic changes such as increased arteriolar shear flow stimulate the phosphatidylinositol-3-kinase/protein kinase B (Akt) pathway leading to activation of endothelial nitric oxide synthase (eNOS) in penile endothelium and further NO release. Occlusion of venous outflow is also required for sinusoidal filling and the maintenance of high intracavernosal pressure and erection. This veno-occlusion is achieved by the compression of the emissary veins that lie between the tunica albuginea and the expanding sinusoidal tissue (Hidalgo-Tamola & Chitaley, 2009).

Since erection is a complex process that involves the participation of vascular, endocrine, cellular and neuronal mechanisms; reason why any damage at these levels, favors the partial or total loss of erection. These damages are not only structural but also functionally. The figure 1 describes the main physiological mechanisms that regulate the erectile function, and the morpho-physiological organizations that might suffer damages during DM.

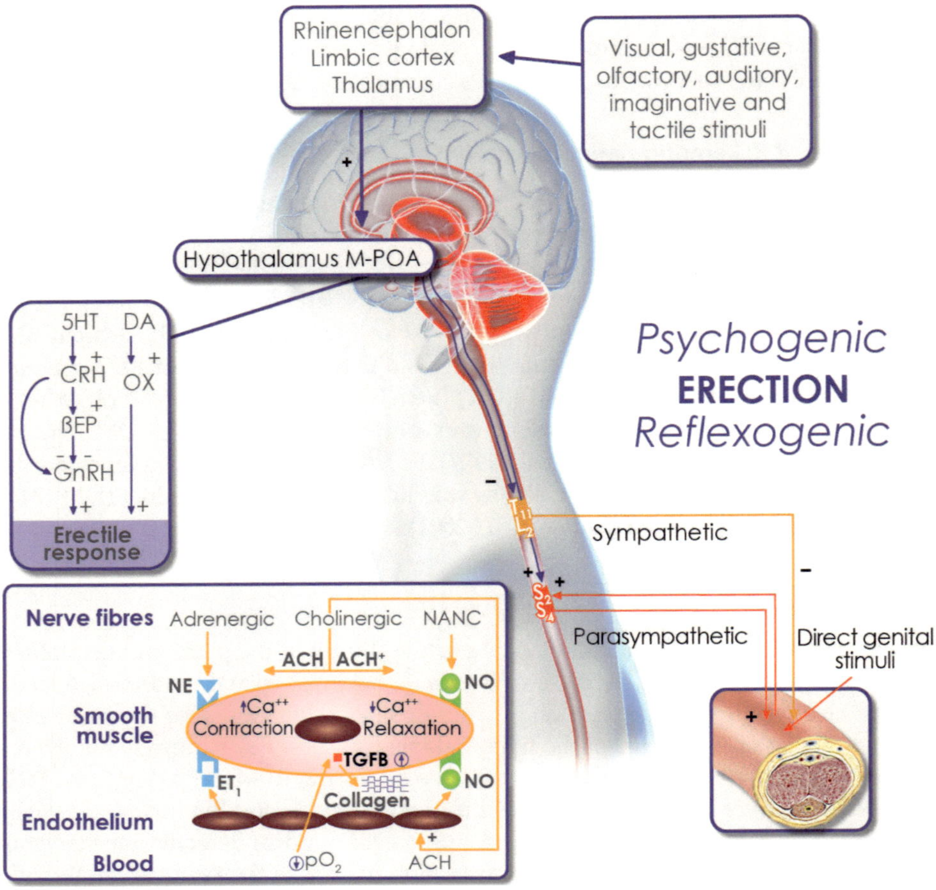

Fig. 1. Schematic representation of central and intracavernosal mechanisms involved in the control of erection. External visual, gustative, auditory, imaginative and tactile are transmitted to the rhinencephalon, the limbic cortex and thalamic nuclei, and are integrated into the hypothalamic medial preoptic area (M-POA) where they stimulate supraspinal erections (psychogenic erection). Up box: serotonin (5HT), corticotrophin-releasing-hormone (CRH) and β-endorphin (βEP) exert inhibitory effects, while gonadotrophin-releasing-hormone (GnRH), dopamine (DA) and oxytocin (OX) are the main stimulators of psychogenic erections. Hypothalamic projections (possibly oxytocinergic) to the spinal cord control thoracolumbar sympathetic (T11-L2) and sacral parasympathetic stimulation from (S2 to S4) fibers which inhibit and stimulate the erection, respectively. Direct genital stimuli initiate a local neural loop leading to parasympathetic stimulation from S2 to S4 and reflexogenic erection. Down box: intracavernosal mechanisms of erection involve cholinergic, adrenergic, and non-adrenergic non-cholinergic (NANC) nervous fibers. The main stimulators of smooth muscle cell contraction (detumescence) are norepinephrine (NE) and endothelin-1 (ET1), while acetylcholine (ACH) and nitric oxide (NO) are the main mediators of smooth muscle cell relaxation and erection via reduction of intracelular calcium (Ca^{+2}) content. Blood oxygen tension (pO_2) in the sinusoids inversely regulates smooth muscle cell transforming growth factor-β (TGFB) expression and collagen accumulation in the pericellular spaces. Modified from Fabbri et al., 1997.

4. Animal models of diabetes employed in the study of ED

In recent years, our understanding of human sexual function and dysfunctions has grown. Sexual responses are complex; therefore, different in vivo models exist, focused on the neurobiology, psychophysiology and different functional components of male sexual responses. When trying to understand how these preclinical models translate to humans, it should also be borne in mind that the primary purpose of sexual activity in animals is reproduction, while in humans it is predominantly recreational. The fact that animal sexual behaviors are highly stereotyped and species specific, it makes difficult to translate results in animal studies to humans (McMurray et al., 2006).

Erectile function monitoring intracavernosal pressure (ICP) is the most common method to preclinical monitoring the quality of an erectile response. ICP has been monitored in both conscious and anaesthetised animal models. The development of electronic data capture systems now allows various aspects of the ICP response to be measured. The typically measured endpoints include basal, peak, and plateau ICP, erection and detumesence time, duration of response, area under the ICP time response curve and the number of erections observed in a given time period. The aim is to use these end points to quantify the different phases and quality of the ICP response and the effect of the actions of drugs upon them (McMurray et al., 2006).

Despite this knowledge, clinical and epidemiological studies seldom separate type-1 (T1DM) and type-2 (T2DM) DM; however, this section will briefly highlight some of the T2DM animal models and animal models of DM induced by chemical treatments (T1DM) used to study the ED.

4.1 Rat models of T2DM

The obese diabetic Zucker rat (OZR) is a model for T2DM with glucose intolerance and an autosomal recessive mutation in the leptin gene. It develops hyperinsulinemia, insulin resistance, and hyperlipidemia at an early age with progression to proteinuria and glomerular injury (Kasiske et al., 1992). Similar characteristics exist between the OZR and patients with T2DM including obesity, hypertension, and impaired vasodilation. The BBZ/WOR rat is a cross between the BB/WOR rat a model for autoimmune diabetes and a Zucker rat. Obese BBZ/WOR rats develop insulin resistance, and hyperglycemia with higher mean serum glucose levels compared with lean T2DM rats (Vernet et al., 1995). Otsuka Long-Evans Tokushima Fatty (OLETF) rats develop spontaneous diabetes by selective breeding. Male rats exhibit late onset hyperglycemia, hypercholesterolemia, and mild obesity. In this model, pancreatic islet cells changes mirror those seen in humans with T2DM (Kawano et al., 1992).

4.2 Mouse models of T2DM

Recently, mouse models of T2DM have been utilized to study ED. The high-fat diet fed mouse model was used as an ED experimental model (Xie et al., 2007). C57BL6 mice were fed a high-fat, high-simple carbohydrate, and low-fiber diet for 22 weeks, and developed obesity with a mean body weight of 39 g, and developed diabetes with a mean fasting serum glucose of 223.6 mg/dL. An additional mouse model of T2DM is the *db/db* mouse (Sharma et al., 2003). The *db/db* mouse has a mutation in the leptin receptor, and develops spontaneous obesity, hyperglycemia, hyperphagia, hyperinsulinemia, and diabetic neuropathy, occurring from 10 days to 8 weeks of age.

4.3 Rabbit and rat models of T1DM induced by chemical treatment

The models of Alloxan-induced in rabbit (Chang et al., 2003; Vignozzi et al., 2007) and Streptozotocin-induced in rat (Vignozzi et al., 2007) of T1DM have been also used to study the ED.

Other animal models of T2DM and insulin resistance exist but have not been used to date to study mechanisms of ED during diabetes (Hidalgo-Tamola & Chitaley, 2009).

Findings gained from the study of some of these animal models have shed light on mechanisms underlying the cause of ED during DM. These factors include impaired vasodilatory signaling, cavernosal hypercontractility, and veno-occlusion, among others.

Although hyperglycemia is a common defining feature both: type-1 and type-2 DM, many unique characteristics distinguish these conditions, including insulin and lipid levels, obesity status, and inflammatory agent profiles. In the laboratory, the presence of ED has been established in animal models of both type-1 and type-2 DM. Impaired cavernosal vasodilation has been established in type-1 diabetic rodents. This dysfunction appears to be mediated by a severe defect in non-adrenergic-non-cholinergic nerve signaling, as well as impairment in penile endothelial function. In contrast, type-2 diabetic animals appear to have minimal impairment in parasympathetic-mediated dilatory function, but do have evidence of endothelial dysfunction. Type-2 diabetic models also exhibit a significant and striking increase in cavernosal contractile sensitivity, and a significant veno-occlusive disorder, neither of which is consistently reported in type-1 diabetic animals. With the distinct mechanisms underlying the ED phenotype in animal models of type-1 and type-2 diabetes, tailoring therapeutic treatments for diabetic-ED to the specific mechanisms underlying this disease complication may be warranted. Further examination of mechanisms underlying ED in DM patients may thus lead to significant changes in the way urologists diagnose, code, and treat diabetic-ED (Chitaley, 2009).

5. Mechanisms proposed to explain the ED in DM

From a historical perspective, theories pertaining to the pathophysiology of ED have changed as time has gone by. In the 1960´s, the prevailing wisdom was that most ED had a psychogenic origin, and it was only in the second half of the 20th century, as we have gained increasing knowledge of the physiology of normal erectile function, that we have begun to understand the importance of vascular, endocrine, cellular and neural mechanisms in the development of ED (Eardley, 2002).

There are several ways of classifying the erectile dysfunction causes, for example as organic, psychogenic or mixed organic and psychogenic, with organic erectile dysfunction being the most common form (Maas et al., 2002). However, take into account the way in which disease can interfere with erection, the classification can be: psychogenic, vascular, neural, cellular, endocrine, and iatrogenic (Eardley, 2002). As was showed above by epidemiological studies (Feldman et al., 1994; Saigal et al., 2006), the risk of erectile dysfunction increases with diabetes and it is in relation with several pathogenic mechanisms in diabetes disease involved in precipitating and maintaining the ED.

As it is showed in the figure 2, the physiopathology of ED in DM is multifactorial and in the following section, we address some of these pathophysiological mechanisms being so far taken into account to explain the development of ED in DM.

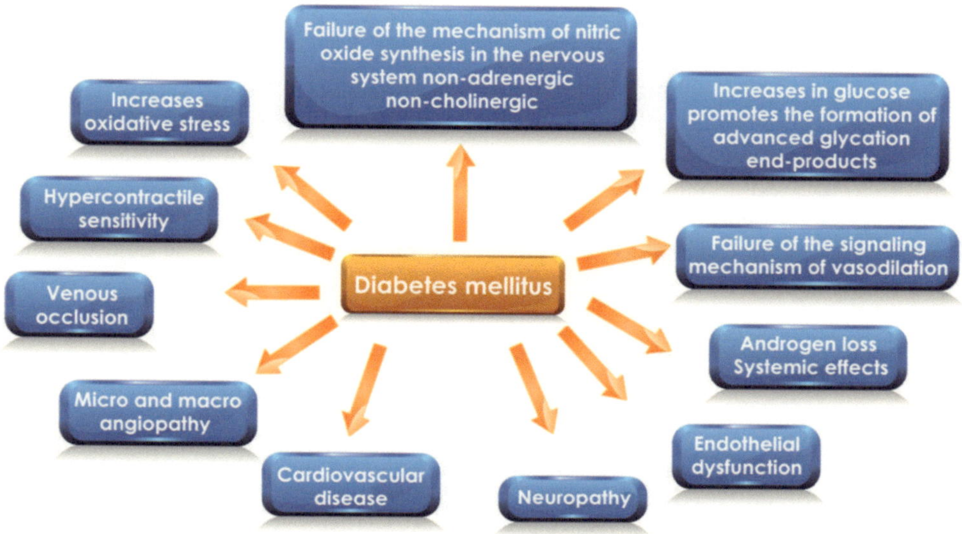

Fig. 2. Mechanisms of diabetes-associated erectile dysfunction.

5.1 Endothelial dysfunction

Several clinical and laboratory studies demonstrate that endothelial dysfunction is an important mechanism for the development of ED associated with T2DM. ED is usually described as a decrease in the bioavailability of NO, as a result of decreased expression and/or activity of eNOS, including increased removal of NO. Damage to the endothelium-dependent vasoreactivity has been demonstrated in various animal models of T2DM. Myograph in vitro studies in mice fed with a high fat diet, db/db diabetic mice and obese Zucker rats have shown that the ability of muscle relaxation of the cavernous tissue decreases even when stimulated with acetylcholine (Luttrell et al., 2008; Wingard et al., 2007; Xie et al., 2007). Jesmin et al., observed a decrease of the immunofluorescent staining of eNOS and the expression of this enzyme in the penile tissue of Long-Evans Tokushima Otsuka obese rats, with respect to controls (Jesmin et al., 2003). The decrease in eNOS mRNA expression suggests that reduced expression of eNOS is initiated at the gene transcription level. The alteration in the eNOS activation is another mechanism that contributes to decreased bioavailability of NO. eNOS activation occurs through phosphorylation of serine-177 residue by serine/threonine protein kinase Akt. In turn, the Akt-dependent pathway regulates the phosphorylation of eNOS mediated by the vascular endothelial growth factor (VEGF). The effects of VEGF include proliferation, migration, angiogenesis, and antiapoptosis in endothelial cells. VEGF increased the phosphorylation and expression of antiapoptotic proteins, mediated by eNOS. It is considered that in the ED, vascular repair mechanisms mediated by VEGF are damaged, probably because the expression of the VEGF and its receptors are altered in the cavernous endothelium, conditioning its angiogenic functions (Costa & Vendeira, 2007). In addition to the decreased eNOS activity, the increased removal of NO by free radicals and oxidative agents has been shown to be important in the cavernous endothelial dysfunction in diabetes-associated ED models (Hidalgo-Tamola & Chitaley, 2009). Endothelins (ET) are potent vasoconstrictor peptides that stimulate the contraction of trabecular smooth muscle of the corpus cavernosum. No one knows the exact involvement of ET on the pathogenesis of ED. High levels of ET-1 observed in diabetic patients could be enough to cause ED, although this does not happen. However, the high intracellular calcium concentration resulting from this condition modulates gene expression sufficiently to cause the proliferation of smooth muscle. Alternatively, alterations in ET receptor sensitivity in conditions such as diabetes and hypertension can enhance the processes of vasoconstriction. It is possible that the ET system may be relevant in ED, but under certain conditions where there is global endothelial dysfunction, such as diabetes and systemic sclerosis, the use of ET antagonists in these patients could be beneficial (Ritchie & Sullivan, 2010).

5.1.1 Failure of the signaling mechanism of vasodilation

Maintenance of cavernosal vasodilation has been hypothesized to occur through the activation of eNOS in endothelial cells, presumably in response to shear stress. Data from animal models of T2DM support the findings of impaired vasodilation in T2DM humans. Accompanying the impaired vasodilatory response, total penile NOS activity was found to be decreased in the BBZ/WOR rat model (Vernet et al., 1995). Similar result was showed by an age-matched case controlled study of 30 patients with T2DM and ED, where was found impaired the cavernosal vasodilation (De Angelis et al., 2001).

Vascular disease is probably the most common cause of ED, and of all the vascular causes, the commonest is atherosclerosis; however, DM joined with other risk factors, namely smoking, hypertension and hyperlipidaemia are also indirectly associated with the development of ED (Fig.3). A reduced arterial inflow leads to relative hypoxia within the penis with subsequent cellular effects. The crucial cellular mediator appears to be TGF-β1, which is increased in hypoxia and induces trophic changes in the cavernosal smooth muscle, and failure of the venous-occlusive mechanism (Feldman et al., 1994; Johannes et al., 2000).

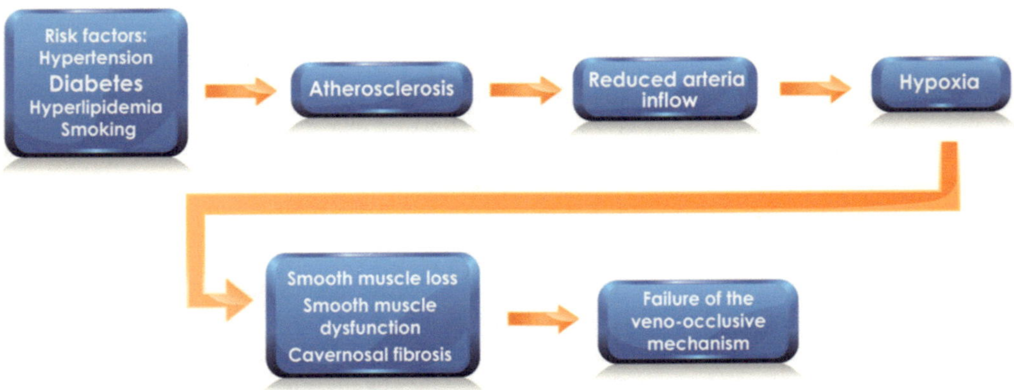

Fig. 3. Schematic representation of the relationship between the DM and other risks factors, with the development of vascular damages that favor the ED in the diabetic patient.

On the other hand, DM can injure cells and cause ED in a direct way. Diabetes damage the endothelium impairs the vascular response of the penis to neural stimuli. The structural changes in the endothelium that are produced by diabetes are accompanied by functional changes that result in impaired smooth muscle relaxation (Cartledge et al., 2001a; Saenz de Tejada et al., 1989). In the figure 4, it is possible observe the alteration of penile vascular endothelium of the rabbit with DM.

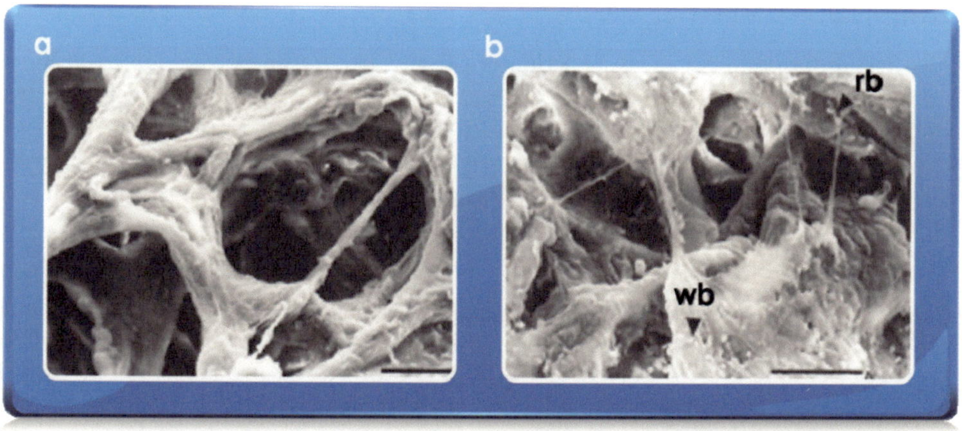

Fig. 4. Electron micrographs of normal penile vascular endothelium (a) and the effect of diabetes in the rabbit (b). Note the ragged appearance of the endothelium and the deposition of red (rb) and white (wb) blood cells in diabetes. (Micrographs published by the Dr. Ian Eardley in Pathophysiology of erectile dysfunction. (2002). *British Journal of Diabetes and Vascular Disease,* Vol. 2, No. 4, pp. 272-6, ISSN 1474-6514, by courtesy of Sullivan, M.

5.1.2 Venous-occlusive dysfunction

In ED, venous-occlusive dysfunction or venous leakage, involves the premature escape of blood inside the corpuses cavernous by incompetence of their drainage system and subsequent inability to reach the intracavernous pressure necessary to provide an effective stiffness. By Doppler studies and Pharmacocavernosometry, it has been observed that a high percentage of patients with T2DM present venous leak (Colakoglu et al., 1999; Metro & Broderick, 1999). Evidence from animal studies has demonstrated the importance of venous-occlusive dysfunction in the development of ED in T2DM. It is considered that the alteration in the process of veno-occlusion may be caused by changes in the structure of the penis, the cells and/or the content of the extracellular matrix. In this regard, the expression of VEGF has broad implications in the structure of the penis, resulting in changes in the rate of apoptosis. The decrease in VEGF expression correlates with elevated levels of pro-apoptotic proteins such as Bcl-2, so it is suggested that the decrease of VEGF in penile tissue in T2DM increases apoptosis and loss of erectile cells. In other studies with animal models of T2DM, there has been observed an alteration in the expression of collagen and the rate of smooth muscle/collagen in cavernous tissue. Likewise, decreased elastin has been found in the corpus cavernosum, specifically, decreased expression of tropoelastin mRNA, precursor protein of elastin and fibrillin-1. Structural alterations in the tunica albuginea caused by T2DM, could affect the compliance of the corpus cavernosum, required for veno-occlusion and intracavernous pressure maintenance (Hidalgo-Tamola & Chitaley, 2009).

5.1.3 Diabetic micro and macro angiopathy

Clinical and biochemical evidence support the participation of the microangiopathic complications of diabetes in the pathogenesis of ED. Multiple studies have shown that chronic hyperglycemia (which is the main determinant of the microangiopathic complications) is a strong risk factor for ED. Diabetes duration and other microvascular complications (i.e. retinopathy, neuropathy and nephropathy) are predictors of the occurrence of ED (Bhasin et al., 2007).

Somatic and autonomic nerve dysfunction is present in a large percentage of individuals with diabetes-associated ED (Chitaley et al., 2009). Its presence is demonstrated by the existence of both, longer latencies in the evoked potentials of pudendal nerves and abnormal bulbar urethral and urethroanal reflexes. Diabetes causes degeneration of the nitrergic nerves, which participates in the nitric oxide-dependent cavernosal smooth muscle relaxation. A central neuropathic mechanism has been postulated by several authors (Costabile, 2003).

Some of the biochemical mechanisms that induce endothelial dysfunction and decreased generation of nitric oxide participate also in the pathogenesis of diabetic neuropathy (Gur et al., 2009). An example is the oxidative stress. Superoxide radicals are present in high amount in cavernosal tissues. Superoxide anion reacts with nitric oxide to form peroxynitrite resulting in decreased nitric oxide bioavailability (Boulton et al., 2004). In addition peroxynitrite is a highly toxic compound for vascular cells and neurons. It causes mitochondrial dysfunction, oxidative DNA damage and apoptosis. Other examples are the activation of protein kinase C and the presence of advance glycation end-products (AGEs). 1,2-Diacylglycerol (DAG), a metabolite responsible of lipotoxicity in obesity and T2DM, activates protein kinase C (in particular the β isoform (PKC-β). These enzymes participate in multiple biological networks. This enzyme is activated also by free radicals. Experimental data suggest that activated PKC-β plays a major role in the hyperglycemia-related tissular damage; one of the possible explanations is the induction of the nuclear kappa B pathway. It is also involved in the carvernosal corpus smooth muscle contraction. On the other hand, chronic hyperglycemia causes the formation of AGEs which induces tissue damage by modifying molecules, activating inflammation and stimulating the synthesis of growth factors. AGEs modify cytoskeletal and myelin structure (England & Asbury, 2004). These changes correlate with a reduction in myelinated fiber density in peripheral nerves. Also, AGEs quench endothelium derived nitric oxide. As result, AGEs decreases smooth muscle relaxation and impairs erectile function (Thorve et al., 2011).

The macrovascular complications during the DM contribute to the development of ED (Chai et al., 2009). Vascular atherosclerotic disease of penile arteries is present in 70-80% of cases with ED. Occlusion of the cavernosal arteries could be a contributing factor in the long term. However, recent studies have shown that structural arterial changes in the penile vascular bed could exist even in cases with ED free of coronary heart disease.

5.2 Diabetic neuropathy

Neuropathy is a common complication of diabetes, in which there is nerve damage as a result of hyperglycemia. The damage involves both somatic and autonomic nerves. Autonomic nerves of the parasympathetic division stimulate relaxation of the muscles in the penis; with the resulting erection, those of the sympathetic division are responsible for the contraction of muscles in the penis and thus maintain penile flaccidity. Although the mechanisms by which it occurs are not completely clear, it is known that nerve fibers are structurally modified by the effect of substances derived from the metabolism of excess glucose, which determines the loss of myelin. The loss of myelin promotes delayed nerve transmission, both reception of motor commands and other. Likewise, it is considered that the damage is caused in turn by the injury of blood vessels supplying the nerves. Neuropathy is another important mechanism responsible for diabetes-associated ED (Costabile, 2003). Diabetes is notorious for its microvascular complications, particularly autonomic neuropathy and peripheral neuropathy (Agarwal et al., 2003). It has been noted that patients with diabetic and neuropathic ED have similar frequencies of somatic and autonomic nervous system neuropathies, suggesting that neuropathy contributes significantly to the diabetes-associated ED. A recent study showed the connection between diabetic and neuropathic ED, demonstrating the presence of apoptotic pathways in the cavernous nerves in both disease processes (Mc Vary et al., 2006). The underlying cause of ED, which is the result of diabetic neuropathy, might be linked to selective nitrergic degeneration, which has been observed in the diabetic rat penis. This selective neurodegeneration seems to result in decreased nNOS activity and decreased NO production, which leads to damage nitrergic relaxation of corpus cavernosum in diabetic patients (Cellek et al., 1999). Additionally, NO could participate in the selective nitrergic degeneration through the formation of oxygen free radicals. It has been suggested that oxidative damage secondary to the production of peroxynitrite derived from NO may contribute to neurodegeneration (Cartledge et al., 2001a; Cellek et al., 1999). Several studies have shown that inhibition of NO synthase and NO production; prevent nitrergic degeneration, suggesting that this is a NO dependent process (Cellek et al., 1999).

5.2.1 Failure of the mechanism of nitric oxide synthesis in the nervous system non-adrenergic non-cholinergic

DM is one of the major risk factors to develop ED. Hyperglycemia is considered the cause of many vascular complications and metabolic alterations associated with both T1DM and T2DM. Diabetes-associated ED has been attributed to a reduction in the number of NOS-containing nerves, the impairment of NOS activity, and both neurogenic- and endothelium-mediated smooth muscle relaxation, and also to downregulation of the mediators downstream from NO, such as cGMP and PKG-1, in the corpus cavernosum (Musicki & Burnett, 2006).

In the cell, NO synthases have to compete, with other enzymes with activity of arginases, for the substrate L-arginine. Inhibition of arginase activity by 2(S)-amino-6-boronohexonic acid (ABH) has been shown to cause significant enhancement of non-adrenergic, non-cholinergic nerve-mediated relaxation of penile corpus cavernosum smooth muscle, suggesting that arginase inhibition sustains L-arginine concentrations for be used in the NO synthesis (Cox et al., 1999). Moreover, another study demonstrated that diabetic corpus cavernosum from humans with ED had higher levels of arginase II protein, gene expression and enzyme activity than normal human cavernosal tissue. The impaired ability of diabetic tissue to synthesize NO was reversed by the selective inhibition of arginase activity by ABH. Increased expression of arginase II in diabetic cavernosal tissue may therefore contribute to the diabetes-associated ED (Bivalacqua et al., 2001). Another explanation for decreased eNOS activity in the diabetic penis can be due to a reduced penile L-arginine content. Oral administration of L-arginine to diabetic rabbits increases endothelium-dependent relaxation of cavernosal tissue by improving the NO biosynthesis (Yildirim et al., 1999).

5.3 Oxidative stress

Oxidative stress occurs when there is an imbalance between pro-oxidants and the ability of the antioxidants to scavenge excess reactive oxygen species. However, its role in ED has not been investigated comprehensively but, significant associations between the production of reactive oxygen species and ED have been showed, especially in diabetic animal models.

NO is a highly reactive free radical that undergoes nonenzymatic reaction with oxyhemoglobin or that reacts with free radicals, such as superoxide anion, to form peroxynitrite (Beckman & Koppenol, 1996). This observation first highlighted the importance of oxidative stress in ED.

Reactive oxygen species (ROS) are formed during regular metabolism due to the univalent reduction of oxygen molecule. Superoxide (O_2^-) is the most important among the ROS. Hydrogen peroxide (H_2O_2), hypochlorous acid (HOCL), and peroxynitrite ($OONO^-$) are other important free radicals implicated in the pathophysiological mechanism of vascular disease. The vascular endothelium is the major source for these free radicals (Beckman & Koppenol, 1996). Superoxide dismutase (SOD) is an important enzyme that removes the superoxide radicals from the human body. There are 3 types of SOD isoenzymes: cytosolic, mitochondrial, and extracellular. Extracellular SOD reportedly plays a critical role in maintaining the redox state of vascular interstitium and thereby prevents the pathophysiological effects of superoxide in the vasculature.

The interaction between NO and reactive oxygen species (ROS) is one of the important mechanisms implicated in the pathophysiological process of ED. NO interacts with superoxide to form peroxynitrite, which has been reported to play a central role in atherogenesis. Peroxynitrite reacts with the tyrosyl residue of proteins, which inactivates superoxide dismutase and leads to decreased removal of superoxide. This further increases the formation of peroxynitrite and reduces the available NO concentration. Peroxynitrite causes smooth-muscle relaxation but is less potent than NO. Also, peroxynitrite and superoxide have been reported to increase the incidence of apoptosis in the endothelium. This leads to denudation of endothelium and further reduction of available NO (Agarwal et al., 2006). On the other hands a reduced NO concentration aggravates the adhesion of platelets to the endothelium, and the co-adhesion of neutrophils to platelets as well as the endothelium through the expression of adhesion molecules, releasing large amounts of superoxide which reduces more the available NO by the formation of peroxynitrite, countering erectile drive as well as promoting further more adhesion of platelets and neutrophils. Under this condition, is favored the releasing of substances (thromboxane A2 and serotonin) that cause vasoconstriction (Jeremy et al., 2000), taking place a vicious circle that generates the vasculopathic erectile dysfunction.

Another mechanism has been implicated in diabetes-associated ED is the activation of protein kinase C, this is an enzyme that modulates several cellular events, and increased levels of this enzyme are associated with increased production of ROS and reduced levels of NO, which can be prevented by administration of antioxidants (Ganz & Seftel, 2000).

The studies demonstrate that oxidative stress has a vital role in the development of diabetes-associated ED. Hyperglycemia is an important mediator of increased production of ROS leading to impaired endothelial function and structural impairment in the diabetic corpus cavernosum. The corpus cavernosum of diabetic rats and diabetic men with ED exhibits increased lipid peroxidation, upregulation of superoxide anion, and decreased antioxidants levels, suggestive of oxidative stress (Bivalacqua et al., 2005).

5.4 Involvement of advanced glycation end-products

The proposed mechanisms for ED in DM patients include: damage in the synthesis of NO, reduction in the activity of PKG-1, increased endothelin and endothelin B (ETB) receptor binding sites; ultrastructural changes in the endothelium, upregulation of the RhoA/Rho-kinase pathway, neuropathy, increased levels of oxygen free radicals and elevated concentration of advanced glycation end-products (AGEs) (Jiaan et al., 1995; Moore & Wang, 2006; Sullivan et al., 1997; Thorve et al., 2011).

Hyperglycemia in DM leads to AGEs, which are derived from non-enzymatic glycosylation reactions, actually known as glycation. Glucose reacts with amino groups, producing what is known as a Schiff base. Schiff base is modified to form more stable Amadori products. Some of these Amadori products undergo irreversible chemical changes and become AGEs (Brownlee et al., 1988; Cárdenas-León et al., 2009; Cartledge et al., 2001b) (Fig. 5). The action of AGEs is mostly via cell surface receptors, such as the receptor for AGEs (RAGE), P60/OST48 protein (R-1), 80KH phosphoprotein (R-2) and galectin-3 (R-3), scavenger receptor II, lactoferrin-like polypeptide, and CD-36 (Basta et al., 2004). Some of the receptors are likely to contribute to clearance of AGEs, whereas others may mediate many of the adverse effects, such as quenching of NO, impairment of extracellular matrix and tissue remodeling, modification of circulating proteins, and receptor-mediated production of ROS. AGEs can also form covalent bonds with collagen vascular, leading to thickening of blood vessels, decreased elasticity, endothelial dysfunction and atherosclerosis (Bucala et al., 1991; Singh et al., 2001). AGEs are accumulated during aging (Jiaan et al., 1995) and diabetes. They are formed abundantly when glucose remains high for prolonged periods (Bucala et al., 1991; Seftel et al., 1997). AGEs have been found elevated in the corpus cavernosum and tunica albuginea of the penis of diabetics rats and humans (Cartledge et al., 2001b; Cirino et al., 2006; Jiaan et al., 1995; Seftel et al., 1997). It is thought that AGEs may contribute to diabetes-associated ED, generating oxygen free radicals, which induce cell damage by oxidative processes and also remove NO, culminating with the decrease of cGMP and affecting the cavernous smooth muscle relaxation (Bivalacqua et al., 2005; Cartledge et al., 2001b). AGEs may take effect at the molecular level on different channels and receptors in cavernous smooth muscle cells, particularly on potassium channels, which facilitate the release of intracellular calcium and subsequent cavernous smooth muscle relaxation. Damage to the potassium channels could lead to lost of the relaxation capacity of the cavernous smooth muscle and to early onset of diabetes-associated ED (Cartledge et al., 2001b; Costabile, 2003). Also, AGEs are considered to be related to ED during diabetes by increasing the expression of mediators of vascular damage such as VEGF and ET-1, which have mitogenic and vasoconstrictor activities (Morano, 2003). Several studies have shown damage to smooth muscle relaxation in the corpus cavernosum and penile ED in diabetic rat in the presence of AGEs (Cartledge et al., 2001b; Usta et al., 2003). Also, it has been observed that under conditions of diabetes, the combined effect of AGEs and their receptor (RAGE), may increase the activity of ET-1 in the cavernous tissue and thus promote the development of diabetes-associated ED (Chen et al., 2008). The involvement of AGEs in diabetes-associated ED has been demonstrated by using aminoguanidine, an inhibitor of AGEs formation (Usta et al., 2004) and ALT-711, a compound that breaks down formed AGEs (Usta et al., 2006), and observing improvement in endothelium-dependent cavernosal smooth muscle relaxation in vitro (Cellek et al., 2004) and erectile responses in vivo (Usta et al., 2003).

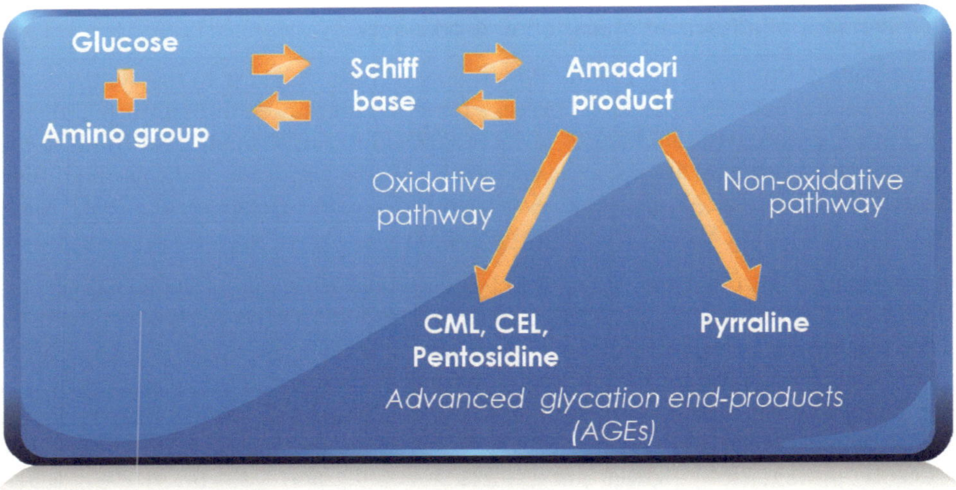

Fig. 5. Schematic representation: mechanisms of main Advanced Glycation End-products (AGEs) formation. CML: Carboxymethyl lysine; CEL: Carboxyethyl lysine.

5.5 Hyper-contractility of the cavernous body

ED is more common in diabetic patients. Hyperglycemia among others, leads to an altered vasodilator neural impulse, causing smooth muscle hyperkinesis and altered veno-occlusion process (Hidalgo-Tamola & Chitaley, 2009). Hypercontractility of corpus cavernosum may occur as a result of heightened sympathetic nervous system activity and/or increase in signaling to smooth muscle. The role of hyperkinesis of smooth muscle cells during T2DM-associated ED is difficult to discern from clinical studies, since most of them combine patients with T1DM and T2DM in the same group of evaluation. However, several animal studies suggest the importance of hyperkinesis in T2DM-associated ED.

Hyperinsulinemia and insulin resistance are associated with overactive sympathetic nervous system, which increases smooth muscle tone and keeps the penis in flaccid state. Currently it is unclear whether the increase in contractility is only due to sympathetic overactivity or the gloom of the signaling pathways in smooth muscle play a predominant role (Carneiro, 2008). The results obtained by using diabetic obese Zucker rats as an experimental model, suggest that increased smooth muscle tone is mediated by protein kinase C and RhoA/Rho-kinase pathway (Wingard et al., 2007). During normal erection, this pathway is inhibited by NO (Mills, 2002), but during diabetes the RhoA/Rho-kinase pathway activity is elevated and suppresses eNOS gene expression and enzyme activity in the penis (Bivalacqua et al., 2004). It has been reported that corpus cavernosal tissue, obtained from alloxan-induced diabetic rabbits, exhibits increased RhoA and Rho-kinase ß expression (Chang et al., 2003). It is considered that other modulators of tone of smooth muscle cells might be involved in T2DM-associated ED. In addition to the altered vasodilator stimuli and increased contractility of the corpus cavernosum, which limit the flow of blood into the penis, the inability to limit the outflow of blood due to a disorder of veno-occlusion, may also be a factor in T2DM-associated ED. ED during diabetes is associated among others with decreased PKG-1. In smooth muscle a major target of the PKG-1 are the calcium-sensitive potassium channels (BK_{Ca}), the overactivation of which hyperpolarizes smooth muscle cells, causing relaxation. But during diabetes the activity of PKG-1 and therefore the activity of the BK_{Ca} are low and the relaxation mechanism is affected. It has been observed that the elimination of BK_{Ca} channels in an experimental model causes hypercontractility of the smooth muscle and ED (Werner et al., 2008).

5.5.1 Relationship between glycaemia, dyslipidemia, hypertension and its medical treatment with ED in DM patients

The hyperglycemia and dyslipidemia associated to DM favors the mechanisms of oxidative stress, endothelial damage and the development of atherosclerosis (Li, et al., 2011; Kumar, et al., 2010) leading to hypertension as consequence of endothelial dysfunction and loss of vascular relaxation. Due to these considerations, it is extremely important the metabolic control of DM subjects to avoid the appearance of ED.

Weight loss is the prime objective of therapy. Several studies in which intensive lifestyle programs or bariatric surgery were implemented to lose weight have shown that erectile function improves in direct proportion with the difference in body weight. The potential mechanisms include improved endothelial function and nitric oxide bioavailability, decreased inflammation, increased testosterone plasma levels, and improved mood and self-esteem. In addition, weight loss is the cornerstone for the treatment of hyperglycemia, hypertriglyceridemia, arterial hypertension and hypoalphalipoproteinemia (Khatana et al., 2008). Patients should be encouraged to quit smoking, to reduce their alcohol intake and to give up recreational drugs. Prescription drugs and over the-counter medications should be checked for possible contributors to ED. Relationship counseling and a psychiatric medication is useful to treat anxiety and depression.

An association exists between glycemic control and ED in men with diabetes. Hermans et al., analyzed 221 consecutive male outpatients with T2DM in whom ED was assessed using the International Index of Erectile Function (IIEF-5) questionnaire (Hermans et al., 2009). Patients with ED (n=83) were compared with an age-matched controls (n=51). Patients with poor control have increased risk for ED compared to patients with good control. Body weight and adiposity are significantly associated with ED. Obesity is associated with an odds ratio of 1.5 to 3 for having ED. Other measures of adiposity, including the waist-to-hip ratio and abdominal circumference, are also independently associated with ED. A sedentary life style increases the risk, independently of its effect on body mass index. Arterial hypertension and abnormal plasma lipid level, common co-morbidities of T2DM, are associated with ED. Both are linked with endothelial dysfunction, reduced nitric oxide synthesis and increased free radicals synthesis.

Several authors have proposed that treatment of hyperglycemia and cardiovascular risk factors should be part of the treatment of ED. Although this proposal is clinically sound, no major randomized controlled studies are available to support it. Only the EDIC trial (Epidemiology of Diabetes Intervention and Complications study) have partially evaluated it. The EDIC study is an extension of the DDCT trial, a landmark study that demonstrated that the correction of hyperglycemia reduces the incidence of microvascular complications. A substudy of the EDIC trial (Uro-EDIC) was designed to evaluate the impact of the correction of hyperglycemia on the incidence of urologic complications. ED was assessed using the IEFF questionnaire. The effect of treatment was evaluated separately in cases (n=280) with or without (n=291) microvascular complications. No difference was observed in the incidence of ED between men randomized to intensive *vs.* conventional therapy (OR 1.24, 95% CI 0.68-2.28) in cases free of microvascular complications at the beginning of the study. In contrast, intensive therapy resulted in a smaller incidence of ED among men with microvascular complications (OR 0.33, 95% CI 0.18-0.60). Regrettably, ED was not included among the study outcomes of the main trials that have evaluated the effect of intensive treatment of hyperglycemia (i.e. ACCORD trial) in men with T2DM. Future studies including validated ED measurements, adequate sample size and important potential confounders are needed to measure the benefit of intensive glycemic control in men with poorly controlled diabetes.

5.6 Androgen loss systemic effects

The erectile response in mammals is regulated by androgens; in particular it has been confirmed that testosterone is an important regulator of the erectile function (Yassin & Saad, 2008). Is known that 6-12% of men between 40 and 69 years old suffer from hypogonadism. In adult men the disease is manifested by erectile dysfunction, among others. Male hypogonadism, which is also called testosterone deficiency syndrome, is characterized by failure of testicular testosterone production and is especially common in men with T2DM, affecting one third of them. Testosterone acts on the penile tissues involved in the mechanism of erection, so deficiency of this hormone, impairs erectile capacity. The pathophysiological mechanisms of low circulating testosterone concentrations are unknown, but it has been suggested that obesity associated with T2DM, helps to reduce testosterone levels by increasing the conversion of testosterone to estradiol in adipose tissue. The increase in the concentration of estradiol leads in turn to a suppression of hipothalamic gonadotrophin releasing hormone (GnRH), which is evidenced by a reduced secretion of pituitary gonadrotropins (luteinizing hormone, LH and follicle stimulating hormone, FSH), which reduces in turn the secretion of testosterone by the Leydig cells and spermatogenesis in the seminiferous tubules, thus manifesting as hypogonadism. This may explain the inverse relationship between BMI and plasma concentrations of testosterone (Dhindsa et al., 2004; Grossmann et al., 2008; Kapoor et al., 2007; Rhoden et al., 2005; Traish et al., 2009). Male hypogonadism is associated with increased adipose tissue. In men with more than 160% of ideal body weight, concentrations of plasma testosterone and sex hormone-binding globulin (SHBG) are usually low while estrogen levels, from the conversion of adrenal androgens in adipose tissue, increase. In men with morbid obesity weighing more than 200% over the ideal weight, free testosterone may decrease. The concentrations of free testosterone and SHBG show an inverse relationship with waist circumference (WC) (Osuna et al., 2006; Pasquali et al., 1997; Svartberg, 2007). With the increase in adipose tissue also increases the production of leptin; favors the insulin resistance and therefore the appearance of hyperinsulinemia. Under these conditions, both leptin and insulin act on Leydig cells and inhibit testosterone synthesis (Pitteloud et al., 2005; Soderberg et al., 2001) (Fig. 6).

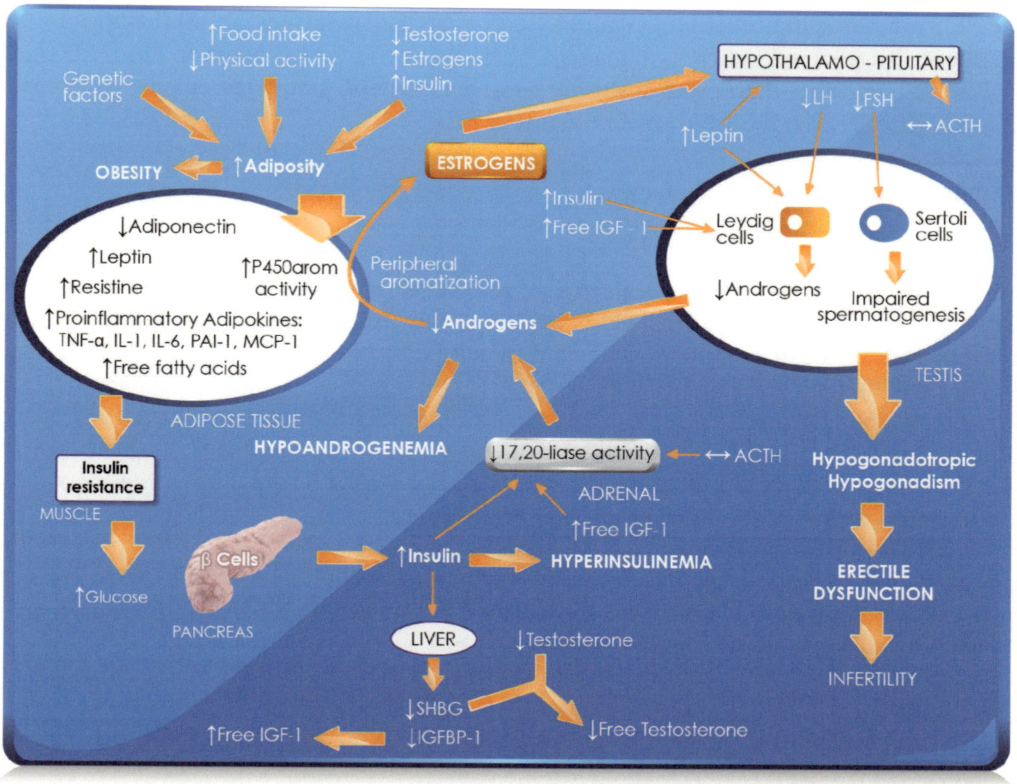

Fig. 6. Relationship between obesity, androgen deficiency (hypogonadism), metabolic syndrome and ED. The increase in adipose tissue and its accumulation in abdominal region, increases the production of adipokines and free fatty acids, this in turn, generates insulin resistance and hyperinsulinemia. The excess of insulin reduces the hepatic synthesis of SHBG and IGFBP-1 with the consequent increase of free IGF-1. The high concentrations of IGF-I and insulin act synergically on the testis and the adrenals glands, reducing the androgens secretion. In the testis, moreover, because of the limited effect that the reduced LH concentration exerts on the synthesis of testosterone, the effect is more marked. Probably, the increase in aromatization of androgens by adipose tissue, contributes to the hypoandrogenemia, together with the low levels of FSH which limit the spermatic development, lead to ED and the hypogonadotropic hypogonadism condition, which is an infertility factor.

Androgen deficiency contributes to pathologies associated with the metabolic syndrome, such as obesity, T2DM, hypertension and hyperlipidemia, which affect the endothelium, resulting in multiple vascular diseases, including ED, representing the latter, an infertility factor (Akishita et al., 2007; Traish et al., 2009; Tripathy et al., 2003) (Fig. 6). Also, several studies have shown that low testosterone levels predict development of T2DM in men (Tomar et al., 2006). There is evidence that the treatment with testosterone to DM animal models improves erectile function by influencing the NO/cGMP/PDE5 pathway (Vignozzi et al., 2005). Testosterone supplementation to diabetic animals also down regulates RhoA/Rho-kinase signaling (Vignozzi et al., 2007) improving also erectile function. The use of PDE 5 inhibitors like Sildenafil (Viagra), Tadalafil (Cialis) and Vardenafil (Levitra) for ED treatment has allowed a better management of this condition (Yassin & Saad, 2008). In particular, combined therapy of testosterone and sildenafil, improves erectile function in patients with T2DM (Hidalgo-Tamola & Chitaley, 2009).

5.7 Other causes of ED in diabetes

5.7.1 Viral and Bacterial pathogens

A role for viral and bacterial pathogens in the development of atherosclerosis has been suggested by multiple studies. Most evidence for this infection theory comes from seroepidemiological and experimental studies with *cytomegalovirus* (CMV) and *Chlamydia pneumonia* (CP), which are intracellular pathogens and can directly infect vascular wall cells, including endothelial cells and smooth muscle cells. Although still under debate, there appears to be an association of CMV and CP with the presence or development of atherosclerotic vascular disease in diabetes. Direct infection of endothelial cells leads to pro-coagulant activity and a local vascular pro-inflammatory response. Although the exact pathogenesis of ED in men with DM is still unclear, endothelial dysfunction plays a pivotal role and some studies suggested an association between ED and CMV and/or CP seropositivity in men with diabetes. Also, levels of the inflammatory markers as C-reactive protein and fibrinogen were elevated in patients with diabetes-associated ED (Blans et al., 2006).

5.7.2 Drugs used in the diabetic patient

A large number of drugs used in the managing of the DM patients may impair sexual function, either by an effect upon erectile and ejaculatory function or sex drive. Some of them are used as part of the diabetes treatment or others associated conditions like hypertension, anxiety and depression. The use of these drugs very rarely produces ED by themselves. Side effects usually appear adjunct to another pathophysiological mechanism (Eardley, 2002; Elías-Calles & Licea, 2003) (Table 1).

Type of drug:	**Secondary sexual effect:**
Antihypertensive (Diuretics):	
Spironolactone	Diminution of the libido, ED
Thiazide	Diminution of the libido, ED
Agents of central action:	
Methyldopa	Diminution of the libido, ED
Clonidine	ED
Reserpine	Diminution of the libido, ED and depression
Alpha-adrenergic blocking agents:	
Prazosin	Retrograde ejaculation

Type of drug:	**Secondary sexual effect:**
Terazosin	Retrograde ejaculation
Beta-adrenergic blocking agents:	
Propranolol	Diminution of the libido, ED
Metoprolol	Diminution of the libido, ED
Alpha and Beta Blocking Agents:	
Labetalol	Inhibition of the ejaculation
Blocking of the sympathetic ganglia:	
Guanethidine	ED, Retrograde ejaculation
Inhibitor of the angiotensin-converting enzyme:	
Lisinopril	ED in 1% of the cases
Psychiatric drugs (Tricyclic Antidepressants):	
Amitriptyline	ED, Inhibition of the ejaculation
Amoxapine	Diminution of the libido, ED
Desipramine	Inhibition of the ejaculation
Imipramine	Inhibition of the ejaculation
Maprotiline	Inhibition of the ejaculation
Nortriptyline	Inhibition of the ejaculation
Protriptyline	ED, Inhibition of the ejaculation
Atypical agent:	
Trazodone	Priapism
Inhibitors of Monoamine oxidase:	
Isocarboxazid	Inhibition of the ejaculation
Phenelzine	ED, Inhibition of the ejaculation
Antipsychotic:	
Thioridazine	Diminution of the libido, Inhibition of the ejaculation
Chlorpromazine	Inhibition of the ejaculation
Mesoridazine	Diminution of the libido, Inhibition of the ejaculation

Type of drug:	**Secondary sexual effect:**
Fluphenazine	Diminution of the libido, Inhibition of the ejaculation
Serotonin reuptake inhibitor:	
Fluoxetine	Anorgasmia
Trifluoperazine	Inhibition of the ejaculation
Chlorprothixene	Inhibition of the ejaculation
Haloperidol	Inhibition of the ejaculation
Anti-mania:	
Lithium carbonate	Possible ED
Anti-ulcer:	
Cimetidine	Diminution of the libido, ED, Gynecomastia

Table 1. Drugs used in the managing of the metabolic and psychological state of the diabetic patients with potential capacity to induce sexual dysfunctions including ED.

6. Conclusions

DM is one of the more important risk factors to the development ED. The uncontrolled metabolic state (characterized by hyperglycaemia, dyslipidemia, insulin resistance, hyperinsulinemia) induce oxidative stress, failure in the signaling mechanism of vasodilation, venous-occlusive dysfunction, atherosclerosis, angiopathy, neuropathy, alterations of the NO-mediated pathways, the formation of advanced glycation end-products, hypercontractility of the cavernous body, overweight and androgen loss systemic effects, and ED as consequence.

Although hyperglycemia is a common defining feature in type-1 and type-2 DM, many unique characteristics distinguish these diseases, including insulin and lipid levels, obesity status, and inflammatory agent profiles. Impaired cavernosal vasodilation has been established in T1DM rodents. This dysfunction appears to be mediated by a severe defect in non-adrenergic-non-cholinergic nerve signaling, as well as impairment in penile endothelial function. In contrast, T2DM animals appear to have minimal impairment in parasympathetic-mediated dilatory function, but do have evidence of endothelial dysfunction. T2DM models also exhibit a significant and striking increase in cavernosal contractile sensitivity, and a significant veno-occlusive disorder, neither of which is consistently reported in T1DM animals. With the distinct mechanisms underlying the ED phenotype in animal models of type-1 and type-2 DM, the therapeutic treatments for diabetes-associated ED most be adjustment to the specific mechanisms underlying this disease complication. Further examination of mechanisms underlying ED in DM patients may thus lead to significant changes in the way urologists diagnose, code, and treat diabetes-associated ED. An adequate metabolic and psychological control is the more effective way to avoid the ED in DM; for these reasons it is of extreme importance the opportune and specialized medical intervention and support.

7. References

[1] Agarwal, S.K., Prakash, A., & Singh, N.P. (2003). Erectile dysfunction in diabetes mellitus: Novel treatments. *International Journal of Diabetes in Developing Countries*, Vol. 23, pp. 94-8, ISSN 0973-3930.

[2] Agarwal, A., Nandipati, K.C., Sharma, R.K., Zippe, C.D., & Raina, R. (2006). Role of oxidative stress in the pathophysiological mechanism of erectile dysfunction. *Journal of Andrology*, Vol. 27, No. 3, pp. 335-47, ISSN 0196-3635.

[3] Akishita, M., Hashimoto, M., Ohike, Y., Ogawa, S., Iijima, K., Eto, M., & Ouchi, Y. (2007). Low testosterone level is an independent determinant of endothelial dysfunction in men. *Hypertension Research*, Vol. 30, No. 11, pp. 1029-34, ISSN 0916-9636.

[4] Basta, G., Schmidt, A.M., & De Caterina, R. (2004). Advanced glycation end products and vascular inflammation: implications for accelerated atherosclerosis in diabetes. *Cardiovascular Research*, Vol. 63, No. 4, pp. 582-92, ISSN 0008-6363.

[5] Beckman, J.S. & Koppenol, W.H. (1996). Nitric oxide, superoxide, and peroxynitrite: the good, the bad, and ugly. *The American journal of physiology*, Vol. 271, No. 5 Pt 1, pp. C1424-37, ISSN 0002-9513.

[6] Benet, A.E., & Melman, A. (1995). The epidemiology of erectile dysfunction. *Urologic Clinics of North America*, Vol. 22, No. 4, pp. 699-709, ISSN 0094-0143.

[7] Bhasin, S., Enzlin, P., Coviello, A., & Basson, R. (2007). Sexual dysfunction in men and women with endocrine disorders. *The Lancet*, Vol. 369, No. 9561, pp. 597-611, ISSN 0140-6736.

[8] Bivalacqua, T.J., Champion, H.C., Usta, M.F., Cellek, S., Chitaley, K., Webb, R.C., Lewis, R.L., Mills, T.M., Hellstrom, W.J., & Kadowitz, P.J. (2004). RhoA/Rho-kinase suppresses endothelial nitric oxide synthase in the penis: a mechanism for diabetes-associated erectile dysfunction. *Proceedings of the National Academy of Sciences of the United States of America*, Vol. 101, No. 24, pp. 9121-6, ISSN 0027-8424.

[9] Bivalacqua, T.J., Hellstrom, W.J., Kadowitz, P.J., & Champion, H.C. (2001). Increased expression of arginase II in human diabetic corpus cavernosum: in diabetic-associated erectile dysfunction. *Biochemical and Biophysical Research Communications*, Vol. 283, No. 4, pp. 923-7, ISSN 0006-291X.

[10] Bivalacqua, T.J., Usta, M.F., Kendirci, M., Pradhan, L., Alvarez, X., Champion, H.C., Kadowitz, P.J., & Hellstrom, W.J. (2005). Superoxide anion production in the rat penis impairs erectile function in diabetes: influence of in vivo extracellular superoxide dismutase gene therapy. *The Journal of Sexual Medicine*, Vol. 2, No. 2, pp. 187-97; discussion 197-8, ISSN 1743-6095.

[11] Blans, M.C., Visseren, F.L., Banga, J.D., Hoekstra, J.B., van der Graaf, Y., Diepersloot, R.J., & Bouter, K.P. (2006). Infection induced inflammation is associated with erectile dysfunction in men with diabetes. *European Journal of Clinical Investigation*, Vol. 36, No. 7, pp. 497-502, ISSN 0014-2972.

[12] Bloomgarden, ZT. (1998). American Diabetes Association Annual Meeting. Endothelial dysfunction, neuropathy and the diabetic foot, diabetic mastopathy, and erectile dysfunction. *Diabetes Care*, Vol. 21, No. 1, pp. 183-9, ISSN 0149-5992.

[13] Bortolotti, A., Fedele, D., Chatenoud, L., Colli, E., Coscelli, C., Landoni, M., Lavezzari, M., Santeusanio, F., & Parazzini, F. (2001). Cigarette smoking: a risk factor for erectile dysfunction in diabetics. *European Urology*, Vol. 40, No. 4, pp. 392-6; discussion 397, ISSN 0302-2838.

[14] Boulton, A.J., Malik, R.A., Arezzo, J.C., & Sosenko, J.M. (2004). Diabetic somatic neuropathies. *Diabetes Care*, Vol. 27, No. 6, pp. 1458-86; ISSN 0149-5992.

[15] Brownlee, M., Cerami, A., & Vlassara, H. (1988). Advanced glycosylation end products in tissue and the biochemical basis of diabetic complications. *The New England Journal of Medicine*, Vol.318, No.20, pp. 1315-21, ISSN 0028-4793.

[16] Bucala, R., Tracey, K.J., & Cerami, A. (1991). Advanced glycosylation products quench nitric oxide and mediate defective endothelium-dependent vasodilatation in experimental diabetes. *The Journal of Clinical Investigation*, Vol. 87, No. 2, pp. 432-8, ISSN 0021-9738.

[17] Cárdenas-León, M., Díaz-Díaz, E., Argüelles-Medina, R., Sánchez-Canales, P., Díaz-Sánchez, V., & Larrea, F. (2009). Glycation and protein crosslinking in the diabetes and ageing pathogenesis. *Revista de Investigación Clínica*. Vol. 61, No. 6, pp. 505-520, (online), www.imbiomed.com.mx, ISSN 0034-8376.

[18] Carneiro, F.S., Giachini, F.R., Lima, V.V., Carneiro, Z.N., Leite, R., Inscho, E.W., Tostes, R.C., & Webb, R.C. (2008). Adenosine actions are preserved in corpus cavernosum from obese and type II diabetic db/db mouse. *The Journal of Sexual Medicine*, Vol. 5, No. 5, pp. 1156-66, ISSN 1743-6095.

[19] Cartledge, J.J., Eardley, I., & Morrison, J.F. (2001a). Nitric oxide-mediated corpus cavernosal smooth muscle relaxation is impaired in ageing and diabetes. *British Journal of Urology International*, Vol. 87, No. 4, pp. 394-401, ISSN 1464-4096.

[20] Cartledge, J.J., Eardley, I., & Morrison, J.F. (2001b). Advanced glycation end-products are responsible for the impairment of corpus cavernosal smooth muscle relaxation seen in diabetes. *British Journal of urology international*, Vol. 87, No. 4, pp. 402-7, ISSN 1464-4096.

[21] Cellek, S., Qu, W., Schmidt, A.M., & Moncada, S. (2004). Synergistic action of advanced glycation end products and endogenous nitric oxide leads to neuronal apoptosis in vitro: a new insight into selective nitrergic neuropathy in diabetes. *Diabetologia*, Vol. 47, No. 2, pp. 331-9, ISSN 0012-186X.

[22] Cellek, S., Rodrigo, J., Lobos, E., Fernandez, P., Serrano, J., & Moncada, S. (1999). Selective nitrergic neurodegeneration in diabetes mellitus - a nitric oxide-dependent phenomenon. *British Journal of Pharmacology*, Vol. 128, No. 8, pp. 1804-12, ISSN 0007-1188.

[23] Chai, S.J., Barrett-Connor, E., & Gamst, A. (2009) Small-vessel lower extremity arterial disease and erectile dysfunction: The Rancho Bernardo study. *Atherosclerosis*, Vol. 203, No. 2, pp. 620-5, ISSN 0021-9150.

[24] Chang, S., Hypolite, J.A., Changolkar, A., Wein, A.J., Chacko, S., & DiSanto, M.E. (2003). Increased contractility of diabetic rabbit corpora smooth muscle in response to endothelin is mediated via Rho-kinase beta. *International Journal of Impotence Research*, Vol. 15, No. 1, pp. 53-62, ISSN 0955-9930.

[25] Chen, D., Shan, Y.X., & Dai, Y.T. (2008). Advanced glycation end products and their receptors elevate the activity of endothelin-1 in rat cavernosum. *Zhonghua Nan Ke Xue*, Vol. 14, No. 2, pp. 110-5, ISSN 1009-3591.

[26] Chitaley, K. (2009). Type 1 and Type 2 diabetic-erectile dysfunction: same diagnosis (ICD-9), different disease?. *The Journal of Sexual Medicine*, Vol. 6, No. Supplement 3, pp. 262-8, ISSN 1743-6095.

[27] Chitaley, K., Kupelian, V., Subak, L., & Wessells, H. (2009). Diabetes, obesity and erectile dysfunction: field overview and research priorities. *The Journal of Urology*, Vol. 182, No. 6 Suppl, pp. S45-50, ISSN 0022-5347.

[28] Cirino, G., Fusco, F., Imbimbo, C., & Mirone, V. (2006). Pharmacology of erectile dysfunction in man. *Pharmacology & Therapeutics*, Vol. 111, No. 2, pp. 400-23, ISSN 0163-7258.

[29] Colakoglu, Z., Kutluay, E., Ertekin, C., Altay, B., Killi, R., & Alkis, A. (1999). Autonomic nerve involvement and venous leakage in diabetic men with impotence. *British Journal of Urology International*, Vol. 83, No. 4, pp. 453-6, ISSN 1464-4096.

[30] Costa, C., & Vendeira, P. (2007). The penis and endothelium. Extragenital aspects of erectile dysfunction. *Revista Internacional de Andrología*, Vol. 5, No. 1, pp. 50-8, ISSN 1698-031X.

[31] Costabile, R.A. (2003) Optimizing treatment for diabetes mellitus induced erectile dysfunction. *The Journal of Urology*, Vol. 170, No. 2 Pt 2, pp. S35-8; discussion S39, ISSN 0022-5347.

[32] Cox, J.D., Kim, N.N., Traish, A.M., & Christianson, D.W. (1999). Arginase-boronic acid complex highlights a physiological role in erectile function. *Nature Structural Biology*, Vol. 6, No. 11, pp. 1043-7, ISSN 1072-8368.

[33] De Angelis, L., Marfella, M.A., Siniscalchi, M., Marino, L., Nappo, F., Giugliano, F., De Lucia, D., & Giugliano, D. (2001). Erectile and endothelial dysfunction in Type II diabetes: a possible link. *Diabetologia*, Vol. 44, No. 9, pp. 1155-60, ISSN 0012-186X.

[34] Dhindsa, S., Prabhakar, S., Sethi, M., Bandyopadhyay, A., Chaudhuri, A., & Dandona, P. (2004). Frequent occurrence of hypogonadotropic hypogonadism in type 2 diabetes. *The Journal of Clinical Endocrinology and Metabolism*, Vol. 89, No. 11, pp. 5462-8, ISSN 0021-972X.

[35] Eardley, I. (2002). Pathophysiology of erectile dysfunction. *British Journal of Diabetes and Vascular Disease*, Vol. 2, No. 4, pp. 272-6, ISSN 1474-6514.

[36] Elías-Calles, L.C., & Licea M.E. (2003). Disfunción sexual eréctil y diabetes mellitus. Aspectos etiopatogénicos. *Revista Cubana de Endocrinología*, Vol. 14, No. 2, (online), http://bvs.sld.cu/revistas/end/vol14_2_03/end07203.htm, ISSN 1561-2953.

[37] England, J.D., & Asbury, A.K. (2004). Peripheral neuropathy. *The Lancet*, Vol. 363, No. 9427, pp. 2151-61, ISSN 0140-6736.

[38] Fabbri, A., Aversa, A., & Isidori, A. (1997). Erectile dysfunction: an overview. *Human Reproduction Update*, Vol. 3, No. 5, pp. 455-66, ISSN 1355-4786.

[39] Fedele, D., Bortolotti, A., Coscelli, C., Santeusanio, F., Chatenoud, L., Colli, E., Lavezzari, M., Landoni, M., & Parazzini, F. (2000). Erectile dysfunction in type 1 and type 2 diabetics in Italy. On behalf of Gruppo Italiano Studio Deficit Erettile nei Diabetici. *International Journal of Epidemiology*, Vol. 29, No. 3, pp. 524-31, ISSN 0300-5771.

[40] Fedele, D., Coscelli, C., Cucinotta, D., Forti, G., Santeusanio, F., Viaggi, S., Fiori, G., Velona, T., & Lavezzari, M. (2001). Incidence of erectile dysfunction in Italian men with diabetes. *The Journal of Urology*, Vol. 166, No. 4, pp. 1368-71, ISSN 0022-5347.

[41] Feldman, H.A., Goldstein, I., Hatzichristou, D.G., Krane, R.J., & McKinlay, J.B. (1994). Impotence and its medical and psychosocial correlates: results of the Massachusetts Male Aging Study. *The Journal of Urology*, Vol. 151, No. 1, pp. 54-61, ISSN 0022-5347.

[42] Ganz, M.B., & Seftel, A. (2000). Glucose-induced changes in protein kinase C and nitric oxide are prevented by vitamin E. *American Journal of Physiology - Endocrinology and Metabolism*, Vol. 278, No. 1, pp. E146-52, ISSN 0193-1849.

[43] Grossmann, M., Thomas, M.C., Panagiotopoulos, S., Sharpe, K., Macisaac, R.J., Clarke, S., Zajac, J.D., & Jerums, G. (2008). Low testosterone levels are common and

associated with insulin resistance in men with diabetes. *The Journal of Clinical Endocrinology and Metabolism*, Vol. 93, No. 5, pp. 1834-40, ISSB 0021-972X.

[44] Gur, S., Kadowitz, P.J. , & Hellstrom, W.J. (2009). A critical appraisal of erectile function in animal models of diabetes mellitus. *International Journal of Andrology*, Vol. 32, No. 2, pp. 93-114, ISSN 0105-6263.

[45] Hermans, M.P., Ahn, S.A., & Rousseau, M.F. (2009). Erectile dysfunction, microangiopathy and UKPDS risk in type 2 diabetes. *Diabetes & Metabolism*, Vol. 35, No. 6, pp. 484-9, ISSN 1262-3636.

[46] Hidalgo-Tamola, J., & Chitaley, K. (2009). Review type 2 diabetes mellitus and erectile dysfunction. *The Journal of Sexual Medicine*, Vol. 6, No. 4, pp. 916-26, ISSN 1743-6095.

[47] Jeremy, J.Y., Angelini, G.D., Khan, M., Mikhailidis, D.P., Morgan, R.J., Thompson, C.S., Bruckdorfer, K.R., & Naseem, K.M. (2000). Platelets, oxidant stress and erectile dysfunction: an hypothesis. *Cardiovascular Research*, Vol. 46, No. 1, pp. 50-4, ISSN 0008-6363.

[48] Jesmin, S., Sakuma, I., Salah-Eldin, A., Nonomura, K., Hattori, Y., & Kitabatake, A. (2003). Diminished penile expression of vascular endothelial growth factor and its receptors at the insulin-resistant stage of a type II diabetic rat model: a possible cause for erectile dysfunction in diabetes. *Journal of Molecular Endocrinology*, Vol. 31, No. 3, pp. 401-18, ISSN 0952-5041.

[49] Jiaan, D.B., Seftel, A.D., Fogarty, J., Hampel, N., Cruz, W., Pomerantz, J., Zuik, M., & Monnier, V.M. (1995). Age-related increase in an advanced glycation end product in penile tissue. *World Journal of Urology*, Vol. 13, No. 6, pp. 369-75, ISSN 0724-4983.

[50] Johannes, C.B., Araujo, A.B., Feldman, H.A., Derby, C.A., Kleinman, K.P., & McKinlay, J.B. (2000). Incidence of erectile dysfunction in men 40 to 69 years old: longitudinal results from the Massachusetts male aging study. *The Journal of Urology*, Vol. 163, No. 2, pp. 460-3, ISSN 0022-5347.

[51] Kadioglu, A., Memisoglu, K., Sazova, O., Erdogru, T., Karsidag, K., & Tellaloglu, S. (1994). The effects of diabetes on penile somato-afferent system. *Archivos Españoles de Urología*, Vol. 47, No. 1, pp. 100-3, ISSN 0004-0614.

[52] Kapoor, D., Aldred, H., Clark, S., Channer, K.S., & Jones, T.H. (2007). Clinical and biochemical assessment of hypogonadism in men with type 2 diabetes: correlations with bioavailable testosterone and visceral adiposity. *Diabetes Care*, Vol. 30, No. 4, pp. 911-7, ISSN 1935-5548.

[53] Kasiske, B.L., O'Donnell, M.P., & Keane, W.F. (1992). The Zucker rat model of obesity, insulin resistance, hyperlipidemia, and renal injury. *Hypertension*, Vol. 19, No. 1 Supplement, pp. I110-5, ISSN 0194-911X.

[54] Kawano, K., Hirashima, T., Mori, S., Saitoh, Y., Kurosumi, M., & Natori, T. (1992) Spontaneous long-term hyperglycemic rat with diabetic complications. Otsuka Long-Evans Tokushima Fatty (OLETF) strain. *Diabetes*, Vol. 41, No. 11, pp. 1422-8, ISSN 0012-1797.

[55] Khatana, S.A., Taveira, T.H., Miner, M.M., Eaton, C.B., & Wu, W.C. (2008). Does cardiovascular risk reduction alleviate erectile dysfunction in men with type II diabetes mellitus?. International Journal of Impotence Research, Vol. 20, No. 5, pp. 501-6, ISSN 0955-9930.

[56] Klein, R., Klein, B.E., Lee, K.E., Moss, S.E., & Cruickshanks, K.J. (1996). Prevalence of self-reported erectile dysfunction in people with long-term IDDM. Diabetes Care, Vol. 19, No. 2, pp. 135-41, ISSN 0149-5992.

[57] Kleinman, K.P., Feldman, H.A., Johannes, C.B., Derby, C.A., & McKinlay, J.B. (2000). A new surrogate variable for erectile dysfunction status in the Massachusetts male aging study. Journal of Clinical Epidemiology, Vol. 53, No. 1, pp. 71-8. ISSN 0895-4356.

[58] Kubin, M., Wagner, G., & Fugl-Meyer, A.R. (2003). Epidemiology of erectile dysfunction. *International Journal of Impotence Research*, Vol. 15, No. 1, pp. 63-71, ISSN 0955-9930.

[59] Kumar, V., Madhu, S.V., Singh, G., & Gambhir, J.K. (2010). Post-prandial hypertriglyceridemia in patients with type 2 diabetes mellitus with and without macrovascular disease. *The Journal of the Association of Physicians of India*, Vol. 58, p.p. 603-7, ISSN 0004-5772.

[60] Laumann, E.O., Paik, A., & Rosen, R.C. (1999). Sexual dysfunction in the United States: prevalence and predictors. *The Journal of the American Medical Association*, Vol. 281, No. 6, pp. 537-44, ISSN 0098-7484.

[61] Li, X.X., Qiu, X.F., Yu, W., Zhu, W.D., Chen, Y., & Dai, Y.T. (2011). Mechanisms of oxidative stress-induced damage and its protection in cavernous mitochondria of diabetic rats. *Beijing Da Xue Xue Bao*, Vol. 43, No. 2, p.p. 189-93, ISSN 1671-167X.

[62] Lundberg, P.O., Ertekin, C., Ghezzi, A., Swash, M., & Vodusek, D. (2001). Neurosexology. Guidelines for Neurologists: European Federation of Neurological Societies Task Force on Neurosexology. *European Journal of Neurology*, Vol. 8, No. Supplement 3, pp. 2-24, ISSN 1351-5101.

[63] Luttrell, I.P., Swee, M., Starcher, B., Parks, W.C., & Chitaley, K. (2008). Erectile dysfunction in the type II diabetic db/db mouse: impaired venoocclusion with altered cavernosal vasoreactivity and matrix. *American Journal of Physiology Heart and Circulatory Physiology*, Vol. 294, No. 5, pp. H2204-11, ISSN 0363-6135.

[64] Maas, R., Schwedhelm, E., Albsmeier, J., & Boger, R.H. (2002). The pathophysiology of erectile dysfunction related to endothelial dysfunction and mediators of vascular function. *Vascular Medicine*, Vol. 7, No. 3, pp. 213-25, ISSN 1358-863X.

[65] Martin-Morales, A., Sanchez-Cruz, J.J., Saenz de Tejada, I., Rodriguez-Vela, L., Jimenez-Cruz, J.F., & Burgos-Rodriguez, R. (2001). Prevalence and independent risk factors for erectile dysfunction in Spain: results of the Epidemiología de la Disfunción Eréctil Masculina Study. *The Journal of Urology*, Vol. 166, No. 2, pp. 569-74; discussion 574-5, ISSN 0022-5347.

[66] Mc Vary, K.Y., Podlasek, C.A., McKenna, K.E., & Wood, D. (2006). Intrinsic and extrinsic apoptotic pathways are employed in neuropathic and diabetic models of erectile dysfunction. *The Journal of Sexual Medicine*, Vol. 3, No. Supplement 1, pp. 45, ISSN 1743-6095.

[67] McCulloch, D.K., Campbell, I.W., Wu, FC., Prescott, R.J., & Clarke, B.F. (1980). The prevalence of diabetic impotence. *Diabetologia*, Vol. 18, No. 4, pp. 279-83, ISSN 0012-186X.

[68] McMurray, G., Casey, J.H. & Naylor, A.M. (2006). Animal models in urological disease and sexual dysfunction *British Journal of Pharmacology*, Vol. 147, No. Supplement 2, pp. S62-79, ISSN 0007-1188.

[69] Meena, B.L., Kochar, D.K., Agarwal, T.D., Choudhary, R., & Kochar, A. (2009). Association between erectile dysfunction and cardiovascular risk in individuals with type-2 diabetes without overt cardiovascular disease. *International Journal of Diabetes in Developing Countries*, Vol. 29, No. 4, pp. 150-4, ISSN 1998-3832.

[70] Metro, M.J. & Broderick, G.A. (1999). Diabetes and vascular impotence: does insulin dependence increase the relative severity?. *International Journal of Impotence Research*, Vol. 11, No. 2, pp. 87-9, ISSN 0955-9930.
[71] Miccoli, R., Giampietro, O., Tognarelli, M., Rossi, B., Giovannitti, G., & Navalesi, R. (1987). Prevalence and type of sexual dysfunctions in diabetic males: a standardized clinical approach. *Journal of Medicine*, Vol. 18, No. 5-6, pp. 305-21, ISSN 0025-7850.
[72] Mills, T.M., Chitaley, K., Lewis, R.W., & Webb, R.C. (2002). Nitric oxide inhibits RhoA/Rho-kinase signaling to cause penile erection. *European Journal of Pharmacology*, Vol. 439, No. 1-3, pp. 173-4, ISSN 0014-2999.
[73] Moore, C.R. & Wang, R. (2006). Pathophysiology and treatment of diabetic erectile dysfunction. *Asian Journal of Andrology*, Vol. 8, No. 6, pp. 675-84, ISSN 1008-682X.
[74] Morano, S. (2003). Pathophysiology of diabetic sexual dysfunction. *Journal of Endocrinology Investigation*, Vol. 26, No. Supplement 3, pp. 65-9, ISSN 0391-4097.
[75] Morley, J.E. (1986). Impotence. *The American Journal of Medicine*, Vol. 80, No. 5, pp. 897-905. ISSN 0002-9343.
[76] Musicki, B. & Burnett, A.L. (2006). eNOS function and dysfunction within the penis. *Experimental Biology and Medicine*, Vol. 231, No. 2, pp. 154-65, ISSN 1535-3702.
[77] National Institutes of Health (NIH) Consensus Conference. (1993). Impotence. NIH Consensus Development Panel on Impotence. *The Journal of the American Medical Association*, Vol. 270, No. 1, pp. 83-90, ISSN 0098-7484.
[78] Osuna, J.A., Gomez-Perez, R., Arata-Bellabarba, G., & Villaroel, V. (2006). Relationship between BMI, total testosterone, sex hormone-binding-globulin, leptin, insulin and insulin resistance in obese men. *Archives of Andrology*, Vol. 52, No. 5, pp. 355-61, ISSN 0148-5016.
[79] Pasquali, R., Macor, C., Vicennati, V., Novo, F., De lasio, R., Mesini, P., Boschi, S., Casimirri, F., & Vettor, R. (1997). Effects of acute hyperinsulinemia on testosterone serum concentrations in adult obese and normal-weight men. *Metabolism*, Vol. 46, No. 5, pp. 526-9, ISSN 0026-0495.
[80] Pitteloud, N., Hardin, M., Dwyer, A.A., Valassi, E., Yialamas, M., Elahi, D., & Hayes, F.J. (2005). Increasing insulin resistance is associated with a decrease in Leydig cell testosterone secretion in men. *The Journal of Clinical Endocrinology and Metabolism*, Vol. 90, No. 5, pp. 2636-41, ISSN 0021-972X.
[81] Rhoden, E.L., Ribeiro, E.P., Teloken, C., & Souto, C.A. (2005). Diabetes mellitus is associated with subnormal serum levels of free testosterone in men. *British Journal of Urology International*, Vol. 96, No. 6, pp. 867-70, ISSN 1464-4096.
[82] Ritchie, R. & Sullivan, M. (2010). Endothelins & erectile dysfunction. *Pharmacological Research*, Vol. 63, No. 6, pp. 496-501, ISSN 1096-1186.
[83] Romeo, J.H., Seftel, A.D., Madhun, Z.T., & Aron, D.C. (2000). Sexual function in men with diabetes type 2: association with glycemic control. *The Journal of Urology*, Vol. 163, No. 3, pp. 788-91, ISSN 0022-5347.
[84] Romero, J.C., Hernández, A., Licea, M.E., & Márquez, A. (1997). Evaluación electrofisiológica, vascular y hormonal en diabéticos tipo 1 con disfunción sexual eréctil. *Revista de la Asociación Latinoamericana de Diabetes*, Vol. 3, pp. 147-53, ISSN 0327-9154.
[85] Roth, A., Kalter-Leibovici, O., Kerbis, Y., Tenenbaum-Koren, E., Chen, J., Sobol, T., & Raz, I. (2003). Prevalence and risk factors for erectile dysfunction in men with

diabetes, hypertension, or both diseases: a community survey among 1,412 Israeli men. *Clinical Cardiology*, Vol. 26, No. 1, pp. 25-30, ISSN 0160-9289.

[86] Saenz de Tejada, I., Goldstein, I., Azadzoi, K., Krane, R.J., & Cohen, R.A. (1989). Impaired neurogenic and endothelium-mediated relaxation of penile smooth muscle from diabetic men with impotence. *The New England Journal of Medicine*, Vol. 320, No. 16, pp. 1025-30, ISSN 0028-4793.

[87] Saigal, C.S., Wessells, H., Pace, J., Schonlau, M., & Wilt, T.J. (2006). Predictors and prevalence of erectile dysfunction in a racially diverse population. *Archives of Internal Medicine*, Vol. 166, No. 2, pp. 207-12, ISSN 0003-9926.

[88] Seftel, A.D., Vaziri, N.D., Ni, Z., Razmjouei, K., Fogarty, J., Hampel, N., Polak, J., Wang, R.Z., Ferguson, K., Block, C., & Haas, C. (1997). Advanced glycation end products in human penis: elevation in diabetic tissue, site of deposition, and possible effect through iNOS or eNOS. *Urology*, Vol. 50, No. 6, pp. 1016-26, ISSN 0090-4295.

[89] Sharma, K., McCue, P. & Dunn, S.R. (2003). Diabetic kidney disease in the db/db mouse. *The American Journal of Physiology: Renal Physiology*, Vol. 284, No. 6, pp. F1138-44, ISSN 0363-6127.

[90] Singh, R., Barden, A., Mori, T., & Beilin, L. (2001). Advanced glycation end-products: a review. *Diabetologia*, Vol. 44, No. 2, pp. 129-46, ISSN 0012-186X.

[91] Soderberg, S., Olsson, T., Eliasson, M., Johnson, O., Brismar, K., Carlstrom, K., & Ahren, B. (2001). A strong association between biologically active testosterone and leptin in non-obese men and women is lost with increasing (central) adiposity. *International Journal of Obesity and Related Metabolic Disorders*, Vol. 25, No. 1, pp. 98-105, ISSN 0307-0565.

[92] Sullivan, M.E., Dashwood, M.R., Thompson, C.S., Muddle, J.R., Mikhailidis, D.P., & Morgan, R.J. (1997). Alterations in endothelin B receptor sites in cavernosal tissue of diabetic rabbits: potential relevance to the pathogenesis of erectile dysfunction. *The Journal of Urology*, Vol. 158, No. 5, pp. 1966-72, ISSN 0022-5347.

[93] Svartberg, J. (2007). Epidemiology: testosterone and the metabolic syndrome. *International Journal of Impotence Research*, Vol. 19, No. 2, pp. 124-8, ISSN 0955-9930.

[94] Thorve, V.S., Kshirsagar, A.D., Vyawahare, N.S., Joshi, V.S., Ingale, K.G., & Mohite, R.J. (2011). Diabetes-induced erectile dysfunction: epidemiology, pathophysiology and management. *Journal of diabetes and its complications*, Vol. 25, No. 2, pp. 129-36, ISSN 1056-8727.

[95] Tomar, R., Dhindsa, S., Chaudhuri, A., Mohanty, P., Garg, R., & Dandona, P. (2006). Contrasting testosterone concentrations in type 1 and type 2 diabetes. *Diabetes Care*, Vol. 29, No. 5, pp. 1120-2, ISSN 0149-5992.

[96] Traish, A.M., Guay, A., Feeley, R., & Saad, F. (2009). The dark side of testosterone deficiency: I. Metabolic syndrome and erectile dysfunction. *Journal of Andrology*, Vol. 30, No. 1, pp. 10-22, ISSN 1939-4640.

[97] Tripathy, D., Dhindsa, S., Garg, R., Khaishagi, A., Syed, T., & Dandona, P. (2003). Hypogonadotropic hypogonadism in erectile dysfunction associated with type 2 diabetes mellitus: a common defect?. *Metabolic Syndrome and Related Disorders*, Vol. 1, No. 1, pp. 75-80, ISSN 1557-8518.

[98] Usta, M.F., Bivalacqua, T.J., Koksal, I.T., Toptas, B., Surmen, S., & Hellstrom, W.J. (2004). The protective effect of aminoguanidine on erectile function in diabetic rats is not related to the timing of treatment. *British Journal of Urology International*, Vol. 94, No. 3, pp. 429-32, ISSN 1464-4096.

[99] Usta, M.F., Bivalacqua, T.J., Yang, D.Y., Ramanitharan, A., Sell, D.R., Viswanathan, A., Monnier, V.M., & Hellstrom, W.J. (2003). The protective effect of aminoguanidine on erectile function in streptozotocin diabetic rats. *The Journal of Urology*, Vol. 170, No. 4 Pt 1, pp. 1437-42, ISSN 0022-5347.

[100] Usta, M.F., Kendirci, M., Gur, S., Foxwell, N.A., Bivalacqua, T.J., Cellek, S., & Hellstrom, W.J. (2006). The breakdown of preformed advanced glycation end products reverses erectile dysfunction in streptozotocin-induced diabetic rats: preventive versus curative treatment. *The Journal of Sexual Medicine*, Vol. 3, No. 2, pp. 242-50; discussion 250-2, ISSN 1743-6095.

[101] Vernet, D., Cai, L., Garban, H., Babbitt, M.L., Murray, F.T., Rajfer, J., & Gonzalez-Cadavid, N.F. (1995). Reduction of penile nitric oxide synthase in diabetic BB/WORdp (type I) and BBZ/WORdp (type II) rats with erectile dysfunction. *Endocrinology*, Vol. 136, No. 12, pp. 5709-17, ISSN 0013-7227.

[102] Vignozzi, L., Corona, G., Petrone, L., Filippi, S., Morelli, A.M., Forti, G., & Maggi, M. (2005). Testosterone and sexual activity. *Journal of Endocrinological Investigation*, Vol. 28, No. supplement 3, pp. 39-44, ISSN 0391-4097.

[103] Vignozzi, L., Morelli, A., Filippi, S., Ambrosini, S., Mancina, R., Luconi, M., Mungai, S., Vannelli, G.B., Zhang, X.H., Forti, G., & Maggi, M. (2007). Testosterone regulates RhoA/Rho-kinase signaling in two distinct animal models of chemical diabetes. *The Journal of Sexual Medicine*, Vol. 4, No. 3, pp. 620-30; discussion 631-32. ISSN 1743-6095.

[104] Werner, M.E., Meredith, A.L., Aldrich, R.W., & Nelson, M.T. (2008). Hypercontractility and impaired sildenafil relaxations in the BKCa channel deletion model of erectile dysfunction. *American Journal of Physiology-Regulatory, Integratives and Comparative Physiology*, Vol. 295, No. 1, pp. R181-8, ISSN 0363-6119.

[105] Wingard, C., Fulton, D., & Husain, S. (2007). Altered penile vascular reactivity and erection in the Zucker obese-diabetic rat. *The Journal of Sexual Medicine*, Vol. 4, No. 2, pp. 348-62; discussion 362-3, ISSN 1743-6095.

[106] World Health Organization. (2000). Erectil Dysfunction. *Health Publication Ltd. Plymouth*. Oxford. United Kindom.

[107] Xie, D., Odronic, S.I., Wu, F., Pippen, A., Donatucci, C.F., & Annex, B.H. (2007). Mouse model of erectile dysfunction due to diet-induced diabetes mellitus. *Urology*, Vol. 70, No. 1, pp. 196-201, ISSN 1527-9995.

[108] Yassin, A.A. & Saad, F. (2008). Testosterone and erectile dysfunction. *Journal of Andrology*, Vol. 29, No. 6, pp. 593-604, ISSN 1939-4640.

[109] Yildirim, S., Ayan, S., Sarioglu, Y., Gultekin, Y., & Butuner, C. (1999). The effects of long-term oral administration of L-arginine on the erectile response of rabbits with alloxan-induced diabetes. *British Journal of Urology International*, Vol. 83, No. 6, pp. 679-85, ISSN 1464-4096.

6

Premature Ejaculation Re-Visited: Definition and Contemporary Management Approaches

Tariq F. Al-Shaiji
University Health Network, University of Toronto
Canada

1. Introduction

Interest in the definition and management of premature ejaculation (PE) has been increasing significantly among all healthcare professionals and its clinical perceptions continue to evolve in recent years. Accumulating evidence suggests that it is considered to be the most common male sexual disorder (Metz & Pryor, 2000). Obtaining a universally accepted definition for PE has been problematic. Nevertheless, all definitions to date have repeatedly included two basic components which are the inability to control or delay ejaculation, and the resultant distress to one or both partners. Based on these components, the currently accepted definitions have been reported by a number of authorities which are authority-based rather than evidence-based (Table 1). In addition, PE can be divided into primary, that begins when the patient becomes sexually active, and secondary, which by definition is acquired later in life (Godpodinoff, 1989). Further subdivisions include global PE presenting in all circumstances, versus situational PE which occurs only with certain partners and situations (Donatucci, 2006). Intravaginal ejaculatory latency time (IELT) refers to the time between vaginal penetration and ejaculation, usually measured with a stopwatch or simply estimated in retrospect (Payne & Sadovsky, 2007). There has been no widely accepted standard for 'normal' IELT. In 2005, Patrick et al. found on a large community-based population of men and their partners that the median IELT, recorded using a partner-held stopwatch, was 7.3 min for men without PE, whereas men with PE had a median IELT of 1.8 min (Patrick et al., 2005). A multinational population survey of IELT by Waldinger et al. showed that 90% of 110 men with self-reported lifelong PE had an IELT of less than 60 seconds (Waldinger et al., 2005). IELT of less than 2 minutes is generally accepted as defining PE (Waldinger et al, 1998). A small percentage of men will ejaculate even before penetration. Others have advocated not to define the disorder with a specific time duration and instead suggested that a diagnosis is made when the man ejaculates too early for female partner satisfaction in greater than one-half of encounters (Masters & Johnson, 1970).

World Health Organization (WHO), 1994 (Lue & Broderick, 2007):

Inability to delay ejaculation sufficiently to enjoy lovemaking manifests as either of the following: occurrence of ejaculation before or very soon after the beginning of intercourse (if a time limit is required: before or within 15 seconds of the beginning of intercourse);

occurrence of ejaculation in the absence of sufficient erection to make intercourse possible. The problem is not the result of prolonged absence from sexual activity.
American Psychiatric Association, the diagnostic and statistical manual of mental disorders-fourth edition (DSM-IV), 2000 (American Psychiatric Association, 2000): A. Persistent or recurrent ejaculation with minimal sexual stimulation before, on, or shortly after penetration and before the person wishes it. The clinician must take into account factors that affect duration of the excitement phase, such as age, novelty of the sexual partner or situation, and recent frequency of sexual activity. B. The disturbance causes marked distress or interpersonal difficulty. C. The premature ejaculation is not due exclusively to the direct effects of a substance (eg, withdrawal from opioids). Specify type: Lifelong vs acquired Specify type: Generalized vs situational
European Urology Association (EUA), 2001(Colpi et al., 2001): The inability to control ejaculation for a "sufficient" length of time before vaginal penetration. It does not involve any impairment of fertility, when intravaginal ejaculation occurs.
Second International Consultation on Sexual Dysfunctions (ICSD), 2003 (World Health Organization [WHO], 2004): Ejaculation with minimal stimulation and earlier than desired, before or soon after penetration, which causes bother or distress and over which the sufferer has little or no voluntary control.
American Urological Association (AUA), 2004 (Montague et al., 2004): Ejaculation that occurs sooner than desired, either before or shortly after penetration, causing distress to either one or both partners.
International Society for Sexual Medicine (ISSM), 2007 (International Society for Sexual Medicine [ISSM], 2007): A male sexual dysfunction characterized by ejaculation which always or nearly always occurs prior to or within about one minute of vaginal penetration, and the inability to delay ejaculation on all or nearly all vaginal penetrations, and negative personal consequences, such as distress, bother, frustration and/or the avoidance of sexual intimacy.

Table 1. Definitions of PE

2. Epidemiology

PE is considered as a culture-dependent symptom which is self-identified, self-reported, and self rated with respect to severity, a fact that has influenced the reported prevalence in the literature. Laumann et al. performed analysis of the National Health and Social Life Survey (NHSLS) which was a probability-based household survey in 1992 that included 1,410 men aged 18 to 59 years (Laumann et al., 1999b). The authors found that approximately 30% of surveyed men reported what they described as "climaxing too soon." Interestingly, the analysis showed that the likelihood of PE was not affected by age, marital status, or race/ethnicity. Similarly, analysis the Global Study of Sexual Attitudes and Behaviours (GSSAB), an international survey of various aspects of sex and relationships among adults aged 40-80 y, was carried out to estimate the prevalence and correlates of sexual problems in 13,618 men from 29 countries representing seven geographic regions (Laumann et al., 2005). The majority of the prevalence rates reported in these seven regions were very similar to the one reported by the NHSLS, with four of the seven regions reporting prevalence rates from 27.4 to 30.5%. One exception was the Middle East region, in which the rate was 12.4%, however lack of sampling standardization from country to country could have led to such a result. In a more recent data by Porst et al. (Porst et al., 2007), the PE Prevalence and Attitudes (PEPA) internet-based survey of 12,133 men aged 18–70 in Germany, Italy, and the United States reported a prevalence of 22.7%. PE prevalence as reported by female partners has also been examined. In a preliminary report of a survey undertaken on 129 women presenting to a community practice, 23.2% of women reported that their partner had PE (defined as ejaculating before she desired at least half of the time they had sex) (Rosenberg et al., 2006).

Some have argued that despite the relatively high reported prevalence rates of PE, men do not frequently offer it as a medical complaint, raising the distinct possibility that the problem may be more prevalent than currently estimated(Grenier & Byers, 1995; Spector & Carey, 1990). In addition, most physicians do not inquire about the condition which support the above argument (Payne & Sadovsky, 2007). Underreporting of PE can be attributable to a number of patient or physician related factors (Table 2).

Patient factors	Physician factors
• Embarrassment/Stigma • Loss of self-esteem • Belief that the condition is psychological • Belief that the condition is transient • Perception of no medical treatment exists • Lack of routine screening	• Lack of knowledge with the condition • Lack of comfort discussing sexual issues • Lack of expertise • Consideration of PE as quality of life (QoL) not medical issue • Low prioritization of the condition by the medical system • Time constraints • Lack of training/motivation • lack of effective treatment options

Table 2. Factors affecting PE reporting (McMahon, 2005; Moreira et al., 2005; Payne & Sadovsky, 2007; Shabsigh, 2006; Symonds et al., 2003)

3. Risk factors

PE by its nature is dependent on subjective description as reported by patients or their partners. The condition has significant heterogeneity with regards to classification and etiology. Several investigators have attempted to pin point specific risk factors or risk association pertaining to PE. Some of these factors show persistent association or co-existence whereas others show modest or conflicting one calling for further well designed studies to determine the impact of these factors on PE. Suggested risk factors for PE are shown in Table 3.

- Erectile dysfunction (ED) (Corona et al., 2004; Laumann et al., 1999b)
- Hypoactive sexual desire (Rowland et al., 2010)
- Low libido (Payne & Sadovsky, 2007)
- Youth (Carson & Gunn, 2006)
- Limited sexual experience (American Psychiatric Association, 2000)
- Low frequency of sexual intercourse (Grenier & Byers, 2001; Laumann et al., 2005)
- Longer period of sexual abstinence (Jannini & Lenzi, 2005)
- Poor overall health and/or a simultaneous urological condition (Carson & Gunn, 2006; Screponi et al., 2001)
- Type II diabetes mellitus, especially with poor metabolic control (El-Sakka, 2003)
- Emotional disturbances and stress (Laumann et al., 1994; Laumann et al., 1999b)
- Generalized clinical anxiety (Dunn et al., 1999)
- Anxiety over sexual encounters (Dunn et al., 1998)
- Familial/genetic predisposition (Waldinger et al., 1997)
- Previous traumatic sexual experiences (Laumann et al., 1999b)
    - Any same sex activity ever
    - Partner had an abortion ever
    - Sexually touched before puberty
    - Sexually harassed ever
- Ethnic group (hispanic/black > white) (Carson & Gunn, 2006; Laumann et al., 1999b)
- Low education status (Laumann et al., 2005)
- Financial problems (Nicolosi et al., 2004)
- Hidden female partner arousal difficulties (Levine, 1975)
- Substance abuse (Payne & Sadovsky, 2007)

Table 3. PE risk factors

4. Physiology of ejaculation and pathophysiology of PE

The normal male sexual response results from a complex integrated neurophysiologic pathway with four components: excitement, plateau, ejaculation and orgasm followed by resolution (McMahon & Samali, 1999). Normal antegrade ejaculation involves the processes of emission and expulsion of semen, which are coordinated by a network of afferent and efferent neural pathways (Coolen et al., 2004; Waldinger, 2002). Three distinct physiological phases of the ejaculatory process have been described including emission, ejaculation, and orgasm. During emission, the smooth muscles in the prostate, seminal vesicles, and vas deferens undergo rhythmic contractions that result in seminal fluid being deposited into the posterior urethra. At the same time, the bladder neck contracts to prevent retrograde flow of seminal fluid into the bladder (Bohlen et al., 2000). The ejaculation phase involves relaxation of the external urinary sphincter and pulsatile contractions of the bulbocavernosus and pelvic floor muscles. Ejaculatory inevitability occurs in response to distention of the posterior urethra. Orgasm, which is the centrally experienced conclusion of sexual excitation, may or may not follow the ejaculatory phase (Donatucci, 2006).

In case of PE, there appears to be a blunting of the normal curve of ejaculatory response, characterized by a steep excitement phase with a shortened plateau phase followed by ejaculation/orgasm and a rapid resolution phase (Payne & Sadovsky, 2007). Historically, attempts to explain the etiology of PE have included a diverse range of psychological and biological factors. Psychological factors include anxiety, an unpleasant introductory or early sexual experience, infrequent sexual intercourse, poor ejaculatory control techniques, and evolutionary as well as psychodynamic factors (Sadeghi-Nejad & Watson, 2008). On the other hand, biological factors include penile hypersensitivity, hyperexcitable ejaculatory reflex, hyperarousability, endocrinopathy, genetic predisposition, and 5 hydroxytryptamine (5-HT)-receptor dysfunction (Donatucci, 2006). Increasing interest is focused on neurobiological explanations, such as hyposensitivity of 5-hydroxytryptamine 2C (5-HT2c) receptors or hypersensitivity of 5-HT1a receptors (Diaz & Close, 2010). It has been suggested that the ejaculatory threshold for men with low 5-HT levels and/or 5-HT 2C receptor hyposensitivity may be genetically 'set' at a lower point, resulting in a more rapid ejaculation (Abdel-Hamid et al., 2009). On the contrary, men with a very high set point may experience delayed or absent ejaculation despite prolonged sexual stimulation and despite achieving a full erection (Abdel-Hamid et al., 2009). Injection of a selective serotonin reuptake inhibitor (SSRI) into rat hypothalamus has been shown to delay ejaculation, whereas administration of a selective serotonin receptor agonist has been shown to cause PE in the rat (Ahlenius et al., 1981). This idea is supported in humans by the successful use of SSRIs, which increase 5-HT levels, in patients with PE (Diaz & Close, 2010). It has been postulated that men with PE have a hyperexcitable ejaculatory reflex that prevents them from controlling ejaculation (Donatucci, 2006).

5. Evaluation

It is universally accepted that a validated instrument to diagnose PE does not exist as yet. In its absence, when men present with PE, a thorough sexual history is of paramount importance to the evaluation. In 2004, the American Urological Association (AUA) Guideline on the Pharmacologic Management of Premature Ejaculation recommends that the diagnosis of PE be based solely upon information gathered through the taking of a sexual history (Montague et al., 2004). Nevertheless, discussion about one's private sexual life is usually not easy for anybody and even more difficult for a person who feels stigmatized for having a sexual-related problem. This embarrassment, especially in case of a male patient interacting with a female healthcare provider, is likely to prevent an open and a frank discussion about sexual problems. The evaluation of the problem should be grounded in recognition that the patient is placing great trust in his physician to treat his problem with respect and sensitivity. A skilled interviewer can help the patient clearly describe his true concerns. This should be carried out in a manner that avoids invasion of privacy, embarrassment, stigmatizing, and guilt. Patients are usually relieved when the healthcare provider acts on subtle cues that give permission for the patient to discuss the issue. Active listening and a compassionate acceptance of the patient are key components to melt the ice and of allow the patient to discuss a sensitive issue such as PE. Including the partner in the discussion is often helpful, but this should be at the patient's discretion. If the patient does not offer it as a complaint, it is useful to perform the sexual history in the context of the review of symptoms, often during discussion of urinary tract symptoms or with the behavioural/relationship questions that are appropriate in the social history.

Four key factors need to be considered when making the diagnosis of PE, three of which are subjective, in essence that they are self-reported, and one factor is objective. The former include poor control over ejaculation, dissatisfaction with intercourse by the patient or partner, and perceived distress about the condition by the patient or partner. Indeed not all of these factors need to be present to identify PE (Diaz & Close, 2010). The latter is decreased IELT. IELT has been assessed by patient and partner recall, and by stopwatch evaluation. There appears to be considerable overlap in times between PE and non-PE groups, suggesting that, until better normative values are available, the diagnosis cannot be made on an individual's IELT alone. Waldinger suggested that in daily clinical practice, diagnosis PE is not difficult, and thus, evaluation with questionnaires or the use of a stopwatch is not required (Waldinger, 2007). Nevertheless, the importance of history taking cannot be overlooked and the above factors should be enquired about.

Establishing an accurate sexual and psychosocial history is critical in identifying the etiology of PE and establishing an effective treatment regimen. There are several key areas that should be addressed when taking the history of a patient with possible PE and these areas has summarized by the AUA Guideline on the Pharmacologic Management of PE (Table 4).

- Frequency and duration of PE
- Proportion of sexual attempts with PE
- Relationship to specific partners
- Frequency and nature of sexual activity
- Aggravating or alleviating factors
- Impact of PE on sexual activity
- Effect on relationships and QoL
- Relationship to drug use/abuse
- Other considerations
    - Lifelong vs. acquired
    - Situational vs. universal/global
    - Because of psychological or combined psychological/biological factors
    - Any links to ED?

AUA: American Urological Association; PE: premature ejaculation; QoL: quality of life; ED: erectile dysfunction.

Table 4. AUA Guideline: sexual history for PE (Montague et al., 2004)

Examples of direct questions that clinicians can ask initially to assist in the process of diagnosing PE have been suggested by Laumann et al. (Laumann et al., 2005):

1. How well are you enjoying your sex life?

2. Do you ejaculate too soon or earlier than desired? If so, can you estimate the amount of time before you ejaculate?
3. Do you feel you have control over the timing of your ejaculation?
4. Does ejaculating early bother/distress you and/ or your partner?

Since a full sexual history may be difficult to incorporate into the timeframe of a typical office visit, the development of brief screening tools to assist in diagnosis and minimize patient and provider embarrassment is warranted (Althof, 2006). Questionnaires in development include the 36-item Premature Ejaculation Questionnaire, the 10-item Index of Premature Ejaculation (IPE), the 10-item Chinese IPE, and the 2-part question used by Rowland et al. (Althof, 2004, 2006; Rowland et al., 2004).

A comprehensive urological and medical history is equally important in evaluating PE patients because of the established relationship between some medical conditions, such as diabetes and other neuropathies, with ejaculatory dysfunction (El-Sakka, 2003). A medical history should include thorough information regarding current medications that might influence sexual functioning (Perelman et al., 2004). Physical examination should include a complete general examination and a genital examination. The examiner should look for signs of underlying chronic disease, endocrine dysfunction, and neurological impairment. Infection in the urethra, prostate, or epididymis should also be ruled out. There is no laboratory test currently available to assist clinicians with the diagnosis of PE. In fact, Laboratory evaluation is rarely necessary in men with lifelong PE, unless there are complicating factors or concerning physical examination findings (Laumann et al., 2005). The physician should always bear in mind that a mixture of decreased libido and ejaculatory problems, or a mixture of ED and PE, is possible. Acquired PE, especially if secondary to ED, may need additional laboratory work, specifically focused on relevant risk factors such as vascular disease, obesity, diabetes, and depression (Palmer & Stuckey, 2008).

6. Treatment

The ultimate aim of PE treatment is to increase the overall sexual satisfaction and relationship satisfaction. The goal is to increase ejaculatory latency. It should be emphasized that PE is not a life-threatening condition and that the primary target outcome for PE treatment is patient and partner satisfaction. In general, treatment options include psychological, behavioral, and attempts to alter the sensory input or retard the ejaculatory reflex through pharmacologic means. It is important to review all available treatment options with the patient and preferably with his partner. The risks, benefits and success of each strategy should be delineated clearly. Each treatment modality can be used individually or in combination with others. Therapeutic options should suit both partners and be appropriate to their habit in planning and frequency of their sexual activities. Arranging follow-up at appropriate intervals to judge treatment efficacy and progress is needed.

6.1 Patient self-help measures

Some patients may attempt self-help measures before seeking medical attention. Self-help approaches are usually gained through personal experience, bibliotherapy (books), or online research. The effectiveness of such remedies is not known and rarely long-lasting. Some of the common measures include using distracting thoughts as well as engaging in short foreplay, gentle thrusting, interrupting thrusting and withdrawing for a few moments (Hartmann et al., 2005; Riley & Segraves, 2006). In other instance, young men with a short refractory period can often experience a second and more controlled ejaculation during a subsequent episode of lovemaking (McMahon, 2005). Some men masturbate before sexual intercourse to desensitize the penis and delay subsequent ejaculations. Other remedies include taking alcohol, using thick condoms or multiple condoms, and applying an over-the-counter purchased anaesthetic preparation to the penis (Riley & Segraves, 2006). Many of these tactics, although creative, curtail the pleasures of lovemaking and are unsuccessful for delaying ejaculatory latency (Althof, 2006).

6.2 Psychological treatment

PE exerts a significant psychological burden on men and their partners (Rowland et al., 2001). These men tend to have mental preoccupation with their condition, show general negative affect associated with sexual situations, more intense feelings of embarrassment/guilt, worry/tension and fear of failure (Hartmann et al., 2005). Psychosexual therapy is best used to help the patient cope with the stress and relationship problems that develop secondary to sexual dysfunction (Palmer & Stuckey, 2008). It promotes open discussion between sexual partners, education about the condition, and expression of physical and emotional concerns (Althof, 2006). Counselling may be useful in conjunction with other treatments if it is considered to be helpful in improving self-esteem, but is rarely effective in treating the cause of lifelong PE. It is more likely to be successful in patients with acquired PE, especially those with situational PE.

Cognitive strategies that are relevant to treatment include the man's increased attention to his somatic sensations so he might better monitor his level of physical arousal, and the use of sensate focus, which in turn permit enjoyment of physical sensations without necessarily generating sexual arousal (Carey, 1998). In another word, the treating physician should teach his PE patient to recognize the signs of increased sexual arousal and then teaching him how to keep his level of sexual excitement below the level of intensity that elicits the ejaculatory reflex. Preliminary studies indicate that this approach is superior to a waiting list control (de Carufel & Trudel, 2006). These techniques also deemphasize the focus on intercourse and orgasm within the sexual relationship and can help to decrease the man's performance anxiety, which, because it presumably operates through sympathetic pathways, may serve to prime the ejaculatory response prematurely (Rowland & Rose, 2008).

6.3 Behavioral techniques

Behavioural techniques were once the mainstay of treatment of PE. The cornerstones of behavioral treatment are the 'stop-start' manoeuvre and its modification, the 'squeeze technique'. Both methods are based on the theory that PE occurs because the man fails to pay sufficient attention to pre-orgasmic levels of sexual tension (Masters & Johnson, 1970; Semans, 1956). In addition, the procedures may act to attenuate stimulus–response connections by gradually exposing the patient to progressively more intense and more prolonged stimulation but maintaining the intensity and duration of the stimulus just below the threshold for triggering the response (Guthrie, 1952).

In 1956, Semans described one of the earliest behavioral interventions, namely the "stop -start technique" (Semans, 1956). This method involves the partner stimulating the man's penis until he has the sensation of almost climaxing, at which time stimulation is ceased until this feeling abates. This cycle is repeated until the ejaculation can be controlled voluntarily. Eventually, the length of time before each stop gets gradually longer. Once the couple feels comfortable with vaginal penetration, they may be instructed to engage in "quiet vagina," in which the female partner temporarily stops moving during intercourse when the man indicates that he is approaching ejaculation, resuming once he says that he has regained control (Payne & Sadovsky, 2007). A similar technique was proposed by sex therapists Masters and Johnson in 1970 (Masters & Johnson, 1970). Their technique differed from the previous in that the partner squeezes the frenulum of the penis after cessation of the stimulus, resulting in a partial loss of erection. The female partner resumes sexual stimulation after at least 30 seconds have passed. However, many practitioners and patients report that this technique is unpractical.

Unfortunately most men do not show any lasting improvement using either of these techniques (De Amicis et al., 1985). Hawton et al. reported that 75% of men with PE who initially responded to behavioral therapy showed no long lasting improvement after 3 years of follow-up (Hawton et al., 1986). The ICSD noted that psychological and/or behavioral therapies, have been at least moderately successful in alleviating PE for some men (Sharlip, 2006). Based on their Guidelines, these approaches have no adverse effects, are specific to the problem, and encourage open communication between men and their partners. However, they lack immediacy and can require a substantial investment of time and money. Generally, the best results have been seen in men who are motivated, are hopeful, and are in a stable monogamous relationship with a cooperative partner (Althof, 2005). The popularity of these practices is declining because of their lack of reproducible success and their intrusiveness in normal sexual activity.

Other behavioral measures that have been described including encouraging couples to carry out attempts with the partner superior or lateral positions, as these typically provide men with a greater sense of ejaculatory control (Rowland & Rose, 2008). Other suggestions include moving the pelvis in a circular motion, slowing down during intercourse, breathing deeply, and practicing shallower penile penetration (Rowland & Cooper, 2005).

6.4 Pharmacologic interventions

6.4.1 Locally acting topical therapy

The oldest form of therapy for PE is the use of local anesthetic agents as described by Schapiro in 1943 (Schapiro, 1943). Topical anesthetics are available in cream, ointment, spray formulations and the rational for their application is based on the theory that men with PE are hypersensitive to penile stimulation. Some of these formulations have been shown to improve IELT compared with baseline (Busato & Galindo, 2004; Dinsmore et al., 2007). The advantages of topical therapies are that they can be applied as needed and systemic side effects are likely to be minimal. However, there are several drawbacks that make them a less than ideal therapeutic option. They are associated with inconvenience of use, messiness and interference with spontaneity (as the agents have to be applied and wiped off at specific times before sexual contact). Like all topical medications, there is always a risk of local burning, irritation, or allergic reaction. Significant penile hypoesthesia may occur which in turn can lead to excessive loss of pleasurable sensation and in some instances prevent the patient from achieving an orgasm (McMahon & Samali, 1999). Some reports indicated that the use of local anesthetics can induce mild erectile dysfunction and lowering of sexual arousal (Slob et al., 2000). One of the most feared drawbacks is the potential for transvaginal absorption of the agents used, which could induce vaginal numbness and even female anorgasmia (Morales et al., 2007). However, this can be prevented with condom use. As a general rule, reliable controlled studies have been lacking in this area.

6.4.2 Lidocaine–prilocaine cream

The eutectic mixture of local anesthetic (EMLA™; AstraZeneca, London, UK) is a local anesthetic cream that contains 2.5% of both lidocaine and prilocaine for topical application. This mixture has a 16°C melting point and thus can be formulated into preparations without the use of a non-aqueous solvent (Gurkan et al., 2008). The cream is applied thinly to the glans penis and distal shaft and covered by a condom for 20-30 minutes. If the condom is removed for intercourse, residual cream should be washed off. The high water content of this mixture enables it to penetrate the intact skin of the penis (Atikeleret al., 2002). The AUA 2004 guideline document described the lidocaine–prilocaine cream to be effective in treating PE when applied 20–30 min before intercourse (Montague et al., 2004). Nevertheless, trials using this topically in men with PE are scant. Busato and Galindo performed a double-blind, randomized, placebo-controlled study to determine the efficacy of EMLA cream in treating PE (Busato & Galindo, 2004). The study included 42 men divided in two groups; group A used a lidocaine-prilocaine solution and group B used an inert cream. There was a significant increase in the mean IELT, from 1.49 to 8.45 min ($P < 0.001$) in group A but not in group B following 2 months use. Although 42 patients were initially recruited, only 29 completed the study; however, none of the drop-outs were due to adverse effects. Adverse events were reported in five (17%) patients in the treatment group. In another study, Atikeler et al. randomized 40 patients into four groups, each comprising 10 patients to assess the efficacy and optimum usage of EMLA cream in managing PE (Atikeler et al., 2002). Patients in group 1 applied lidocaine-prilocaine cream 5% for 20 min, the patients in group 2 applied it for 30 min, and the patients in group 3 applied the cream for 45 min before sexual contact, with all patients covering the penis with a condom. Patients in the fourth group applied a base cream to act as placebo. In the placebo group, there was no change in their pre-ejaculation period. In group 1, the pre-ejaculation period increased to 6.71 +/- 2.54 min without any adverse effects. In group 2, the pre-ejaculation period increased in four patients up to 8.70 +/- 1.70 min, however six patients in this group and all patients in group 3 had erection loss because of numbness.

6.4.3 Lidocaine–prilocaine spray (PSD502)

Topical eutectic mixture for premature ejaculation (TEMPE Plethora Solutions PLC, London, UK) is a formulation of lignocaine and prilocaine in a metered dose aerosol-delivery system. Each spray delivers 7.5 mg of lidocaine and 2.5 mg of prilocaine. It is designed to optimize tissue penetration such that the onset of effect is more rapid than with the cream formulations and a condom is not required (Gurkan et al., 2008). The spray does not penetrate keratinized epithelium, and so only anesthetizes the glans; however there still appears to be some risk of hypoesthesia associated with its use (Dinsmore et al., 2007). It has an oily texture that enhances adherence to the penile surface and is easily washed off with water (Henry et al., 2008). TEMPE has been examined in a pilot study (N = 14) , a placebo-controlled phase II study (N = 55) (48), and in two large, placebo-controlled phase III trials, all of which have shown statistically and clinically significant prolongation of IELT compared with placebo (Carson & Wyllie, 2010; Dinsmore et al., 2007; Dinsmore & Wyllie, 2009; Henry & Morales, 2003).

6.4.4 Lignocaine spray

The active ingredient within this spray is the local anesthetic lignocaine (9.6%). It is marketed as Stud 100 or Premjact and applied to the glans penis in 3-6 sprays, 5-15 minutes before sexual intercourse. In theory, this agent works in the same way as other topical anesthetic agents. Although it has been available for more than 25 years and can often be bought over the counter without a prescription, there has been a paucity of data from clinical trials to support its use in the management of PE.

6.4.5 Dyclonine/alprostadil cream

A preparation which combines dyclonine, a local anesthetic usually used in the field of dentistry, with the vasodilator alprostadil has been described in the management of PE by one pilot study published as an abstract (Gittleman et al., 2005). The cream is applied to the tip of the penis in the region of the meatus 5–20 min before intercourse. The study claims some positive results, however the data is limited and further studies are needed before any conclusion can be drawn.

6.4.6 Severance-secret (SS) cream

SS-cream (Cheil Jedan Corporation, Seoul, Korea), developed at the Yong-Dong Severance Hospital in Korea, is made with extracts from nine herbal products including Korean ginseng, bufonoid venom and cinnamon. Some of these products have local anaesthetic as well as vasoactive properties (Morales et al., 2007). It is thought to also act through desensitization , although its exact mechanism is unclear. The cream is applied topically to the glans penis 1 hour prior to intercourse and washed off immediately before coitus begins. It is marked with its unpleasant smell and colour, which makes it unacceptable to many patients. It is available for use only in Korea in which all studies conducted on its efficacy were published there by the same group. Within these clinical trials, SS cream resulted in significant increases in IELT and satisfaction with sexual intercourse in comparison with placebo (Choi et al., 1999, 2000). Because of its unpleasant odour, the original SS-cream was unlikely to be of interest outside of South Korea (Powell & Wyllie, 2009). To compensate for the unpleasant smell and color, a reformulation was designed by the producers that contain only couple of the main ingredients present in the original cream. However, only animal data is available for this new formulation that claims higher efficacy than the original formulation (Tian et al., 2004).

6.5 Systemic therapy

6.5.1 Phosphodiesterase Type 5 (PDE5) Inhibitors

It has been estimated that at least 30% of PE men have concomitant ED (Laumann et al.,1999a). Whether the man with ED ejaculates early during intercourse before his erection fails, or whether the man with PE develops secondary ED due to anxiety regarding his PE is unknown. An alternative view held by other investigators suggests that PE and ED share a vicious circle, in which the level of excitation is instinctively reduced by a man with PE trying to control his ejaculation (thus leading to ED), and on the other hand, a man suffering from ED will try to increase his excitation to achieve an erection, thus leading to a rapid ejaculation (Jannini et al., 2005). Whatever the cause of PE co-existing with ED, the ssuccessful use of PDE-5 inhibitors in this subgroup of patients has raised the question of whether PDE-5 inhibitors can be efficacious in the treatment of primary PE. It has been proposed that the use of a PDE5 inhibitor may increase the level of nitric oxide centrally (reducing sympathetic drive) and peripherally (leading to smooth muscle dilatation of the vas deferens and seminal vesicles, opposing sympathetic vasoconstriction), thus leading to prolongation of IELT in men with PE (Palmer & Stuckey, 2008). Despite this theory, it is deemed unlikely that PDE-5 inhibitors have a significant role in the treatment of primary PE. This argument is supported by McMahon et al. who reviewed all reports on the use PDE-5 inhibitors for PE that were published between 2001 and 2006 (McMahon et al., 2006). The authors analysed 14 studies that reported on sildenafil, vardenafil and tadalafil. They concluded that PDE-5 inhibitors were not effective in the management of men with lifelong PE and normal erectile function. However, Sadeghi-Nejad and Watson suggested that PDE-5 inhibitors may exert a secondary beneficial effect for patients with PE since they (i) allow for a sustained penile erection, even after ejaculation; (ii) facilitate a second coitus after the initial ejaculation, which is likely to be less prone to PE; and/or (iii) help the patient to overcome performance anxiety, that often exacerbates PE (Sadeghi-Nejad & Watson, 2008).

6.5.2 α1-adrenoceptor antagonist

Ejaculation is peripherally controlled by the sympathetic nervous system, and therefore blocking the sympathetic system by α1-blockers may theoretically delay ejaculation. This hypothesis has been supported by a rat model demonstrating a decreased vasal and seminal vesicle pressure in response to hypogastric nerve stimulation (S.W. Kim et al., 2004). Clinically, terazosin and alfuzosin have been investigated in men with PE. Cavallini showed that both terazosin 5 mg/d and alfuzosin 6 mg/d proved effective in approximately 50% of the cases in a placebo-controlled study in 91 men with PE (Cavallini, 1995). Similarly but more recently, Basar et al. demonstrated that daily use of terazosin 5 to 10 mg showed a clinically significant improvement during a short-term follow up in another placebo-controlled study in 90 men with PE and urinary tract symptoms without chronic prostatitis and benign prostatic hyperplasia (Basar et al., 2005). It should be pointed out that the methodology of both studies has been rather weak making their validity under question and calling for additional well-designed controlled studies. Despite these limitations, α-blockers use in the PE patient with concomitant lower urinary track symptoms may be of benefit (Basar et al., 2005).

6.5.3 Tramadol

Tramadol is a centrally acting synthetic on-demand analgesic that has been on the market for a number of years. It has two distinct mechanisms of action: it exerts an effect on the ∝–opioid receptor, but also inhibits noradrenaline and serotonin reuptake (Frink et al., 1996). It is available in generic form in most countries and has been used in an on-demand fashion (off-label and empirically) to treat PE. The exact mechanism by which it delays ejaculation is not well understood, however it is thought to be related to its action on the ∝–opioid receptor, which may reduce sensitivity, in addition to the inhibition of serotonin reuptake, which may delay ejaculation (Linton & Wylie, 2010). It has a short half-life and acceptable safety profile. Since its is rapidly absorbed and eliminated, it makes it desirable for an as needed dosing regimen (Eradiri et al., 2006).

Salem et al. conducted a single-blind, placebo-controlled, crossover, stopwatch monitored two-period study on 60 patients with lifelong PE utilizing 25 mg of tramadol (Salem et al., 2008). The treatment group experienced a 6.3 fold increase in IELT compared to a 1.7 fold increase in the placebo group. Patients uniformly reported satisfaction with their resulting control over ejaculation. Mild side effects were reported in eight patients (13.3%), consisting of mild dyspepsia and somnolence. In another study, Safarinejad and Hosseini performed a double-blind, placebo-controlled, fixed-dose, randomized study to evaluate the efficacy and safety of tramadol (Safarinejad & Hosseini, 2006). They randomly assigned 64 potent men with PE to receive 50 mg tramadol or placebo and showed an increase in IELT from 19 seconds to over 4 minutes in the tramadol arm. The most common adverse events were nausea (15.6%), vomiting (6.2%), and dizziness (6.2%), but they were reported to be mild. A large phase III trials is in progress in Europe and other trials are anticipated (Hellstrom, 2011). Although tramadol is reported to have a decreased risk of dependence compared to traditional opioids, its use as an on-demand treatment for PE is still limited by the potential risk of addiction (Cossmann et al.,1997). In community settings, dependence does occur, albeit minimal (McDiarmid et al., 2005).

6.5.4 Clomipramine

Clomipramine is a tricyclic antidepressant used in the treatment of obsessive compulsive disorders. It inhibits the reuptake of noradrenaline and 5-HT by adrenergic and 5-HT neurones (Gur et al., 1999). In 1973, Eaton published his novel report on the efficacy of clomipramine to manage PE marking the beginning of a new era in the approach to treating this condition and several subsequent publications have confirmed its effectiveness (Eaton, 1973). It has been studied both as a daily dose and as an on-demand medication.

On-demand use of 20 to 40 mg clomipramine can effectively delay ejaculation if taken 3 to 5 hours prior to intercourse (Haensel et al., 1996; Segraves et al., 1993). Waldinger et al. showed a 4-fold increase in the IELT with on demand 25 mg of clomipramine (Waldinger et al., 2004a). The on demand dosing appears to be associated with high incidence of side effects with nausea being the most common, which is experienced on the day of sexual intercourse and the day after (Waldinger et al., 2004a). Rowland et al. indicated that patients with initial ejaculatory latencies over 60 seconds, self-reported sexual satisfaction of 5 or higher (on a seven-point scale) and ejaculation frequency of twice or more per week were more likely to benefit from on-demand 25 mg clomipramine therapy (Rowland et al., 2004). In the 1970s to the 1990s, various studies demonstrated clomipramine efficacy in delaying ejaculation in daily rather low dosages of 10 to 30 mg (Assalian, 1988). For instance, in a randomized, placebo-controlled crossover trial in 36 men with PE, Kim an Seo were able to show that continuous dosing with clomipramine significantly lengthened the IELT compared with placebo ($P < 0.01$), as measured by stopwatch assessment (S. C. Kim & Seo, 1998). In addition, a meta-analysis evaluating the systemic treatments for PE by Waldinger et al found clomipramine to be efficacious, particularly continuous dosing (Waldinger et al., 2004b). The results also showed it to be comparable to the commonly used selective serotonin re-uptake inhibitors (SSRIs) in its effects. Small studies showed that after daily treatment with clomipramine, men with PE reported improved relationship and emotional satisfaction, men and their partners reported increased sexual satisfaction, and the partners reported an increased ability to achieve coital orgasm (Althof et al., 1995). Rowland et al. examined the role of daily treatment with clomipramine in 4 men with PE when the as required regimen was ineffective (Rowland et al., 2001). They recommended a two-tiered approach, initially using a single dose of up to 25 mg, taken from 4 to 24 hours prior to intercourse. If on-demand treatment proved unsatisfactory, a daily, long-term dose of 10–30 mg was instated. The study concluded that men with PE who do not respond to clomipramine 'as required' are probably not insensitive to pharmacological treatment, but may simply require higher doses or a different regimen. All four subjects improved when taking daily clomipramine at varying doses.

Use of clomipramine in men with PE might be limited by its associated adverse events. Common side effects include dry mouth, fatigue, nausea, and dizziness (Haensel et al., 1996). Although these side effects may abate over time, stopping the medication is also associated with a loss of efficacy (Althof et al., 1995). The study by Kim and Seo showed that on continuous dosing, the adverse event profile of clomipramine was found to be significantly worse than with SSRI treatment (S. C. Kim & Seo, 1998). Furthermore, Waldinger et al. reported that the use of an on-demand regimen to reduce exposure to clomipramine did not eliminate potentially annoying nonsexual side-effects, including sleepiness, yawning and nausea, which were significantly worse on the day of dosing and the subsequent day with clomipramine than with SSRI therapy (Waldinger et al., 2004a). Other possible side effects involved with the usage of clomipramine include an increased risk of suicide, especially when initiated in men under the age of 24 (U S Food and Drug Administration [FDA], 2007) and an adverse effect on sperm function when used at higher doses (75 mg for more than 3 months) (Maier & Koinig, 1994). It may impede both sperm motility and vasal/epididymal contractility by blocking calcium channel mechanisms (Mousavizadeh et al., 2002). This potential consequence of long-term, high dose usage should be kept in mind when choosing PE therapy for men who may be contemplating fatherhood in the future (Sadeghi-Nejad & Watson, 2008).

6.5.5 Selective serotonin reuptake inhibitors

Although none of the selective serotonin reuptake inhibitors (SSRIs) are approved by regulatory bodies for the management of PE, their common "side effect" of delaying ejaculation in 30%–50% of otherwise healthy depressed patients has made them the preferred "off-label" treatment option for PE (Balon, 2006). Indicated primarily in the treatment of depression, SSRIs can increase the level of serotonin in the brain, inhibiting the ejaculatory reflex centre, and can prolong IELT for several minutes (Hellstrom, 2006). The extent of this delay varies widely depending upon the type, dose, and frequency of SSRI administration and the genetically determined ejaculatory threshold set point (Sadeghi-Nejad & Watson, 2008). The effect of this class of medication is not restricted to PE patients since its use by otherwise healthy subjects can also significantly delay ejaculation (Wang et al., 2007). Dosing levels of SSRIs are generally lower for PE than for depression, and various dosing regimens have been tested (including continuous, daily or situational). Indeed, this is the most common class of medications used to treat PE nowadays.

Currently four SSRIs are commonly in use in the treatment of PE including fluoxetine, paroxetine, sertraline and citalopram. Paroxetine has been found to have substantially greater efficacy, increasing IELT approximately 8.8-fold above the baseline, followed by sertraline and fluoxetine (Waldinger et al., 2003, 2004). Among the SSRIs, fluvoxamine and venlafaxine have been shown to be ineffective (Kilic et al., 2005; Waldinger et al., 2002). Daily treatment with paroxetine 10–40 mg, sertraline 50–200 mg, fluoxetine 20–40 mg, and citalopram 20–40 mg is usually effective in delaying ejaculation (Rowland et al., 2010). The desired ejaculation delay usually occurs within 5–10 days of starting treatment, however the full therapeutic effect may require 2–3 weeks of treatment and is usually sustained during long-term use (McMahon, 2002). The first publication about the delaying effect of paroxetine was published in 1994 and since then multiple placebo-controlled randomized studies have confirmed the effectiveness of each of the aforementioned SSRIs in treating PE (Biri et al., 1998; Gurkan et al., 2008; Kara et al., 1996; S. C. Kim & Seo, 1998; Waldinger et al., 1998). The argument for daily dosing comes from the fact that the pharmacokinetic profile of conventional antidepressants should be optimized for the treatment of depression which requires their continuous presence in the bloodstream to achieve the maximum effect (Althof, 2006b). Side effects are usually minor, starting in the first week after intake and gradually disappearing within 2–3 weeks of starting the course of treatment which include fatigue, yawning, mild nausea, loose stools and perspiration (McMahon, 2005). Diminished libido and mild erectile dysfunction are reported infrequently (Waldinger, 2007), especially in the absence of concomitant depression (Montejo et al., 2001). Rare side effects that have been reported include bleeding (Halperin & Reber, 2007), weight gain related type II diabetes mellitus (Raeder et al., 2006), bone mineral density loss with prolonged treatment (Haney et al., 2007), and priapism (Dent et al., 2002), however, these events were reported in patients suffering from depression. The use of SSRIs, especially in young depressed patients, is reported to increase impulsive actions and suicide Rate (Cohen, 2007). There is also the potential for the development of a serious drug interaction that can lead to 'serotoninergic syndrome' which manifests as headache, nausea, sweating and dizziness in mild cases, and in hyperthermia, rigidity and delirium in severe cases (Sharlip, 2006). Symptoms can occur following abrupt cessation or reduction of SSRI therapy beginbeginning from 24 to 72 hours after discontinuance and may last more than a week (Linton & Wylie, 2010). This is thought to be more prevalent with the SSRIs that have shorter half lives (Hellstrom, 2009). Based on this, it is generally recommended that SSRIs should not be stopped suddenly but reduced over several weeks (Sadeghi-Nejad & Watson, 2008). Several physicians may consider the reported side effects hard to 'justify' for the treatment of PE, in which the primary outcome is patient satisfaction. However, the AUA has suggested that the level of side effects is acceptable for the benefit derived in the patient with PE, and the type and rate of occurrence of these effects also appears to be acceptable to most patients (Montague et al., 2004).

The side effect profile of the SSRIs taken on a chronic daily basis has led to the suggestion that an "on demand" SSRI may be useful for PE. This is supported by the fact that men may be reluctant to receive an antidepressant to treat a condition other than depression and use it chronically, having known that sexual activity does not generally occur on a daily basis (Althof, 2006b). On-demand administration of paroxetine, sertraline, and fluoxetine 4–6 hours before intercourse is modestly efficacious and well tolerated but is associated with substantially less ejaculatory delay than daily treatment (S. W. Kim & Paick, 1999; McMahon & Touma, 1999; M. D. Waldinger et al., 2004a). McMahon and Touma performed a comparison of 20 mg paroxetine PRN 3 to 4 hours prior to intercourse vs 20 mg paroxetine daily for 4 weeks, followed by PRN paroxetine in those who responded to daily paroxetine (McMahon & Touma, 1999). The authors showed that the schedule of daily dosing followed by PRN dosing was significantly superior to the PRN only schedule. However, sexual side effects were observed in the daily paroxetine group and the initial benefits that they experienced were not sustained with time in men with primary PE (11 of 16 failures). In the PRN only group 15 of 19 men with primary PE failed to respond. Publications focusing on on-demand use of SSRIs for PE continue to be limited and the data available is difficult to compare as it is heterogeneous in terms of medications used, study design and outcome reporting. Paroxetine appears to be the most effective medication again (Gurkan et al., 2008).

Dapoxetine is the first compound specifically developed for the treatment of PE. It is a novel fast-acting SSRI that exerts its effects through the inhibition of the serotonin reuptake transporter (Hellstrom, 2009). Because of its short acting property, it probably better suited as an "on-demand" treatment for PE. In fact, it has received regulatory approval as an on-demand treatment for PE in several parts of the world (McMahon et al., 2010). In contrast to conventional SSRIs, maximum plasma concentrations are achieved 1.01 h after a 30-mg oral dose, initial half-life is 1.42 h and 24 h after administration, plasma concentrations decrease to less than 5% of peak levels (Dresser et al., 2006). Pryor et al. published an integrated analysis of two double-blind, randomised controlled trials to determine the efficacy and tolerability of dapoxetine in the treatment of PE (Pryor et al., 2006). Men with moderate-to-severe premature ejaculation took placebo (n=870), 30 mg dapoxetine (874), or 60 mg dapoxetine (870) on-demand (as needed, 1-3 h before anticipated sexual activity). The primary endpoint was IELT measured by stopwatch. At the completion of the study, 672, 676, and 610 patients completed in the placebo, 30 mg dapoxetine, and 60 mg dapoxetine groups, respectively. Dapoxetine significantly prolonged IELT ($p<0.0001$, all doses vs placebo). Mean IELT at baseline was 0.90 minute, 0.92 minute, and 0.91 minute, and at study endpoint (week 12 or final visit) was 1.75 (2.21) minutes for placebo, 2.78 (3.48) minutes for 30 mg dapoxetine, and 3.32 (3.68) minutes for 60 mg dapoxetine. Both dapoxetine doses were effective on the first dose. Common adverse events (30 mg and 60 mg dapoxetine, respectively) were nausea (8.7%, 20.1%), diarrhoea (3.9%, 6.8%), headache (5.9%, 6.8%), and dizziness (3.0%, 6.2%). More recently, Buvat et al. published results from phase III trial from 22 countries, evaluating dapoxetine 30 mg and 60 mg versus placebo (Buvat et al., 2009). The trial showed that IELT was significantly increased with dapoxetine. At the end of 24 weeks the IELT had increased from 0.9 minutes to 1.9 minutes, 3.1 minutes, 3.5 minutes with placebo, dapoxetine 30 mg and 60 mg. All patients reported outcome measures were significantly improved with dapoxetine versus placebo. The drug was submitted for FDA approval in 2004, however in October 2005, the company developing the drug received a "not approvable" letter from the FDA ("Dapoxetine: LY 210448," 2005; Press release, 2005).The questions raised by the FDA letter were not disclosed, however dapoxetine's developer mentioned that it plans to address the questions and continue the drug's global development program (Press release, 2005).

6.6 Combination therapy

While the choice of PE treatment is essentially between behavioural and pharmacological approaches, physicians should recognize that combination treatment is an option, especially for patients with severe PE or those refractory to mono-therapy. In a study by Atan et al., oral fluoxetine 20 mg/day, when reinforced by the topical application of lidocaine ointment, showed a "cure" or an improvement in 83.3% of men with PE, compared with 72% of those treated with fluoxetine alone (given as 20 mg/day then increased to 40 mg/day) (Atan et al., 2000). Chen et al. examined the efficacy of sildenafil as adjuvant therapy to paroxetine in alleviating PE (Chen et al., 2003). They found that sildenafil combined with paroxetine was effective in 97% of patients, compared to an improvement for only 47% using paroxetine alone. In addition, the best results obtained in this study were observed when sildenafil was combined with SSRIs as well as implementing behavioral counseling. In another study, Salonia et al. have shown in a prospective open-label study that paroxetine combined with sildenafil provided significantly better results in terms of ejaculatory latency time and intercourse satisfaction versus paroxetine alone in potent patients with PE, albeit with a mild increase in drug related side effects (Salonia et al., 2002). Perelman and Althof independently described combination therapy as a "concurrent or stepwise integration of psychological and medical interventions"(Althof, 2006a; Perelman, 2006). Patients with severe PE need more than pharmacotherapy to overcome obstacles to effective sexual activity and require targeted psychoeducational interventions termed "coaching" (S. Althof, 2006a). Steggall et al. speculated that a combination approach may offer both an improvement in ejaculatory delay, but also facilitate engagement with behavioural therapies (Steggall et al., 2008). In a small-scale study, the authors randomised participants with PE either to paroxetine 20 mg daily or to a lidocaine-based spray (Premjact) for 2 months followed immediately by a standardized behavioral therapy programme for a further 2 months. Of the 60 men who consented to participate in this trial, 44 completed the pharmacologic phase and 22 completed both phases of the program. It was found that both paroxetine and premjact Spray provided a statistically significant delay in ejaculation (as measured by stopwatch); which was partially maintained during the behavioral program. However, the improvement induced by medications could only be continued through sex therapy in those men reporting acquired PE; the men with lifelong PE returned to baseline. It was concluded that for acquired PE, combination therapy may offer advantages through an initial stabilizing effect on the couple with subsequent increased acceptance of and adherence to behavioral therapy. There is growing evidence that combination therapy using new pharmaceuticals and psychotherapy will become the treatment of choice (Perelman, 2006).

6.7 Emerging and experimental treatment options for PE

It has been demonstrated that desensitisation of the 5-HT 1A receptor during chronic administration of SSRIs [e.g., combination of robalzotan (NAD-299) with fluoxetine and citalopram (Williamson et al., 2003) and combination of WAY-100635 with citalopram (de Jong et al., 2005) and paroxetine (Looney et al., 2005) induces prolonged delay in ejaculation in the rat. However, when used alone they had no effect on ejaculation. Although this novel pharmacological combination is promising, further clinical research is warranted to evaluate the efficacy and potential adverse effects of this combination. A new avenue being explored in the pharmacological treatment of PE is the use of oxytocin compounds as potential therapeutic agents (Giuliano, 2007), based on immunohistochemical studies that have demonstrated local synthesis of oxytocin and its synthesis-associated protein, neurophysin I, in the epithelial cells of the epididymis (Filippi et al., 2005). Dietary deficiencies, such as low magnesium intake, may prove to play a limited role as well (Aloosh et al., 2006). Although its role in the management of ED is well established, the use of vasoactive intracavernosal injection (ICI) pharmacotherapy for the treatment of PE is not supported by a large body of peer-reviewed literature, and is not commonly used in clinical practice. ICI has been used as a strategy in certain cases to allow men with PE to maintain their erections and continue satisfactory sexual intercourse despite rapid ejaculation (Fein, 1990).

Non-pharmacological approaches are also being explored. Optale et al. showed that immersive virtual reality can speed up the therapeutic psychodynamic process, wherein the patient wears a helmet with miniature television screen and earphones to discuss and summarize his thoughts (Optale et al., 2004). Wise and Watson suggested a novel device based on the penile hypersensitivity hypothesis (Jan Wise & Watson, 2000). This experimental device is a "desensitizing band" which, when worn during masturbation, does not constrict blood flow and helps the PE sufferer gain control over ejaculation. Unfortunately, the device is hardly available for patient use for economic reasons of viability of sales (Linton & Wylie, 2010). Basal et al. described the application of pulsed radio frequency neuromodulation to treat PE by the desensitization of the dorsal penile nerves (Basal et al., 2010). This was a small pilot study consisting of 15 patients and showed a significant increase in the IELT compared to baseline. After the procedure, there were no reported problems with pain, penile hypoesthesia, or ED. Nevertheless, sham-controlled studies with larger numbers of patients are needed. Recently, Sunay et al. performed a randomized, placebo-controlled trial to determine if acupuncture is an effective measure to manage PE (Sunay et al., 2011). Ninety PE patients were randomly assigned into paroxetine 20mg/day, acupuncture or sham-acupuncture (placebo) which was treated twice a week for 4 weeks. The acupuncture points were selected and performed by an experienced acupuncturist according to the publication World Health Organization Standard Acupuncture Point Locations in the Western Pacific Region. Significant differences were found between IELTs of the paroxetine and placebo groups (p=0.001) and the acupuncture and placebo groups (p=0.001) after treatment. Increases of IELTs with paroxetine, acupuncture, and placebo acupuncture were 82.7, 65.7, and 33.1 , respectively. The study is criticized for obvious lack of follow up.

Some authors have reported the use of surgically induced penile hypoanesthesia as a mean to manage PE. A surgical approach consisting of a dorsal neurectomy with or without glandular augmentation using hyaluronic acid gel has been reported (J.J. Kim et al., 2004). Although there are reported positive results with significantly increased IELT, the two groups that underwent dorsal neurectomy or dorsal neurectomy and glandular augmentation, both had significant side effects, including penile numbness, paresthesia and pain. The group that underwent hyaluronic acid augmentation alone reported no adverse side effects. Five years study on the glans augmentation arm of the trial and the hyaluronic acid implants were well maintained, showing long-term efficacy (Kwak et al., 2008). The role of surgery in the management of PE remains unclear, and thus further trials are needed before its role can be established.

6.8 Treatment recommendation

Since the frequency of sexual intercourse is very variable, and spontaneity in sexual intercourse is usually an important factor, an ideal drug for treating PE would be a discrete and 'on-demand' therapy with a predictable therapeutic effect within a few minutes of administration so that it could be taken once sexual foreplay has commenced (Riley & Segraves, 2006). It should have a low incidence of side-effects and have no unwanted effects on the partner (Hellstrom, 2006). Unfortunately, such drug is not currently available. In addition, no drug exists yet that was able to obtain FDA approval as specific treatment for PE. Until such a day is seen, the off-label application of different pharmacotherapy continues to be practiced.

Based on the above mentioned limitations, several authorities have attempted to produce guidelines and algorithms on the management of PE. These guidelines include but are not limited to those published by the American Urological Association (AUA) (Montague et al., 2004), the European Association for Urology (EAU) (Colpi et al., 2004) and the International Consultation on Sexual Dysfunctions (ICSD) (McMahon et al., 2004). These guidelines share common directions and similarities. For example, in terms of treatment modalities, the AUA committee suggested that although oral antidepressants and topical anaesthetic agents are not approved by the FDA for PE, they have been shown to delay ejaculation in men with PE and have a low side effect profile when used at the lower doses commonly used for the treatment of PE (Montague et al., 2004). The commonly used agents in the management of PE as published by the AUA guidelines are shown in Table 5. Additionally, it was suggested that medication could be used to restore confidence together with behavioral treatment, where available, to help men learn to overcome PE on their own (Althof, 2006b; Perelman, 2006). This strategy has become an important part of many of the currently published algorithms (Figure 1).

Drug	Dosage
Topical	
Lidocaine/prilocaine cream	Lidocaine 2.5%/prilocaine 2.5%, 20-30 minutes before intercourse
Oral (Selective serotonin reuptake inhibitors)	
Daily	
Sertaline	25-200 mg/day
Fluoxetine	5-20 mg/day
Paroxetine	10, 20, 40 mg/day
On-demand	
Sertaline	50mg, 4-8 hours before intercourse
Paroxetine	20 mg, 3-4 hours before intercourse
Oral (Tricyclic)	
Daily	
Clomipramine	25-50 mg/day
On-demand	
Clomipramine	25 mg, 4-24 hours before intercourse

Table 5. Pharmacological options for the management of PE (Montague et al., 2004)

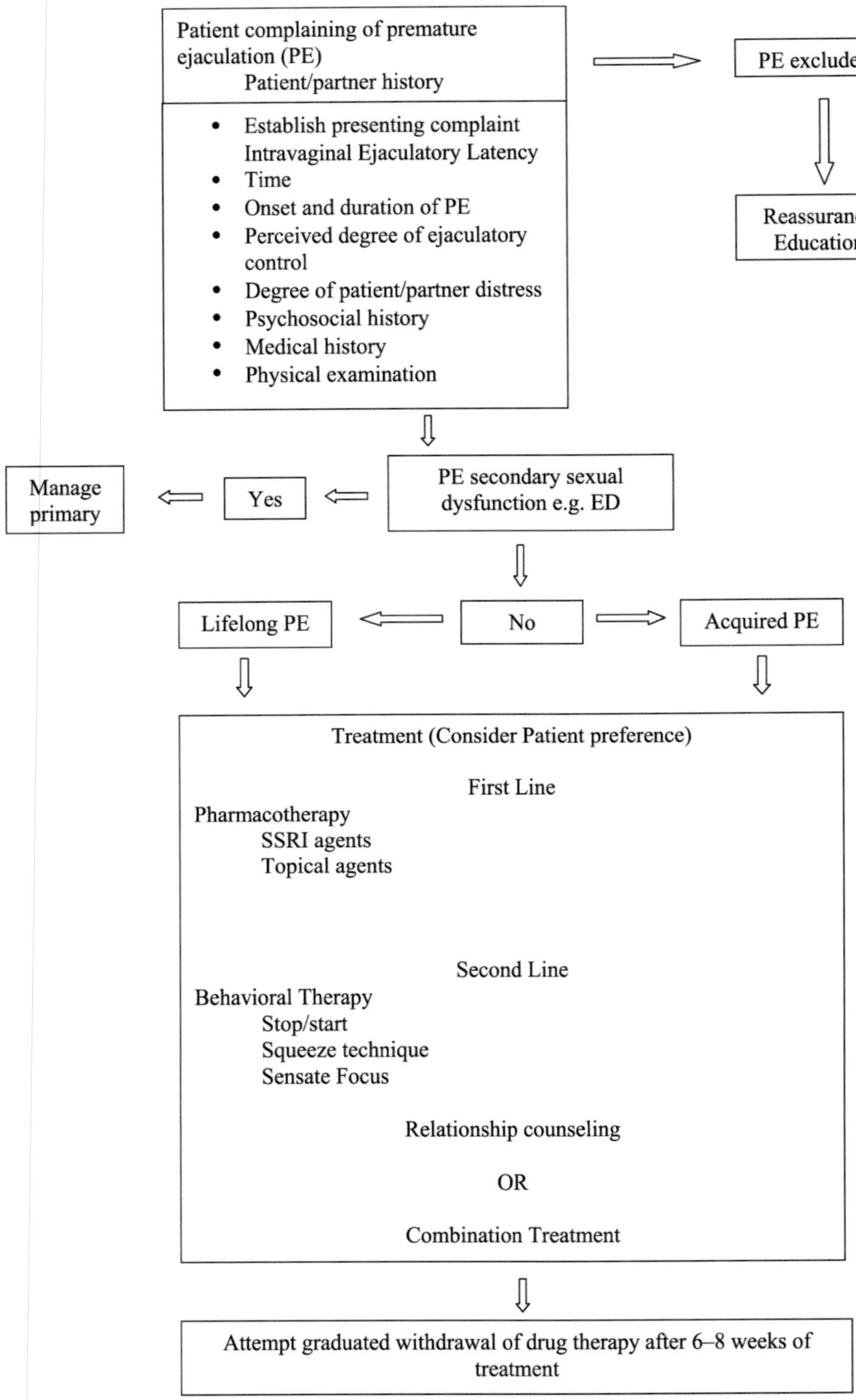

Fig. 1. Algorithm for the management of premature ejaculation (McMahon, 2005; Morales et al., 2007; Rowland et al., 2010).

7. Concluding message

PE is one of the most common male sexual disorders that can have a significant impact on the quality of life of couples. It is a complex disease process that requires clear definition to facilitate research and treatment. It remains substantially under-diagnosed and under-treated, since it is not very well understood by healthcare providers. It is a self reported disorder and one in which the diagnosis is mainly based on history. A sexual history should include all three aspects of PE, namely short IELT, lack of control and distress for both partners. Among the many neurotransmitter systems involved in ejaculatory modulation, central 5-HT has been implicated as a key mediator of ejaculatory control and thus a therapeutic target. Both behavioral and pharmacological options are available to manage PE. Behavioral techniques and psychotherapy can be cumbersome and expensive, with limited long-term efficacy, and therefore are used to complement pharmacotherapy. Currently available pharmaceutical therapy involves the off-label use of SSRIs, Clomipramine, tramadol, PDE-5 inhibitors, as well as topical anaesthetics, each of which have shown varying degrees of efficacy and tolerability. These pharmacotherapies are far from ideal. Their clinical utility is limited by several factors, including a high incidence of adverse events. Each treatment option should be discussed with the PE patient including dosing, the anticipated success rate and possible side effects such that the patient participates in the decision making. Therapy should be tailored for each patient as one treatment does not fit all, as well as preference varies between men. Therapy for PE will continue to develop as the understanding of ejaculation expands and current agents in development may eventually come closer to an ideal and specific therapy for PE.

8. References

Abdel-Hamid, I. A., Jannini, E. A., & Andersson, K. E. (2009). Premature ejaculation: focus on therapeutic targets. *Expert Opin Ther Targets, 13*(2), 175-193.

Ahlenius, S., Larsson, K., Svensson, L., Hjorth, S., Carlsson, A., Lindberg, P., Wikstrom, H., Sanchez, D., Arvidsson, L. E., Hacksell, U., & Nilsson, J. L. (1981). Effects of a new type of 5-HT receptor agonist on male rat sexual behavior. *Pharmacol Biochem Behav, 15*(5), 785-792.

Aloosh, M., Hassani, M., & Nikoobakht, M. (2006). Seminal plasma magnesium and premature ejaculation: a case-control study. *BJU Int, 98*(2), 402-404.

Althof, S. (2006). The psychology of premature ejaculation: therapies and consequences. *J Sex Med, 3 Suppl 4*, 324-331.

Althof, S. E. (2004). Assessment of rapid ejaculation: review of new and existing measures. *Curr Sexual Health Rep, 1*, 61.

Althof, S. E. (2005). Psychological treatment strategies for rapid ejaculation: rationale, practical aspects, and outcome. *World J Urol, 23*(2), 89-92.

Althof, S. E. (2006). Prevalence, characteristics and implications of premature ejaculation/rapid ejaculation. *J Urol, 175*(3 Pt 1), 842-848.

Althof, S. E., Levine, S. B., Corty, E. W., Risen, C. B., Stern, E. B., & Kurit, D. M. (1995). A double-blind crossover trial of clomipramine for rapid ejaculation in 15 couples. *J Clin Psychiatry, 56*(9), 402-407.

American Psychiatric Association. (2000). *The Diagnostic and Statistical Manual of Mental Disorders* (4th ed.). Washington, DC: American Psychiatric Association.

Assalian, P. (1988). Clomipramine in the treatment of premature ejaculation. *J Sex Res, 24*, 213-215.

Atan, A., Basar, M. M., & Aydoganli, L. (2000). Comparison of the efficacy of fluoxetine alone vs. fluoxetine plus local lidocaine ointment in the treatment of premature ejaculation. *Arch Esp Urol, 53*(9), 856-858.

Atikeler, M. K., Gecit, I., & Senol, F. A. (2002). Optimum usage of prilocaine-lidocaine cream in premature ejaculation. *Andrologia, 34*(6), 356-359.

Balon, R. (2006). SSRI-associated sexual dysfunction. *Am J Psychiatry, 163*(9), 1504-1509; quiz 1664.

Basal, S., Goktas, S., Ergin, A., Yildirim, I., Atim, A., Tahmaz, L., & Dayanc, M. (2010). A novel treatment modality in patients with premature ejaculation resistant to conventional methods: the neuromodulation of dorsal penile nerves by pulsed radiofrequency. *J Androl, 31*(2), 126-130.

Basar, M. M., Yilmaz, E., Ferhat, M., Basar, H., & Batislam, E. (2005). Terazosin in the treatment of premature ejaculation: a short-term follow-up. *Int Urol Nephrol, 37*(4), 773-777.

Biri, H., Isen, K., Sinik, Z., Onaran, M., Kupeli, B., & Bozkirli, I. (1998). Sertraline in the treatment of premature ejaculation: a double-blind placebo controlled study. *Int Urol Nephrol, 30*(5), 611-615.

Bohlen, D., Hugonnet, C. L., Mills, R. D., Weise, E. S., & Schmid, H. P. (2000). Five meters of H(2)O: the pressure at the urinary bladder neck during human ejaculation. *Prostate, 44*(4), 339-341.

Busato, W., & Galindo, C. C. (2004). Topical anaesthetic use for treating premature ejaculation: a double-blind, randomized, placebo-controlled study. *BJU Int, 93*(7), 1018-1021.

Buvat, J., Tesfaye, F., Rothman, M., Rivas, D. A., & Giuliano, F. (2009). Dapoxetine for the treatment of premature ejaculation: results from a randomized, double-blind, placebo-controlled phase 3 trial in 22 countries. *Eur Urol, 55*(4), 957-967.

Carey, M. P. (1998). Cognitive behavioral treatment of sexual dysfunction. In V. E. Caballo (Ed.), *International Handbook of Cognitive and Behavioural Treatments for Psychological Disorders* (pp. 251-280). Kidlington, Oxford: Pergamon.

Carson, C., & Gunn, K. (2006). Premature ejaculation: definition and prevalence. *Int J Impot Res, 18 Suppl 1*, S5-13.

Carson, C., & Wyllie, M. (2010). Improved ejaculatory latency, control and sexual satisfaction when PSD502 is applied topically in men with premature ejaculation: results of a phase III, double-blind, placebo-controlled study. *J Sex Med, 7*(9), 3179-3189.

Cavallini, G. (1995). Alpha-1 blockade pharmacotherapy in primitive psychogenic premature ejaculation resistant to psychotherapy. *Eur Urol, 28*(2), 126-130.

Chen, J., Mabjeesh, N. J., Matzkin, H., & Greenstein, A. (2003). Efficacy of sildenafil as adjuvant therapy to selective serotonin reuptake inhibitor in alleviating premature ejaculation. *Urology, 61*(1), 197-200.

Choi, H. K., Jung, G. W., Moon, K. H., Xin, Z. C., Choi, Y. D., Lee, W. H., Rha, K. H., Choi, Y. J., & Kim, D. K. (2000). Clinical study of SS-cream in patients with lifelong premature ejaculation. *Urology, 55*(2), 257-261.

Choi, H. K., Xin, Z. C., Choi, Y. D., Lee, W. H., Mah, S. Y., & Kim, D. K. (1999). Safety and efficacy study with various doses of SS-cream in patients with premature ejaculation in a double-blind, randomized, placebo controlled clinical study. *Int J Impot Res, 11*(5), 261-264.

Cohen, D. (2007). Should the use of selective serotonin reuptake inhibitors in child and adolescent depression be banned? *Psychother Psychosom, 76*, 5-14.

Colpi, G., Weidner, W., Jungwirth, A., Pomerol, J., Papp, G., Hargreave, T., & Dohle, G. (2004). EAU guidelines on ejaculatory dysfunction. *Eur Urol, 46*(5), 555-558.

Colpi, G. M., Hargreave, T. B., Papp, G. K., Pomerol, J. M., & Weidner, W. (2001). *Guidelines on Disorders of Ejaculation*. Retrieved July 17, 2011, from http://www.uroweb.org/files/uploaded_files/guidelines/ejaculationdisor.pdf

Coolen, L. M., Allard, J., Truitt, W. A., & McKenna, K. E. (2004). Central regulation of ejaculation. *Physiol Behav, 83*(2), 203-215.

Corona, G., Petrone, L., Mannucci, E., Jannini, E. A., Mansani, R., Magini, A., Giommi, R., Forti, G., & Maggi, M. (2004). Psycho-biological correlates of rapid ejaculation in patients attending an andrologic unit for sexual dysfunctions. *Eur Urol, 46*(5), 615-622.

Cossmann, M., Kohnen, C., Langford, R., & McCartney, C. (1997). [Tolerance and safety of tramadol use. Results of international studies and data from drug surveillance]. *Drugs, 53 Suppl 2*, 50-62.

Dapoxetine: LY 210448. (2005). *Drugs R D, 6*(5), 307-311.

De Amicis, L. A., Goldberg, D. C., LoPiccolo, J., Friedman, J., & Davies, L. (1985). Clinical follow-up of couples treated for sexual dysfunction. *Arch Sex Behav, 14*(6), 467-489.

de Carufel, F., & Trudel, G. (2006). Effects of a new functional-sexological treatment for premature ejaculation. *J Sex Marital Ther, 32*(2), 97-114.

de Jong, T. R., Pattij, T., Veening, J. G., Dederen, P. J., Waldinger, M. D., Cools, A. R., & Olivier, B. (2005). Citalopram combined with WAY 100635 inhibits ejaculation and ejaculation-related Fos immunoreactivity. *Eur J Pharmacol, 509*(1), 49-59.

Dent, L. A., Brown, W. C., & Murney, J. D. (2002). Citalopram-induced priapism. *Pharmacotherapy, 22*(4), 538-541.

Diaz, V. A., Jr., & Close, J. D. (2010). Male sexual dysfunction. *Prim Care, 37*(3), 473-489, vii-viii.

Dinsmore, W. W., Hackett, G., Goldmeier, D., Waldinger, M., Dean, J., Wright, P., Callander, M., Wylie, K., Novak, C., Keywood, C., Heath, P., & Wyllie, M. (2007). Topical eutectic mixture for premature ejaculation (TEMPE): a novel aerosol-delivery form of lidocaine-prilocaine for treating premature ejaculation. *BJU Int, 99*(2), 369-375.

Dinsmore, W. W., & Wyllie, M. G. (2009). PSD502 improves ejaculatory latency, control and sexual satisfaction when applied topically 5 min before intercourse in men with premature ejaculation: results of a phase III, multicentre, double-blind, placebo-controlled study. *BJU Int, 103*(7), 940-949.

Donatucci, C. F. (2006). Etiology of ejaculation and pathophysiology of premature ejaculation. *J Sex Med, 3 Suppl 4*, 303-308.

Dresser, M. J., Kang, D., Staehr, P., Gidwani, S., Guo, C., Mulhall, J. P., & Modi, N. B. (2006). Pharmacokinetics of dapoxetine, a new treatment for premature ejaculation: Impact of age and effects of a high-fat meal. *J Clin Pharmacol, 46*(9), 1023-1029.

Dunn, K. M., Croft, P. R., & Hackett, G. I. (1998). Sexual problems: a study of the prevalence and need for health care in the general population. *Fam Pract, 15*(6), 519-524.

Dunn, K. M., Croft, P. R., & Hackett, G. I. (1999). Association of sexual problems with social, psychological, and physical problems in men and women: a cross sectional population survey. *J Epidemiol Community Health, 53*(3), 144-148.

Eaton, H. (1973). Clomipramine in the treatment of premature ejaculation. *J Int Med Res, 1*, 432.

El-Sakka, A. I. (2003). Premature ejaculation in non-insulin-dependent diabetic patients. *Int J Androl, 26*(6), 329-334.

Eradiri, O., Sista, S., Lai, J. C.-K., Danyluk, A., & Brett, V. (2006). Bioavailability of extendedrelease and immediate-release formulations of tramadol HCI. *J Clin Pharmacol, 46*, 1091.

FDA. (2007). *FDA proposes new warnings about suicidal thinking, behavior in young adults who take antidepressant medications*. Retrieved July 17, 2011, from http://69.20.19.211/bbs/topics/NEWS/2007/ NEW01624.html

Fein, R. L. (1990). Intracavernous medication for treatment of premature ejaculation. *Urology, 35*(4), 301-303.

Filippi, S., Morelli, A., Vignozzi, L., Vannelli, G. B., Marini, M., Ferruzzi, P., Mancina, R., Crescioli, C., Mondaini, N., Forti, G., Ledda, F., & Maggi, M. (2005). Oxytocin mediates the estrogen-dependent contractile activity of endothelin-1 in human and rabbit epididymis. *Endocrinology, 146*(8), 3506-3517.

Frink, M. C., Hennies, H. H., Englberger, W., Haurand, M., & Wilffert, B. (1996). Influence of tramadol on neurotransmitter systems of the rat brain. *Arzneimittelforschung, 46*(11), 1029-1036.

Gittleman, M. C., Mo, J., & Lu, M. (2005, December 4-7). *Synergistic effect of meatal application of dyclonine/alprostadil cream for the treatment of early ejaculation (EE) in a double-blind and crossover study*. Paper presented at the the 8th Congress of the European Society for Sexual Medicine, Copenhagen, Denmark.

Giuliano, F. (2007). Interview with Dr Francois Giuliano (by Christine McKillop). New avenues in the pharmacological treatment of premature ejaculation. *Eur Urol, 52*(4), 1254-1257.

Godpodinoff, M. L. (1989). Premature ejaculation: clinical subgroups and etiology. *J Sex Marital Ther, 15*(2), 130-134.

Grenier, G., & Byers, E. S. (1995). Rapid ejaculation: a review of conceptual, etiological, and treatment issues. *Arch Sex Behav, 24*(4), 447-472.

Grenier, G., & Byers, E. S. (2001). Operationalizing premature or rapid ejaculation. *J Sex Res, 38*, 169-178.

Gur, E., Lerer, B., & Newman, M. E. (1999). Chronic clomipramine and triiodothyronine increase serotonin levels in rat frontal cortex in vivo: relationship to serotonin autoreceptor activity. *J Pharmacol Exp Ther, 288*(1), 81-87.

Gurkan, L., Oommen, M., & Hellstrom, W. J. (2008). Premature ejaculation: current and future treatments. *Asian J Androl, 10*(1), 102-109.

Guthrie, E. (1952). *The Psychology of Learning*. New York: Harper.

Haensel, S. M., Rowland, D. L., & Kallan, K. T. (1996). Clomipramine and sexual function in men with premature ejaculation and controls. *J Urol, 156*(4), 1310-1315.

Halperin, D., & Reber, G. (2007). Influence of antidepressants on hemostasis. *Dialogues Clin Neurosci, 9*(1), 47-59.

Haney, E. M., Chan, B. K., Diem, S. J., Ensrud, K. E., Cauley, J. A., Barrett-Connor, E., Orwoll, E., & Bliziotes, M. M. (2007). Association of low bone mineral density with selective serotonin reuptake inhibitor use by older men. *Arch Intern Med, 167*(12), 1246-1251.

Hartmann, U., Schedlowski, M., & Kruger, T. H. (2005). Cognitive and partner-related factors in rapid ejaculation: differences between dysfunctional and functional men. *World J Urol, 23*(2), 93-101.

Hawton, K., Catalan, J., Martin, P., & Fagg, J. (1986). Long-term outcome of sex therapy. *Behav Res Ther, 24*(6), 665-675.

Hellstrom, W. J. (2006). Current and future pharmacotherapies of premature ejaculation. *J Sex Med, 3 Suppl 4*, 332-341.

Hellstrom, W. J. (2009). Emerging treatments for premature ejaculation: focus on dapoxetine. *Neuropsychiatr Dis Treat, 5*, 37-46.

Hellstrom, W. J. (2011). Update on treatments for premature ejaculation. *Int J Clin Pract, 65*(1), 16-26.

Henry, R., & Morales, A. (2003). Topical lidocaine-prilocaine spray for the treatment of premature ejaculation: a proof of concept study. *Int J Impot Res, 15*(4), 277-281.

Henry, R., Morales, A., & Wyllie, M. G. (2008). TEMPE: Topical Eutectic-Like Mixture for Premature Ejaculation. *Expert Opin Drug Deliv, 5*(2), 251-261.

International Society for Sexual Medicine. (2007). *ISSM definition of premature ejaculation*. Retrieved July 17, 2007, from http://www.issm.info/

Jan Wise, M. E., & Watson, J. P. (2000). A new treatment for premature ejaculation: case series for a desensitizing band. *Sex and Relation Ther, 15*, 345-350.

Jannini, E. A., & Lenzi, A. (2005). Epidemiology of premature ejaculation. *Curr Opin Urol, 15*(6), 399-403.

Jannini, E. A., Lombardo, F., & Lenzi, A. (2005). Correlation between ejaculatory and erectile dysfunction. *Int J Androl, 28 Suppl 2*, 40-45.

Kara, H., Aydin, S., Yucel, M., Agargun, M. Y., Odabas, O., & Yilmaz, Y. (1996). The efficacy of fluoxetine in the treatment of premature ejaculation: a double-blind placebo controlled study. *J Urol, 156*(5), 1631-1632.

Kilic, S., Ergin, H., & Baydinc, Y. C. (2005). Venlafaxine extended release for the treatment of patients with premature ejaculation: a pilot, single-blind, placebo-controlled, fixed-dose crossover study on short-term administration of an antidepressant drug. *Int J Androl, 28*(1), 47-52.

Kim, J. J., Kwak, T. I., Jeon, B. G., Cheon, J., & Moon, D. G. (2004). Effects of glans penis augmentation using hyaluronic acid gel for premature ejaculation. *Int J Impot Res, 16*(6), 547-551.

Kim, S. C., & Seo, K. K. (1998). Efficacy and safety of fluoxetine, sertraline and clomipramine in patients with premature ejaculation: a double-blind, placebo controlled study. *J Urol, 159*(2), 425-427.

Kim, S. W., Lee, S. H., & Paick, J. S. (2004). In vivo rat model to measure hypogastric nerve stimulation-induced seminal vesicle and vasal pressure responses simultaneously. *Int J Impot Res, 16*(5), 427-432.

Kim, S. W., & Paick, J. S. (1999). Short-term analysis of the effects of as needed use of sertraline at 5 PM for the treatment of premature ejaculation. *Urology, 54*(3), 544-547.

Kwak, T. I., Jin, M. H., Kim, J. J., & Moon, D. G. (2008). Long-term effects of glans penis augmentation using injectable hyaluronic acid gel for premature ejaculation. *Int J Impot Res, 20*(4), 425-428.

Laumann, E. O., Gagnon, J. H., Michael, R. T., & Michaels, S. (1994). The Social Organization of Sexuality. *University of Chicago Press.*

Laumann, E. O., Nicolosi, A., Glasser, D. B., Paik, A., Gingell, C., Moreira, E., & Wang, T. (2005). Sexual problems among women and men aged 40-80 y: prevalence and correlates identified in the Global Study of Sexual Attitudes and Behaviors. *Int J Impot Res, 17*(1), 39-57.

Laumann, E. O., Paik, A., & Rosen, R. C. (1999a). The epidemiology of erectile dysfunction: results from the National Health and Social Life Survey. *Int J Impot Res, 11 Suppl 1*, S60-64.

Laumann, E. O., Paik, A., & Rosen, R. C. (1999b). Sexual dysfunction in the United States: prevalence and predictors. *Jama, 281*(6), 537-544.

Levine, S. B. (1975). Premature ejaculation: some thoughts about its pathogenesis. *J Sex Marital Ther, 1*(4), 326-334.

Linton, K. D., & Wylie, K. R. (2010). Recent advances in the treatment of premature ejaculation. *Drug Des Devel Ther, 4*, 1-6.

Looney, C., Thor, K. B., Ricca, D., & Marson, L. (2005). Differential effects of simultaneous or sequential administration of paroxetine and WAY-100,635 on ejaculatory behavior. *Pharmacol Biochem Behav, 82*(3), 427-433.

Lue, T., & Broderick, G. (2007). Evaluation and nonsurgical management of erectile dysfunction and premature ejaculation. In P. C. Walsh, A. B. Retik, E. D. Vaughan, A. J. Wein, L. R. Kavoussi, A. C. Novick, A. W. Partin & C. A. Peters (Eds.), *Campbell-Walsh urology* (9th ed., pp. 750-787). Philadelphia, PA: Saunders-Elsevier.

Maier, U., & Koinig, G. (1994). Andrological findings in young patients under long-term antidepressive therapy with clomipramine. *Psychopharmacology (Berl), 116*(3), 357-359.

Masters, W., & Johnson, V. (1970). *Premature ejaculation: Human sexual inadequacy*. Boston: Little Brown & Co.

McDiarmid, T., Mackler, L., & Schneider, D. M. (2005). Clinical inquiries. What is the addiction risk associated with tramadol? *J Fam Pract, 54*(1), 72-73.

McMahon, C. (2005). Premature ejaculation: past, present, and future perspectives. *J Sex Med, 2 Suppl 2*, 94-95.

McMahon, C., Kim, S. W., Park, N. C., Chang, C. P., Rivas, D., Tesfaye, F., Rothman, M., & Aquilina, J. (2010). Treatment of premature ejaculation in the Asia-Pacific region: results from a phase III double-blind, parallel-group study of dapoxetine. *J Sex Med, 7*(1 Pt 1), 256-268.

McMahon, C. G. (2002). Long term results of treatment of premature ejaculation with selective serotonin re-uptake inhibitors. *Int J Imp Res, 14*, 19.

McMahon, C. G. (2005). The etiology and management of premature ejaculation. *Nat Clin Pract Urol, 2*(9), 426-433.

McMahon, C. G., Abdo, C., Incrocci, L., Perelman, M., Rowland, D., Waldinger, M., & Xin, Z. C. (2004). Disorders of orgasm and ejaculation in men. *J Sex Med, 1*(1), 58-65.

McMahon, C. G., McMahon, C. N., Leow, L. J., & Winestock, C. G. (2006). Efficacy of type-5 phosphodiesterase inhibitors in the drug treatment of premature ejaculation: a systematic review. *BJU Int, 98*(2), 259-272.

McMahon, C. G., & Samali, R. (1999). Pharmacological treatment of premature ejaculation. *Curr Opin Urol, 9*(6), 553-561.

McMahon, C. G., & Touma, K. (1999). Treatment of premature ejaculation with paroxetine hydrochloride as needed: 2 single-blind placebo controlled crossover studies. *J Urol, 161*(6), 1826-1830.

Metz, M. E., & Pryor, J. L. (2000). Premature ejaculation: a psychophysiological approach for assessment and management. *J Sex Marital Ther, 26*(4), 293-320.

Montague, D. K., Jarow, J., Broderick, G. A., Dmochowski, R. R., Heaton, J. P., Lue, T. F., Nehra, A., & Sharlip, I. D. (2004). AUA guideline on the pharmacologic management of premature ejaculation. *J Urol, 172*(1), 290-294.

Montejo, A. L., Llorca, G., Izquierdo, J. A., & Rico-Villademoros, F. (2001). Incidence of sexual dysfunction associated with antidepressant agents: a prospective multicenter study of 1022 outpatients. Spanish Working Group for the Study of Psychotropic-Related Sexual Dysfunction. *J Clin Psychiatry, 62 Suppl 3*, 10-21.

Morales, A., Barada, J., & Wyllie, M. G. (2007). A review of the current status of topical treatments for premature ejaculation. *BJU Int, 100*(3), 493-501.

Moreira, E. D., Jr., Brock, G., Glasser, D. B., Nicolosi, A., Laumann, E. O., Paik, A., Wang, T., & Gingell, C. (2005). Help-seeking behaviour for sexual problems: the global study of sexual attitudes and behaviors. *Int J Clin Pract, 59*(1), 6-16.

Mousavizadeh, K., Ghafourifar, P., & Sadeghi-Nejad, H. (2002). Calcium channel blocking activity of thioridazine, clomipramine and fluoxetine in isolated rat vas deferens: a relative potency measurement study. *J Urol, 168*(6), 2716-2719.

Nicolosi, A., Laumann, E. O., Glasser, D. B., Moreira, E. D., Jr., Paik, A., & Gingell, C. (2004). Sexual behavior and sexual dysfunctions after age 40: the global study of sexual attitudes and behaviors. *Urology, 64*(5), 991-997.

Optale, G., Pastore, M., Marin, S., Bordin, D., Nasta, A., & Pianon, C. (2004). Male sexual dysfunctions: immersive virtual reality and multimedia therapy. *Stud Health Technol Inform, 99*, 165-178.

Palmer, N. R., & Stuckey, B. G. (2008). Premature ejaculation: a clinical update. *Med J Aust, 188*(11), 662-666.

Patrick, D. L., Althof, S. E., Pryor, J. L., Rosen, R., Rowland, D. L., Ho, K. F., McNulty, P., Rothman, M., & Jamieson, C. (2005). Premature ejaculation: an observational study of men and their partners. *J Sex Med, 2*(3), 358-367.

Payne, R. E., & Sadovsky, R. (2007). Identifying and treating premature ejaculation: importance of the sexual history. *Cleve Clin J Med, 74 Suppl 3*, S47-53.

Perelman, M., McMahon, C., & Barada, J. (2004). Evaluation and treatment of the ejaculatory disorders. In T. F. Lue (Ed.), *Atlas of male sexual dysfunction* (pp. 127-157). Philadelphia, PA: Current Medicine, Inc.

Perelman, M. A. (2006). A new combination treatment for premature ejaculation: a sex therapist's perspective. *J Sex Med, 3*(6), 1004-1012.

Porst, H., Montorsi, F., Rosen, R. C., Gaynor, L., Grupe, S., & Alexander, J. (2007). The Premature Ejaculation Prevalence and Attitudes (PEPA) survey: prevalence, comorbidities, and professional help-seeking. *Eur Urol, 51*(3), 816-823; discussion 824.

Powell, J. A., & Wyllie, M. G. (2009). 'Up and coming' treatments for premature ejaculation: progress towards an approved therapy. *Int J Impot Res, 21*(2), 107-115.

Press release. (2005). ALZA Corporation receives letter from FDA on dapoxetine application. *Alza Corporation Press.*

Pryor, J. L., Althof, S. E., Steidle, C., Rosen, R. C., Hellstrom, W. J., Shabsigh, R., Miloslavsky, M., & Kell, S. (2006). Efficacy and tolerability of dapoxetine in treatment of premature ejaculation: an integrated analysis of two double-blind, randomised controlled trials. *Lancet, 368*(9539), 929-937.

Raeder, M. B., Bjelland, I., Emil Vollset, S., & Steen, V. M. (2006). Obesity, dyslipidemia, and diabetes with selective serotonin reuptake inhibitors: the Hordaland Health Study. *J Clin Psychiatry, 67*(12), 1974-1982.

Riley, A., & Segraves, R. T. (2006). Treatment of premature ejaculation. *Int J Clin Pract, 60*(6), 694-697.

Rosenberg, M. T., Sailor, N., Tallman, C. T., & Ohl, D. A. (2006, May 20-25). *Premature ejaculation as reported by female partners: prevalence and sexual satisfaction survey results from a community practice.* Paper presented at the American Urological Association Annual Meeting, Atlanta, GA.

Rowland, D., McMahon, C. G., Abdo, C., Chen, J., Jannini, E., Waldinger, M. D., & Ahn, T. Y. (2010). Disorders of orgasm and ejaculation in men. *J Sex Med, 7*(4 Pt 2), 1668-1686.

Rowland, D., Perelman, M., Althof, S., Barada, J., McCullough, A., Bull, S., Jamieson, C., & Ho, K. F. (2004). Self-reported premature ejaculation and aspects of sexual functioning and satisfaction. *J Sex Med, 1*(2), 225-232.

Rowland, D. L., & Cooper, S. E. (2005). Behavioral and psychological models in ejaculatory function research. In J. P. Mulhall (Ed.), *Current Sexual Health Reports* (Vol. 2, pp. 29-34). Philadelphia, PA: Current Science Inc.

Rowland, D. L., Cooper, S. E., & Schneider, M. (2001). Defining premature ejaculation for experimental and clinical investigations. *Arch Sex Behav, 30*(3), 235-253.

Rowland, D. L., De Gouveia Brazao, C. A., & Koos Slob, A. (2001). Effective daily treatment with clomipramine in men with premature ejaculation when 25 mg (as required) is ineffective. *BJU Int, 87*(4), 357-360.

Rowland, D. L., & Rose, P. (2008). Understanding & treating premature ejaculation. *Nurse Pract, 33*(10), 21-27.

Rowland, D. L., Tai, W. L., Brummett, K., & Slob, A. K. (2004). Predicting responsiveness to the treatment of rapid ejaculation with 25 mg clomipramine as needed. *Int J Impot Res, 16*(4), 354-357.

Sadeghi-Nejad, H., & Watson, R. (2008). Premature ejaculation: current medical treatment and new directions (CME). *J Sex Med, 5*(5), 1037-1050; quiz 1051-1032.

Safarinejad, M. R., & Hosseini, S. Y. (2006). Safety and efficacy of tramadol in the treatment of premature ejaculation: a double-blind, placebo-controlled, fixed-dose, randomized study. *J Clin Psychopharmacol, 26*(1), 27-31.

Salem, E. A., Wilson, S. K., Bissada, N. K., Delk, J. R., Hellstrom, W. J., & Cleves, M. A. (2008). Tramadol HCL has promise in on-demand use to treat premature ejaculation. *J Sex Med, 5*(1), 188-193.

Salonia, A., Maga, T., Colombo, R., Scattoni, V., Briganti, A., Cestari, A., Guazzoni, G., Rigatti, P., & Montorsi, F. (2002). A prospective study comparing paroxetine alone versus paroxetine plus sildenafil in patients with premature ejaculation. *J Urol, 168*(6), 2486-2489.

Schapiro, B. (1943). Premature ejaculation: a review of 1130 cases. *J Urol, 3*, 374-379.

Screponi, E., Carosa, E., Di Stasi, S. M., Pepe, M., Carruba, G., & Jannini, E. A. (2001). Prevalence of chronic prostatitis in men with premature ejaculation. *Urology, 58*(2), 198-202.

Segraves, R. T., Saran, A., Segraves, K., & Maguire, E. (1993). Clomipramine versus placebo in the treatment of premature ejaculation: a pilot study. *J Sex Marital Ther, 19*(3), 198-200.

Semans, J. H. (1956). Premature ejaculation: a new approach. *South Med J, 49*(4), 353-358.

Shabsigh, R. (2006). Diagnosing premature ejaculation: a review. *J Sex Med, 3 Suppl 4*, 318-323.

Sharlip, I. D. (2006). Guidelines for the diagnosis and management of premature ejaculation. *J Sex Med, 3 Suppl 4*, 309-317.

Slob, A., Van Berke, A., & Van der Werff ten Bosch, J. (2000). Premature ejaculation treated by local penile anaesthesia in an uncontrolled clinical replication study. *J Sex Res, 37*, 244-247.

Spector, I. P., & Carey, M. P. (1990). Incidence and prevalence of the sexual dysfunctions: a critical review of the empirical literature. *Arch Sex Behav, 19*(4), 389-408.

Steggall, M. J., Fowler, C. G., & Pryce, A. (2008). Combination Therapy for Premature Ejaculation: Results of a Small-Scale Study. *Sex Rel Ther, 23*, 365-376.

Sunay, D., Sunay, M., Aydogmus, Y., Bagbanci, S., Arslan, H., Karabulut, A., & Emir, L. (2011). Acupuncture versus paroxetine for the treatment of premature ejaculation: a randomized, placebo-controlled clinical trial. *Eur Urol, 59*(5), 765-771.

Symonds, T., Roblin, D., Hart, K., & Althof, S. (2003). How does premature ejaculation impact a man s life? *J Sex Marital Ther, 29*(5), 361-370.

Tian, L., Xin, Z. C., Xin, H., Fu, J., Yuan, Y. M., Liu, W. J., & Yang, C. (2004). Effect of renewed SS-cream on spinal somatosensory evoked potential in rabbits. *Asian J Androl, 6*(1), 15-18.

Waldinger, M. D. (2002). The neurobiological approach to premature ejaculation. *J Urol, 168*(6), 2359-2367.

Waldinger, M. D. (2003). Towards evidence-based drug treatment research on premature ejaculation: a critical evaluation of methodology. *Int J Impot Res, 15*(5), 309-313.

Waldinger, M. D. (2007). Premature ejaculation: definition and drug treatment. *Drugs, 67*(4), 547-568.

Waldinger, M. D., Berendsen, H. H., Blok, B. F., Olivier, B., & Holstege, G. (1998). Premature ejaculation and serotonergic antidepressants-induced delayed ejaculation: the involvement of the serotonergic system. *Behav Brain Res, 92*(2), 111-118.

Waldinger, M. D., Hengeveld, M. W., Zwinderman, A. H., & Olivier, B. (1998). Effect of SSRI antidepressants on ejaculation: a double-blind, randomized, placebo-controlled study with fluoxetine, fluvoxamine, paroxetine, and sertraline. *J Clin Psychopharmacol, 18*(4), 274-281.

Waldinger, M. D., Quinn, P., Dilleen, M., Mundayat, R., Schweitzer, D. H., & Boolell, M. (2005). A multinational population survey of intravaginal ejaculation latency time. *J Sex Med, 2*(4), 492-497.

Waldinger, M. D., Rietschel, M., Nothen, M. M., Hengsveld, M. W., & Olivier, B. (1997). Familial occurrence of primary premature ejaculation. *Psychiatr Genet, 8*, 37-40.

Waldinger, M. D., van De Plas, A., Pattij, T., van Oorschot, R., Coolen, L. M., Veening, J. G., & Olivier, B. (2002). The selective serotonin re-uptake inhibitors fluvoxamine and paroxetine differ in sexual inhibitory effects after chronic treatment. *Psychopharmacology (Berl), 160*(3), 283-289.

Waldinger, M. D., Zwinderman, A. H., & Olivier, B. (2004). On-demand treatment of premature ejaculation with clomipramine and paroxetine: a randomized, double-blind fixed-dose study with stopwatch assessment. *Eur Urol, 46*(4), 510-515; discussion 516.

Waldinger, M. D., Zwinderman, A. H., Schweitzer, D. H., & Olivier, B. (2004). Relevance of methodological design for the interpretation of efficacy of drug treatment of premature ejaculation: a systematic review and meta-analysis. *Int J Impot Res, 16*(4), 369-381.

Wang, W. F., Chang, L., Minhas, S., & Ralph, D. J. (2007). Selective serotonin reuptake inhibitors in the treatment of premature ejaculation. *Chin Med J (Engl), 120*(11), 1000-1006.

Williamson, I. J., Turner, L., Woods, K., & ., e. a. (2003). The 5-HT1A receptor antagonist robalzotan enhances SSRI-induced ejaculation delay in the rat. *Br J Pharmacol, 138 (Suppl. 1)*, PO32.

World Health Organization. (2004). *Second international consultation on sexual dysfunctions.* Paris: World Health Organization.

7

Erectile Dysfunction in Paraplegic Males

Charalampos Konstantinidis
National Institute of Rehabilitation
Greece

1. Introduction

In the U.S. there are over 300,000 people who suffer from spinal cord injuries. This incident increases every year by 10,000 to 12,000 new patients (Harrop et al., 2006). In Canada, about 36,000 people live with spinal cord injuries, while 55% of them, are people in the reproductive phase of their life, aged 16-30 years, and the ratio of men to women is calculated to 4 /1(Mittmann et al., 2005). For several years there was a myth in societies that people with paraplegia or quadriplegia have no sexuality, do not have erectile function and that they are infertile. In fact, sexual expression is a component of personality and it is independent to the erectile function or fertility status. In handicaps lack of sexual interest is associated with social withdrawal and inability to recover while sexual alertness is associated with faster and better recovery. The degree of sexual rehabilitation is directly related to physical rehabilitation, social integration and quality of life (Biering-Sorensen & Sonksen, 2001; Fisher et al., 2002). Last years the medical community emphasizes on quality of life and sexuality of people with spinal cord injuries. It is shown that the 66% of patients with spinal cord injuries consider their erection sufficient for sexual activity. The incidence of injury on the person's sexual function depends on the location and the extent of the damage. After Spinal Cord Lesions (SCL), both men and women are reporting decreased desire and low frequency of sexual activity (Deforge et al., 2006).

2. Pathophysiology of Erectile Dysfunction (ED) after SCL

Erection is a neurovascular phenomenon which takes place under neuro-hormonal control. Sensory data from the eyes and skin are relayed to certain areas within the hypothalamus where appropriate signals are relayed to the penis. The upper centers which regulate the erectile function in the brain are located at the cortex and the hypothalamus, as mentioned above. The main involved nuclei are: paraventicular nucleus, medial preoptic area, paragigantocellular nucleus, and locus coeruleus. The lower centers are located in the spinal cord. These centers are two: the psychogenic, sympathetic erection center which is located at the Th11-12 until L2-3 level of spinal cord and the reflexogenic, parasympathetic erection center which is located at the S2-4 level of spinal cord. The sympathetic erection center is purely autonomous, contains fibers with evoked and others with inhibitory action and travels with the inferior hypogastric plexus. The parasympathetic erection center contains also somatic fibers. The afferent fibers are coming from the pudendal nerve and the dorsal penile nerve, while the efferent fibers involve in the formation of the cavernous nerves and the inferior hypogastric and sacral plexus. Sympathetic innervation provides inhibitory pathways whereas parasympathetic and somatic innervations are crucial for erection. The two centers of the spinal cord are under the control of the brain (Saenz de Tejada et al., 2005).

Erection can be distinguished to reflective and psychogenic according to the origin of its induction and the erection center which is mainly involved. Reflective erection is the outcome of somatoaesthetic stimulation and may be independent of sexual arousal. This erection takes place through the reflexogenic, parasympathetic erection center. Psychogenic erection, which predominates in humans, is the result of sexual desire caused by images, fantasies and thoughts related to previous sexual experiences. The psychogenic, sympathetic erection center is mainly responsible for this kind of erection. The erectile function in patients with SCL depends on the location of the injury and the extent of the lesion. In patients with upper cord lesions, reflexogenic erections are preserved in 95% of them, while in patients with complete lower cord damages this rate is only 25%. The quality of erection is better as higher the lesion is located (Eardley & Kirby, 1991). Derry et al., in their study are reporting that 25% of men with SCL regain their erectile function one month after injury, when 60% and 80% regain their erections in a period of six months and one year respectively after injury (Derry et al., 2002). The preservation of the sacral parasympathetic neurons leads to the maintenance of reflexogenic erection. In case of sacral injury thoracolumbar pathway may take over through synaptic connections. In general, men with cervical and thoracic lesions regain their erections sooner and better than men with lumbar lesions (Courtois et al., 1993).

Reflexive erections, which require the integrity of parasympathetic erectile center (S2-4), have been observed in people with SCL. These arise after irritation of the skin or mucosa below the level of the lesion. Manipulations such as rubbing of the thighs or nipples, squeezing of the glans, suprapubic percussion, irritation of the anal region, proved to be more effective than masturbation or any other stimulation of the genitalia (Saenz de Tejada et al., 2005; Derry et al., 2002). Lesions higher to Th11 level are combined with erection of both corpora cavernosum and corpus spongiosum, while lesions below this level exclude the participation in the erection of the corpus spongiosum (Biering-Sorensen & Sonksen, 2001). This erection is usually sufficient for penetration, but it has short duration. The reflexive erections maintain in 95% of patients with total damage over the sacral center, while in lower level lesions this percentage is up to 25%. The training for the challenge of this reflex is part of the sexual rehabilitation.

Psychogenic erections have been observed in 60% of patients with intact sympathetic erectile center (Th11-L2) and lesion below the L2 level. Psychogenic erections, as mentioned above, are independent from direct physical stimulation and are the result of visual or acoustic stimuli, dreams, fantasies or memories. These erections are usually with low quality and short duration. Objectively, it is more of a swelling of the penis rather than a hard erection, rarely allowing penetration (Derry et al., 2002; Courtois et al., 1999; Smith & Bodner, 1993; Chapelle et al., 1980).

Mixed erection occurs when the SCL is between the two centers. These erections onset after a psychic stimulus and maintain or even are enhanced by a physical stimulus, or they are prolonged reflecting erections which are enhanced by a strong sexual desire.

Nocturnal erections have been also recorded in men with SCL. These erections usually take place during the REM phase of the sleep. The comparison between the erections of quadriplegic and paraplegic patients showed that quadriplegic men had better erections (regarding hardness and duration) than paraplegic patients. Additionally, thoracic spinal lesion was associated with poor nocturnal erections comparing with cervical spinal injuries (Suh et al., 2003).

Patients with lesions above the Th6 level often present the phenomenon of autonomous dysreflexia, which involves reflecting increased sympathetic tone at the level below the lesion. This increased sympathetic response causes vasoconstriction and hypertension. At the levels higher to the spinal lesion, vasodilatation takes place and causes flashing and headache. The more serious symptom is the parasympathetic activation which decreases the heart rate. This situation with excessive hypertension and bradycardia is dangerous for the patient and it was found that sexual arousal may trigger dysreflexia. In these cases sexual activity must be avoided (Rossier et al., 1971; Frankel & Mathias, 1980).

3. Diagnostic approach to patients with SCL

3.1 Sexual history

Sexual history is the first step in the evaluation of patients with ED. Our purpose is to assess the pre-injury and the post-traumatic sexual function and to identify the ED. The absence or presence of erections, under what circumstances they took place, the number and the frequency of them, the quality of erections (regarding hardness and duration) compared with the erectile function before injury and the frequency of sexual intercourse, are some of the questions which have to be answered. Additionally, a good history will assess the mental and psychological status of individuals whereas ED with psychogenic origin described in 10% of men with SCL (Monga et al., 1999; Tay et al., 1996).

3.2 Physical examination and laboratory tests

Physical examination reveals clinical signs which contribute to the diagnostic approach of ED. During the examination of the external genitalia, neurological examination should also be included. Our aim is to identify the level of lesion, according the sacral and the thoracic-lumbar origin of the neurosis of external genital organs. Assess of the sensation of the genitalia, the perineum and the perianal region as well, is essential for the evaluation of parasympathetic erectile center, as the somatic-sensation of these areas reflects to the S2-4 level of the spinal cord. By evaluating the reflex of the cremaster muscle, we can assess the S1-2 reflex arc. By evaluating the reflexes of rectus muscles, we can assess the Th9-12 reflex arcs and the bulbocavernous reflex is suitable to investigate the integrity of S2-4 reflex arc (Vodusek, 2003). Additionally, tendon reflexes of the lower limbs can evaluate the lumbar region of spinal cord.

Apart from control of reflexes, the use of specific neurological tests has been reported in the literature. The measurement of latency time of the bulbocavernous reflex by placing electrodes on the penis and the bulbocavernosal muscles and the measurement of somatosensory cortical evoked potentials by placing electrodes on the scalp, may give an accurate assessment of the nervous lesions (Bird & Hanno, 1998).

3.3 Nocturnal Penile Tumescence and Rigidity (NPTR)

The recording of nocturnal erections in normal subjects is a method for the differential diagnosis of psychogenic from organic erectile dysfunction. The recording of these erections, usually during REM phases of sleep, is made by the Rigiscan (Fig. 1). Rigiscan uses two inflatable rings which are adapted at the base and at the tip of the penile shaft. These rings work as sensors for the increase in the diameter (tumescence) and the hardness during erection. The duration and the quality of these erections represent the erectile capacity of the patient. The findings must be confirmed for at least two nights.

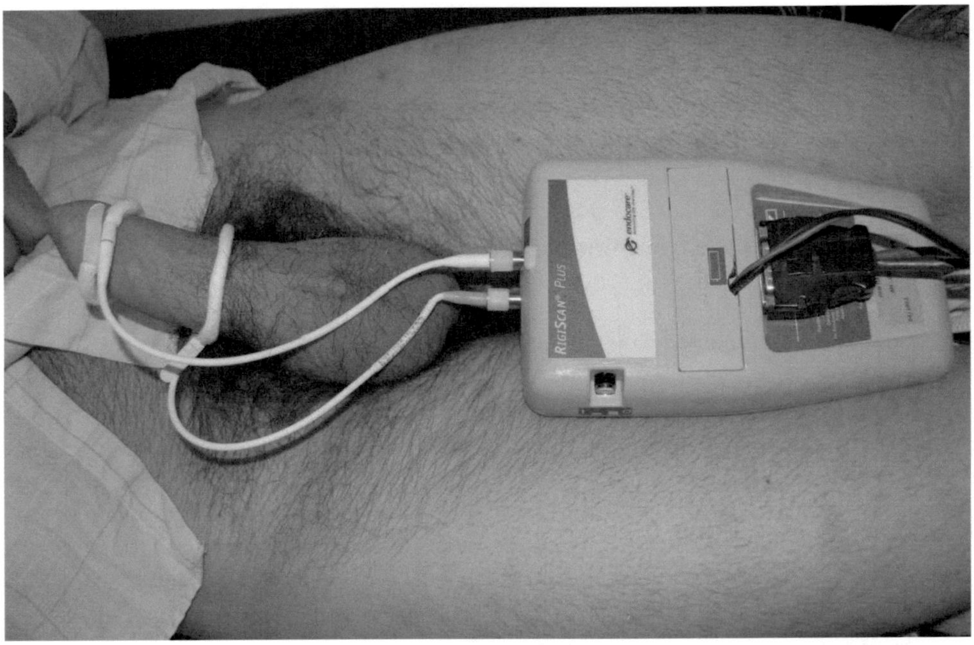

Fig. 1. Rigiscan device uses two inflatable rings which act as transducers in order to study the tumescence and the rigidity during erectile episodes.

Rigiscan studies have shown that the onset of erection does not appear to require intact pathways from the brain towards the spinal cord, while nocturnal erections were observed in men with complete SCL (Suh et al., 2003). Rigiscan studies showed that men with SCL do suffer from psychogenic ED at a rate of up to 10% (Tay et al,. 1996).

3.4 Dynamic Doppler Ultrasound Evaluation

Dynamic Color Doppler ultrasound tomography is a method which can evaluate the vascular potential of the corpora cavernosa and can assess the hemodynamic of the penis. After the administration of vasoactive drugs (intracavernousal injection of alprostadil 10μg), blood flow is studied by measuring the peak-systolic and the end-diastolic velocity (Fig.2). According to these findings, vascular etiology (low arterial inflow or venous escape syndrome), of erectile dysfunction can be identified.

In cases of neurogenic ED, ultrasound findings are usually normal, as the majority of these patients, is young with no vascular pathology. If a reduced blood supply of the cavernous artery is present, probably this occurs due to concomitant vascular inefficiency (Kim et al., 2006). Normal reply to vasoactive drugs is described in 80% of patients with SCL, while there are some other studies which record high rates of vascular lesions in these patients (Robinson et al., 1987).

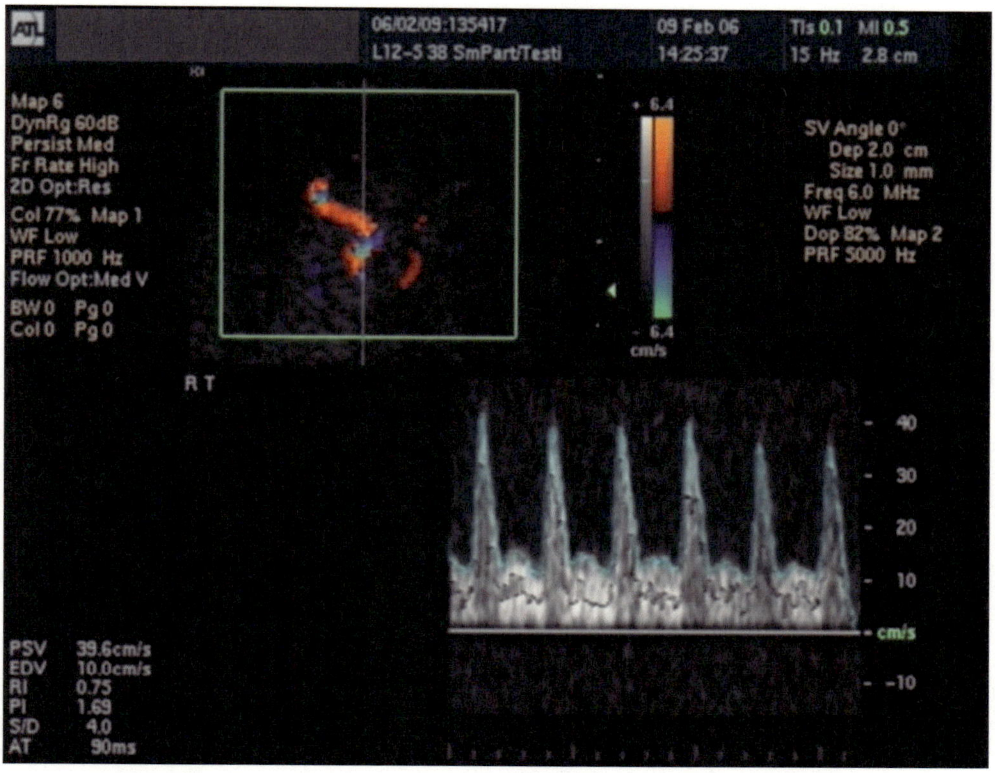

Fig. 2. Color Doppler ultrasound, 10 minutes after intracavernousal injection of 10 μg alprostadil. Due to high End-Diastolic Velocity (EDV) this is an image of venous escape syndrome.

4. ED treatment in men with SCL

The treatment of ED in paraplegic or quadriplegic patients follows the therapeutic strategy of any other case of organic ED. According to that, we can apply stepped treatment of 1st, 2nd and 3rd line. The 1st line of treatment includes oral inhibitors of phosphodiesterase type 5 (PDE-5) and vacuum devices. In the 2nd line of treatment there are penile injections and transurethral application of vasoactive substances. Finally, in the 3rd line of treatment option there is the implantation of penile prosthesis (Ramos & Samso, 2004). Patients should be informed about all the treatment options from the beginning of the therapy, although the treatment is applied step by step. This is very important for neurogenic patients in order to be optimistic for the outcome of the treatment. General considerations regarding blood pressure, lipid profile, hormonal status, diabetes mellitus and stop smoking are necessary to all patients with ED. On the other hand, most of the patients with SCL are young men with excellent sexual function before injury and the etiology of their ED is mostly neurogenic. In these patients psychogenic component is present sometimes and other organic causes, vascular inefficiency for example, occur rarely.

4.1 First line treatment

4.1.1 Oral treatment

Since sildenafil gained the approval of use, it has proved its efficiency against ED, of any organic reason. The efficacy and its safety have been demonstrated in studies in patients with SCL. In bibliography there are two relevant, randomized, prospective, multicenter placebo controlled studies. Giuliano et al. studied 178 patients with SCL and indicated 76% efficacy of sildenafil compared with 4% of placebo (Giuliano et al., 1999). In another similar study by Maytom et al. (with only 27 patients) it was referred efficacy in sildenafil 65% vs. 8% in placebo (Maytom et al., 1999). In the same study the overall satisfaction with their sexual activity reported in 75% in the sildenafil group compared with 7% in the placebo group. In a meta-analysis of eight other studies it was indicated the overall effectiveness of sildenafil in 80% of these patients (Deforge et al., 2006). Derry et al. reviewing the literature indicates that the proportion of patients with SCL showing improvement in their erectile function reaches 94%. The majority of them (72%) indicate successful sexual intercourse, as well. Response rates were generally higher in patients with partial section of the spinal cord (incomplete lesions). However, a significant proportion of patients with complete cross-section, regardless of the location of the lesion, benefited from the administration of sildenafil (Derry et al., 2002; Sanchez Ramos et al., 2001). The existing literature, thus, demonstrates high efficacy and safety of oral treatment with sildenafil in patients with ED after SCL.

There are at least two studies in the literature supporting the efficacy of vardenafil in the treatment of ED for patients with SCL. Giuliano et al. in a multicenter, double-blind and placebo controlled study, with duration of 12 weeks, which included 418 patients, reported erections, sufficient for penetration in 76% of patients in the vardenafil group, compared with 41% of patients in the placebo treatment group (Giuliano et al., 2006). In the same study, 59% of the vardenafil group indicated satisfactory duration of erection, compared to 22% of the placebo group. Another open label study, without control, dealing with vardenafil administration in SCL patients, based on 38 patients, indicated achievement of erection, efficient for penetration in 83% of patients and duration of erection satisfactory for 88% of those (Kimoto et al., 2006).

Regarding tadalafil, there is a comparative study by Del Popolo et al. between sildenafil and tadalafil in patients with ED and SCL (Del Popolo et al., 2004). This was a randomized, blind; cross-over study with 15 patients in each arm and duration of 12 weeks. The study indicated that tadalafil allowed to the majority of patients to achieve a satisfactory erection for up to 24 hours after the administration of the drug, but this was due to pharmacokinetic of tadalafil. Additionally, an improvement of sexual satisfaction of both patients and their sexual partners has been recorded in both groups (sildenafil and tadalafil). In another multicenter, randomized, placebo-controlled study by Giuliano et al. was reported statistical significant improvement, to the tadalafil group, at the erectile function domain of the IIFF questionnaire and at the questions 2 and 3 of the Sexual Encounter Profile (SEP) which regards the achievement of sufficient erection and satisfactory intercourse (Giuliano et al., 2007). These findings were confirmed by another study by Lombardi et al., that reported improvement at the IIFF score and at the ability to achieve an efficient erection (SEP 2) and a satisfactory intercourse (SEP 3), in patients with SCL after the appropriate dose of tadalafil (Lombardi et al., 2008).

There is a comparative study of all PDE-5 inhibitors in patients with SCL which was published in 2007 (Soler et al., 2007). The study consisted of three groups of patients, according the PDE-5 inhibitor which was used. In the group of sildenafil there were 120 patients, in the group of vardenafil there were 66 patients and in the group of tadalafil there were 54 patients. Initially all patients received the lower dose of each drug and there was dose up regulation until the efficacy was sufficient. The overall efficacy was similar for all the drugs (85% for sildenafil, 74% for vardenafil and 72% for tadalafil). The duration of erections was also similar for all (26 - 34 minutes). The higher dose of the drug required in 45% in the group of sildenafil, compared with over 70% of the patients in the other two groups. In another meta-analysis of 18 studies, regarding PDE-5 inhibitors in men with SCL was reported statistical significant improvement of erectile function compared to placebo in 11 studies (Lombardi et al., 2009). The overall amount of patients was 705 in sildenafil, 305 in vardenafil and 224 in tadalafil. Only 15 patients stopped treatment due to adverse events. This meta-analysis came to the conclusion that the relatively small amount of patients and the different methodology of the studies do not allow reliable comparisons between the drugs. On the other hand, there is enough data in the literature supporting that PDE-5 inhibitors are safe and effective treatment option for the ED of men with SCL.

4.1.2 Vacuum devise

The use of vacuum device is an alternative treatment option for the ED of people with SCL, with satisfactory efficacy (Zasler & Katz, 1989; Heller et al., 1992). The vacuum device is a cylinder with an open edge. The penis is placed through the open edge inside the device and by pumping; vacuum is created inside the cylinder. The negative pressure forces the blood to fill the corpora cavernousa, causing erection. After erection a ring which is placed tight around the base of the penis is necessary for the maintenance of the erection (Fig. 3).

Efficacy and complications of these devices were studied in 20 patients and their partners (Denil et al., 1996). After 3 months of use, 93% of men and 83% of women reported erections sufficient for vaginal penetration which lasted for about 18 minutes. After 6 months, however, only 41% of men and 45% of women were satisfied with the use of vacuum device. The most unpleasant fact was the early loss of the rigidity of the erection. Overall, 60% of men and 42% of women reported improvement in their sexual lives by using the vacuum device. Finally, adverse effects such as bruising or swelling and even gangrene of the penis have been recorded (Rivas & Chancellor, 1994). The higher complication rate of vacuum device in men with SCL has to do with the absence of sensation in the area, so a very tight ring remaining for a long time can cause tissue ischemia and necrosis without any pain or disturbance. The appropriate advice for the people using the device is to be careful with the overall use and to avoid the very high negative pressure and the long-lasting strangle of the penile shaft.

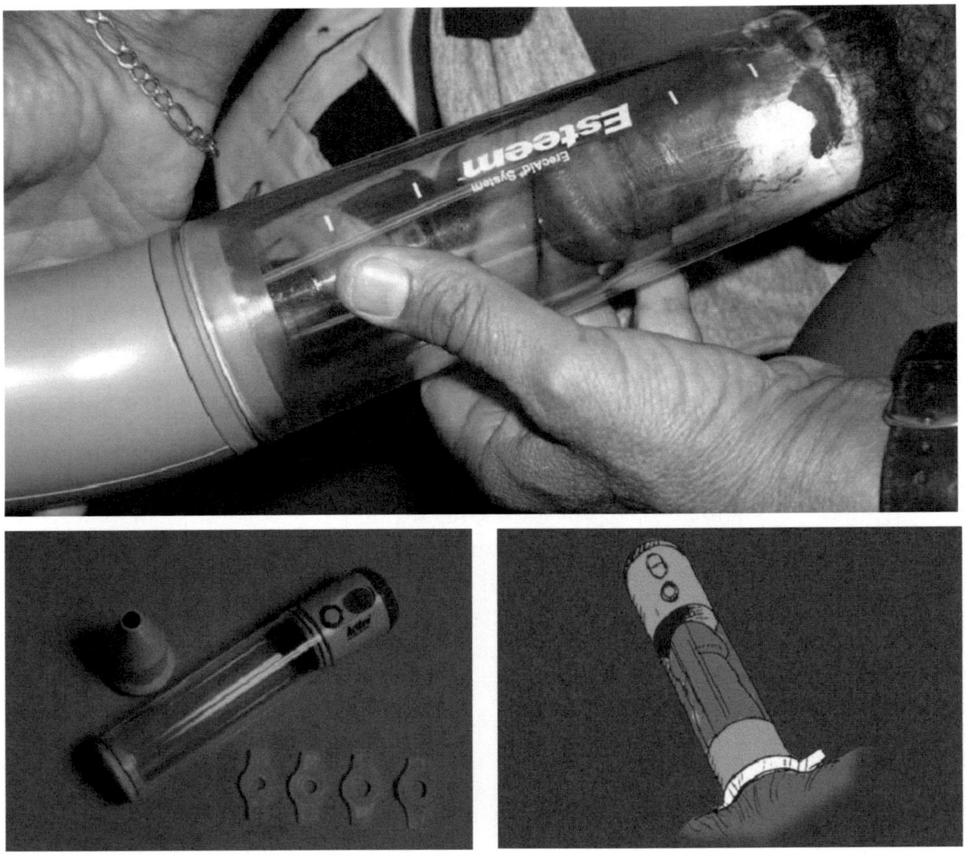

Fig. 3. The vacuum device is a cylinder with an open edge. The penis is placed through the open edge inside the device and by pumping; vacuum is created inside the cylinder.

4.2 Second line treatment

4.2.1 Intracavernousal injections of vasoactive substances

Men with ED after SCL respond very well to intracavernousal injections of vasoactive substances (Hirsch et al., 1994; Deforge et al 2006). This happens, because most of these people are young, with small likelihood of an additional vascular disease. The technique is simple and relatively painless. The high effectiveness of the injections in combination with the absence of sensation at the penis makes this choice friendlier to paraplegics. The injection takes place between the 1st and 3rd or between the 9th and 11th hours of the penile shaft (Fig. 4). A gentle massage of the area helps the drug to be absorbed. The erection begins five to ten minutes later and it is independent from any sexual arousal.

Most studies report high rates, which reach 95% response to vaso-active substances such as papaverine and alprostadil (Lebib Ben Achour et al., 2001; Dietzen & Lloyd, 1992). Side effects and complications described in the literature are: priapism, skin bruises and cavernosal fibrosis. Papaverine is responsible for higher rates of priapism and fibrosis than alprostadil. Patients with SCL develop priapism more often, maybe due to excessive release

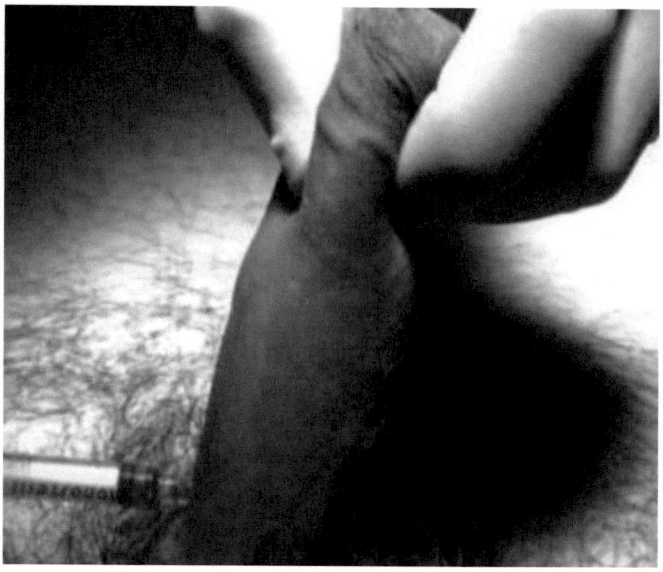

Fig. 4. The injection takes place between the 1st and 3rd or between the 9th and 11th hours of the penile shaft, after penile stretching.

of neurotransmitters which promote erection or due to sympathetic hypertonia. For these reasons in the beginning of the treatment lower doses of vasoactive drugs are used and the dose is entitled for each patient. In a meta-analysis of other studies, there was an overall rate of men with satisfactory erections reaching the 90% of the users of intracavernousal injections (DeForge et al., 2006). In another study there was a comparison between the use of vacuum device and the administration of injections of papaverine (Chancellor et al., 1994). Eighteen men with SCL participated in this study, which was cross-over designed. After both treatment options, half of the patients chose injections and half of them chose vacuum device.

4.2.2 Urethral administration of vasoactive substances

The communication between the corpora cavernosa and the corpus spongiosum was the base for the intra-urethral application of vasoactive drugs. Alprostadil (PGE1) has been used for this purpose. The way of action is the same to intracavernousal injections, without needles and punctures. There is an applicator which places the drug into the urethra (Fig. 5). The overall efficacy rate is reported at 65.9% of 995 men with ED (Padma-Nathan et al., 1997).

In patients with SCL the outcome was not as satisfactory as using intracavernousal injections (Bodner et al., 1999). Regarding adverse events, systemic absorption of alprostadil was responsible for hypotensive episodes. The use of a tight ring at the base of the penis is essential in order to avoid this rapid absorption and to maintain the achieved erection.

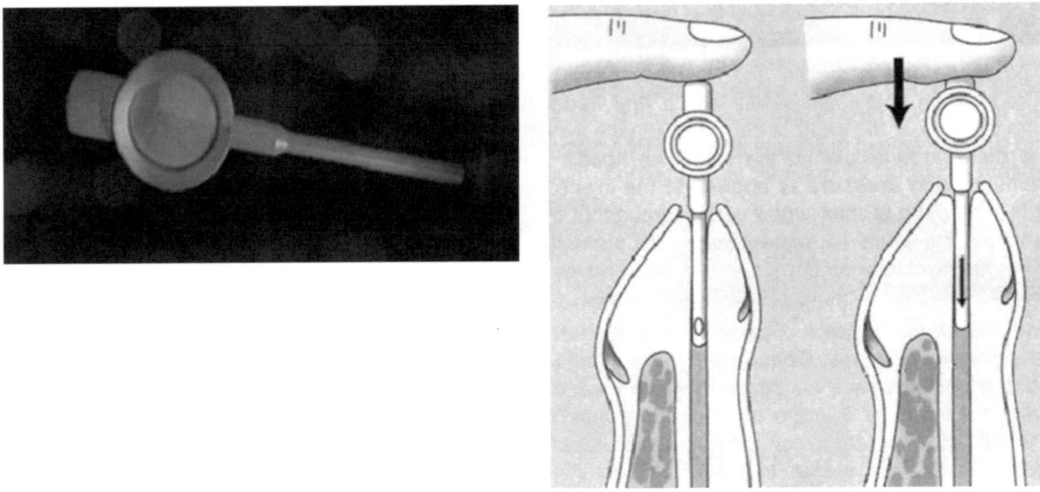

Fig. 5. For the intra-urethral placement of alprostadil a specific applicator is used.

4.3 Third line treatment

The implantation of penile prosthesis is the 3rd line treatment and represents the surgical option for the management of ED. The prosthesis can be malleable or hydraulic. Hydraulic one may consist of two or three pieces (Fig. 6). The application of penile prosthesis in men with SCL accompanied with a high rate of complications, as it was indicated in some older studies (Dietzen & Lloyd, 1992). In these series it was reported mechanical damage in 43%, infection in 37%, erosion in 10% and hematoma 7% of patients. An overall complication rate of 13.3% was also reported in another study (Kimoto & Iwatsubo, 1994).

As the prosthesis models become more contemporary the results improve as well. In a relatively recent study a total number of 245 patients with SCL participated (Zermann et al., 2006). Apart from the restoration of erectile function, penile prosthesis implantation offered a wide enough penis in order to achieve a better fixation of a condom catheter. Regarding erectile function, 82.6% of men and 67.5% of their sexual partners reported the treatment as successful. Complication rate was lower than in older studies. It was reported infection in 5%, and erosion from 0 to 18% depending on the type of prosthesis (none for the three pieces inflatable ones and 18% for the malleable types). In a meta-analysis based on five previous studies where prostheses were implanted in patients with SCL, serious complications were reported in 10% of the cases. On the other hand, patients who experienced no complications were very satisfied (Deforge et al., 2006; Xuan et al., 2007). The higher complication rate which is reported in paraplegics, compare to ambulant, impotent patients probably has to do with the absence of sensation which may lead to excessive use of the prosthesis which is compressing the glans and the other tissues, causing ischemia. This is the first step for erosion. Generally speaking, a penile prosthesis improves the quality of life of patients with SCL significantly; however, erosion and infection are still remarkable problems.

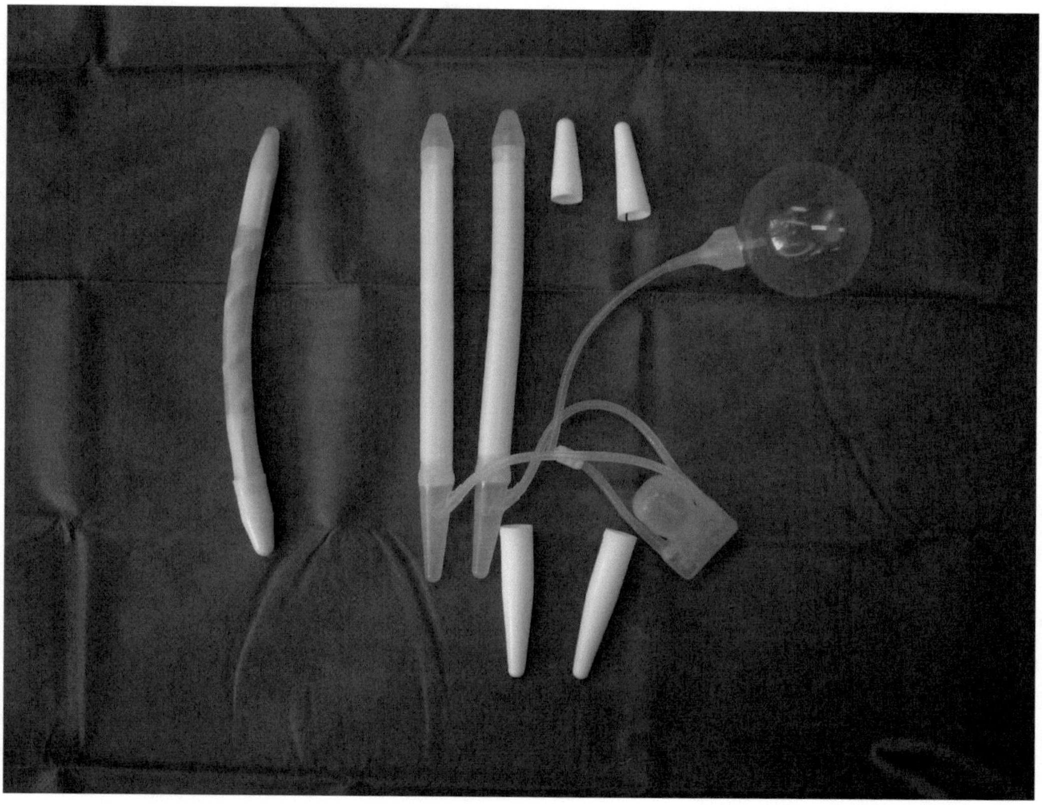

Fig. 6. On the left: a malleable prosthesis (one of the two cylindrical pieces); on the right: a three pieces inflatable prosthesis with some of additional tips. You can distinguish the cylinders, the pump and the reservoir.

5. Therapeutic strategy

The accurate diagnostic for SCL is crucial for choosing an adequate treatment. The level, the extension and the total or partial character of the neural damage may drive to one or other treatment option. Generally, patients with partial section of the spinal cord will respond better to oral or topical treatments. It has been also proven that oral pharmacotherapy with PDE-5 inhibitors is more effective if at least one of the erection centers has maintained. At the begging, PDE-5 inhibitors were used in patients with intact S2-4 reflex arc, which indicated the integrity of parasympathetic erection center. Later on, it was found that this kind of pharmacotherapy is also effective in patients who did not appear any spontaneous erectile function. In general, patients with lesions at higher levels respond better to oral therapy.

The use of vacuum device and penile injections require skill on behalf of the patients. Tetraplegic patients face more difficulties in the appliance of these therapies, which are possible only by the partner's contribution. If the patient is a condom catheter user due to incontinence, penile prosthesis may offer a solution for both erectile dysfunction and incontinence, by supporting a better fixation of the condom catheter.

In our center we use an algorithm for the management of ED in paraplegics. This is described below: If the patient has residual (spontaneous or induced by sexual arousal) erection, which is, in general, not sufficient for vaginal penetration, vacuum device and/or oral pharmacotherapy with PDE-5 inhibitors are offered. If the patient is not satisfied we apply intracavernousal injections of vasoactive drugs, alprostadil in most cases. At this point the majority of our patients is satisfied. In cases that there is fibrosis of the cavernosal tissue, usually after recurrent priapism episodes, penile prosthesis remains the only reliable choice for the management of the ED of these men. The implantation of the penile prosthesis is the ultimate therapeutic option with excellent results. Finally, it has to become clear to all patients that the above treatment options are suitable for the ED and do not solve the ejaculation or/and orgasm disorders they might experienced.

The role of sexual partner is very important as the partner must be part of the therapeutic option. The couple has to "open its mind" regarding the sexual activity. They must compromise, at the beginning, and finally, regulate their sexual lives in a status that penetration is not the main sexual activity.

6. Conclusion

Men with paraplegia suffer from sexual dysfunction which impacts the quality of their life and affects their partners. ED, possible absence of orgasm and infertility are conditions related to paraplegia. Patients with SCL face neurogenic ED. Erection is a neurovascular phenomenon which takes place under neuro-hormonal control. Any lesion at the involved neural pathways is responsible for this dysfunction. On the other hand the vascular element of the erection is, in general, healthy. According to these principals, the treatment strategy is designed and applied. No therapeutic method is efficient and suitable for all patients. Treatment must follow the wishes, the mental level and the skills of the patient according the needs of the couple.

The physicians who treat paraplegic patients must take these conditions into consideration. A team work by rehabilitation doctors, urologists and psychiatrics is needed for the optimal treatment option.Sexual rehabilitation targets in neuromodulation using voluntary release of a reflex erection attempting to use this erection for sexual purpose. This is possible through stimulation of the skin or mucosa below the level of the lesion. If a trigger point which promotes an erection is identified, patient has to get familiar with the onset of this reflex in order to use it during sexual activity.

Treatment options like PDE-5 inhibitors, vacuum devices, intracavernousal injections or intra-urethral administration of vasoactive medications and penile prosthesis are in specialist's armament for the treatment of erectile dysfunction in men with paraplegia.The oral treatment with PDE-5 inhibitors is effective in the majority of paraplegic patients.

Vacuum device is a reliable treatment option with some restrictions. The most effective conservative treatment is the intracavernousal injection of vasoactive drugs, as the erectile dysfunction is not caused by vascular inefficiency. Urethral application of vasoactive drugs is less effective and is associated with high incidence of hypotension. The implantation of penile prosthesis remains the most effective treatment option, which is associated with a relatively high rate of complications (~10%) in this population (Deforge et al., 2006). Sexual rehabilitation remains very important for the physical rehabilitation and the active return of these people to the society.

7. References

Biering-Sorensen F & Sonksen J. Sexual function in spinal cord lesioned men. *Spinal Cord* 2001 Sep; 39(9):455-470

Bird SJ & Hanno PM. Bulbocavernosus reflex studies and autonomic testing in the diagnosis of erectile dysfunction. *J Neurol Sci* 1998 Jan 21; 154(1):8-13

Bodner DR, Haas CA, Krueger B & Seftel AD. Intraurethral alprostadil for treatment of erectile dysfunction in patients with spinal cord injury. *Urology* 1999 Jan; 53(1):199-202

Chancellor MB, Rivas DA, Panzer DE, Freedman MK & Staas WE Jr. Prospective comparison of topical minoxidil to vacuum constriction device and intracorporeal papaverine injection in treatment of erectile dysfunction due to spinal cord injury. *Urology.* 1994 Mar; 43(3):365-9.

Chapelle PA, Durand J & Lacert P. Penile erection following complete spinal cord injury in man. *Br J Urol* 1980 Jun; 52(3):216-219

Courtois FJ, Macdougall JC & Sachs BD: Erectile mechanism in paraplegia. *Physiol Behav* 1993; 53:721-726

Courtois FJ, Goulet MC, Charvier KF & Leriche A. Posttraumatic erectile potential of spinal cord injured men: how physiologic recordings supplement subjective reports *Arch Phys Med Rehabil.* 1999 Oct; 80(10):1268-1272

Deforge D, Blackmer J, Garritty C, Yazdi F, Cronin V, Barrowman N, Fang M, Mamaladze V, Zhang L, Sampson M & Moher D. Male erectile dysfunction following spinal cord injury: a systematic review. *Spinal Cord* 2006 Aug; 44(8):465-473

Del Popolo G, Li Marzi V, Mondaini N & Lombardi G. Time/duration effectiveness of sildenafil versus tadalafil in the treatment of erectile dysfunction in male spinal cord-injured patients. *Spinal Cord* 2004 Nov; 42(11):643-648

Denil J, Ohl DA & Smythe C. Vacuum erection device in spinal cord injured men: patient and partner satisfaction. *Arch Phys Med Rehabil* 1996 Aug; 77(8):750-753

Derry F, Hultling C, Seftel AD & Sipski ML. Efficacy and safety of sildenafil citrate (Viagra) in men with erectile dysfunction and spinal cord injury: a review. *Urology* 2002 Sep; 60(2 Suppl 2):49-57

Dietzen CJ & Lloyd LK. Complications of intracavernous injections and penile prostheses in spinal cord injured men. *Arch Phys Med Rehabil* 1992 Jul; 73(7):652-655

Eardley I & Kirby R: Neurogenic impotence. In: Kirby RS, Carson CC, Webster GD, ed. *Impotence: Diagnosis and Management of Male Erectile Dysfunction,* Oxford: Butterworth-Heinemann; 1991:227-231.

Fisher TL, Laud PW, Byfield MG, Brown TT, Hayat MJ & Fiedler IG. Sexual health after spinal cord injury: a longitudinal study. *Arch Phys Med Rehabil* 2002 Aug; 83(8):1043-1051

Frankel HL & Mathias CJ. Severe hypertension in patients with high spinal cord lesions undergoing electro-ejaculation--management with prostaglandin E2. *Paraplegia.* 1980 Oct; 18(5):293-299

Giuliano F, Hultling C, El Masry WS, Smith MD, Osterloh IH, Orr M & Maytom M. Randomized trial of sildenafil for the treatment of erectile dysfunction in spinal cord injury. Sildenafil Study Group. *Ann Neurol.* 1999 Jul; 46(1):15-21

Giuliano F, Rubio-Aurioles E, Kennelly M, Montorsi F, Kim ED, Finkbeiner AE Pommerville PJ, Colopy MW, Wilkins HJ & Wachs BH; Vardenafil Study Group. Efficacy and safety of vardenafil in men with erectile dysfunction caused by spinal cord injury. *Neurology* 2006 Jan 24; 66(2):210-216

Giuliano F, Sanchez-Ramos A, Löchner-Ernst D, Del Popolo G, Cruz N, Leriche A, Lombardi G, Reichert S, Dahl P, Elion-Mboussa A & Casariego J. Efficacy and safety of tadalafil in men with erectile dysfunction following spinal cord injury. *Arch Neurol.* 2007 Nov;64(11):1584-92. Epub 2007 Sep 10

Harrop JS, Sharan A & Ratliff J. Central cord injury: pathophysiology, management, and outcomes. *Spine J.* 2006 Nov-Dec; 6 (6 Suppl):S198-206

Heller L, Keren O, Aloni R & Davidoff G. An open trial of vacuum penile tumescence: constriction therapy for neurological impotence. *Paraplegia* 1992 Aug; 30(8):550-553

Hirsch IH, Smith RL, Chancellor MB, Bagley DH, Carsello J & Staas WE Jr. Use of intracavernous injection of prostaglandin E1 for neuropathic erectile dysfunction. *Paraplegia.* 1994 Oct;32(10):661-4.

Kim SH. Post-traumatic erectile dysfunction: Doppler US findings. *Abdom Imaging* 2006 Sep-Oct; 31(5):598-609

Kimoto Y & Iwatsubo E. Penile prostheses for the management of the neuropathic bladder and sexual dysfunction in spinal cord injury patients: long term follow up. *Paraplegia.* 1994 May; 32(5):336-9.

Kimoto Y, Sakamoto S, Fujikawa K, Tachibana T, Yamamoto N & Otani T. Up-titration of vardena fi l dose from 10 mg to 20 mg improved erectile function in men with spinal cord injury *Int J Urol* 2006 Nov; 13(11):1428-1433

Lebib Ben Achour S, Laffont I, Boyer F, Boiteau F & Dizien O. Intracavernous injections in the treatment of erectile dysfunction in spinal cord injured patients: experience with 36 patients. *Ann Readapt Med Phys* 2001 Feb; 44(1):35-40

Lombardi G, Macchiarella A, Cecconi F & Del Popolo G. Efficacy and safety of medium and long-term tadalafil use in spinal cord patients with erectile dysfunction. *J Sex Med.* 2009 Feb;6(2):535-43. Epub 2008 Dec 2

Lombardi G, Macchiarella A, Cecconi F & Del Popolo G. Ten years of phosphodiesterase type 5 inhibitors in spinal cord injured patients. *J Sex Med.* 2009 May;6(5):1248-58. Epub 2009 Feb 9.

Maytom MC, Derry FA, Dinsmore WW, Glass CA, Smith MD, Orr M & Osterloh IH. A two-part pilot study of sildenafil (VIAGRA) in men with erectile dysfunction caused by spinal cord injury. *Spinal Cord.* 1999 Feb; 37(2):110-116

Mittmann N, Craven BC, Gordon M, MacMillan DH, Hassouna M, Raynard W, Kaiser A, Lanctôt LK & Tarride JE. Erectile dysfunction in spinal cord injury: a cost-utility analysis. *J Rehabil Med* 2005 Nov; 37(6):358-364

Monga M, Bernie J & Rajasekaran M. Male infertility and erectile dysfunction in spinal cord injury: a review. *Arch Phys Med Rehabil* 1999 Oct; 80(10):1331-1339

Padma-Nathan H, Hellstrom WJ, Kaiser FE, Labasky RF, Lue TF, Nolten WE, Norwood PC, Peterson CA, Shabsigh R, Tam PY, Place VA & Gesundheit N. Treatment of men with erectile dysfunction with transurethral alprostadil. Medicated Urethral System for Erection (MUSE) Study Group. *N Engl J Med* 1997 Jan 2; 336(1):1-7.

Ramos AS & Samso JV. Specific aspects of erectile dysfunction in spinal cord injury. *Int J Impot Res* 2004 Oct; 16 Suppl 2:S42-45

Rivas DA & Chancellor MB. Complications associated with the use of vacuum constriction devices for erectile dysfunction in the spinal cord injured population. *J Am Paraplegia Soc* 1994 Jul; 17(3):136-139

Robinson LQ, Woodcock JP & Stephenson TP. Results of investigation of impotence in patients with overt or probable neuropathy. *Br J Urol* 1987, 60:583–587

Rossier AB, Ziegler WH, Duchosal PW & Meylan J. Sexual function and Dysreflexia. *Paraplegia* 1971 May;9(1):51-63

Saenz de Tejada I, Angulo J, Cellek S, Gonzalez-Cadavid N, Heaton J, Pickard R & Simonsen U. Pathophysiology of erectile dysfunction. *J Sex Med* 2005 Jan; 2(1):26-39

Sánchez Ramos A, Vidal J, Jáuregui ML, Barrera M, Recio C, Giner M, Toribio L, Salvador S, Sanmartín A, de la Fuente M, Santos JF, de Juan FJ, Moraleda S, Méndez JL, Ramírez L & Casado RM. Efficacy, safety and predictive factors of therapeutic success with sildenafil for erectile dysfunction in patients with different spinal cord injuries. *Spinal Cord.* 2001 Dec; 39(12):637-43

Smith EM & Bodner DR. Sexual dysfunction after spinal cord injury. *Urol Clin North Am* 1993 Aug; 20(3):535-542

Soler JM, Previnaire JG, Denys P & Chartier-Kastler E. Phosphodiesterase inhibitors in the treatment of erectile dysfunction in spinal cord-injured men. *Spinal Cord.* 2007 Feb; 45(2):169-173

Suh DD, Yang CC & Clowers DE. Nocturnal penile tumescence and effects of complete spinal cord injury: possible physiologic mechanisms. *Urology* 2003 Jan; 61(1):184-189

Tay HP, Juma S & Joseph AC. Psychogenic impotence in spinal cord injury patients. *Arch Phys Med Rehabil* 1996 Apr; 77(4):391-393

Vodusek DB. Bulbocavernous reflex revisited. *Neurourol Urodyn* 2003; 22(7): 681-682

Xuan XJ, Wang DH, Sun P & Mei H. Outcome of implanting penile prosthesis for treating erectile dysfunction: experience with 42 cases. *Asian J Androl.* 2007 Sep; 9(5):716-9.

Zasler ND & Katz PG. Synergist erection system in the management of impotence secondary to spinal cord injury. Arch Phys Med Rehabil 1989 Sep; 70(9):712-716

Zermann DH, Kutzenberger J, Sauerwein D, Schubert J & Loeffler U. Penile prosthetic surgery in neurologically impaired patients: long-term follow up. J Urol 2006 Mar; 175(3 Pt 1):1041-1044; discussion 1044

Part 3

ED Treatment Options and Perspectives

8

Current Perspectives on Pharmacotherapy Treatments for Erectile Dysfunction

Jason E. Davis, Kenia Pedrosa Nunes,
Inger Stallmann-Jorgensen and R. Clinton Webb
Georgia Health Sciences University, Augusta, Georgia
USA

1. Introduction

Erectile dysfunction (ED) is the most common sexual problem in men [1]. ED is defined as a difficulty in initiating or maintaining penile erection adequate for sexual activity. ED has a weighty effect on intimate relationships, quality of life, and overall self-esteem for men. In addition, ED may also be an early indication of undetected cardiovascular disease [2]. One of the largest current studies of ED, the Massachusetts Male Aging Study, established that the prevalence of ED increases with age as it affects up to half of the male population between 40 and 70 years old [3]. Thus, as the world's older population increases, it is estimated that the prevalence of ED will double from 152 million men in 1995 to 322 million men in 2025, indicating a dire need to reevaluate current ED therapeutic strategies [4]. In most documented cases, ED may also present with comorbidities of hypertension, diabetes mellitus, obesity, and atherosclerosis [3].

During the 1980s, most of the pioneering research in ED was sparked by the introduction of intracavernosal vasoactive drugs, which were very effective as agents inducing penile rigidity [5]. It was not until the late 1990's and early 2000's that oral phosphodiesterase-5 inhibitors were introduced, which were truly instrumental in revolutionizing the sexual medicine field [6]. Today, first-line therapy for the treatment of ED consists of orally as well as sublingually administered drugs, while intracavernosal injection (ICI), therapy, which involves direct injection of vasoactive agents into cavernosal tissue, is considered only as a second-line therapy. This chapter will discuss current perspectives on ED's pharmacotherapy and present a more in-depth review on treatments for ED, based on the works from Andersson, K.E. [7] and Uckert, S. [8].

2. First-line treatment: Oral pharmacotherapy

2.1 PDE5 inhibitors

The family of phosphodiesterases is comprised of 11 catalytic enzymes that regulate the second messenger activity in cells by cleavage of the phosphodiester bond of either cyclic adenosine monophosphate (cAMP) or cyclic guanosine monophosphate (cGMP), or both [9] PDE5 is present in high concentrations in the smooth muscle of corpora cavernosa of the penis and in the smooth muscle of the pudendal arteries; therefore, phosphodiesterase 5 inhibitors (PDE5) are the major initial line of pharmacotherapy for erectile dysfunction (ED). PDEs are orally active agents that are taken, on demand, prior to sexual intercourse [9]. PDE5 was discovered by Corbin and colleagues [3, 4]. The PDE5 enzyme is a homo-dimer with two identical subunits, and each subunit is 100,000 kilo Daltons. Both subunits have a catalytic domain and a regulatory domain; however, it is the catalytic domain that is the main target for PDE5 inhibitors [9]. Nevertheless, it was the discovery of nitric oxide (NO) and cGMP as the major effectors in penile smooth muscle relaxation that led to the identification of PDE5 inhibitors that can further elevate intracellular levels of cGMP [10-11]. Most PDE5 inhibitors have a comparable structure to sildenafil; in addition, a part of the molecular structure of most PDE5 inhibitors bears resemblance to the cGMP structure. This is of significance since PDE5 inhibitors are competitive antagonists of both cGMP and PDE5 [7].

The actions of PDE5 inhibitors are often described in terms of their selectivity when compared to other PDE inhibitors. The selectivity of PDE5 inhibitors is a key factor since studies have shown that some PDE5 inhibitors may cross-react with PDE6, (predominant phosphodiesterase in the retina), causing visual disturbances; for example perception of bluish haze and increased light sensitivity, has occurred in some patients [12-13]. Additionally, some PDE5 inhibitors also cross-react with PDE11; PDE11 is mainly located in cardiac, testicular and pituitary tissues of the heart and testes; however, the consequences of this cross-reaction are unknown [7]. The normal pathway for penile erection is by sexual stimulation, which releases NO at nerve endings in the penis whereby increasing the blood supply to the penis. NO, the major vasodilatory agent causes this increase in blood by diffusing into vascular smooth muscle cells in both the penile corpus cavernosum and the pudendal arteries to cause stimulation of guanylyl cyclase (GS). Elevation of cGMP in these cells leads to the activation of cGMP-dependent protein kinase (PKG), a lowering of intracellular calcium, resulting in smooth muscle relaxation. PDE5 inhibitors act by selectively enhancing erectile function by penetrating into smooth muscle cells and inhibiting PDE5, resulting in decreased breakdown of cGMP, thus PDE5 inhibitors increase blood flow of the smooth muscle by increasing relaxation, allowing for an erection to occur [9, 14]. PDE5 inhibitors are degraded in the liver, since they are not metabolized by any other enzymes in the smooth muscle cells of the corpus cavernosum. So, PDE5 inhibitors must be transported to the liver in order to be degraded. This is important to note, as it determines the duration of action, because the disappearance of the inhibitor from the plasma may indicate, but does not always prove, its clearance from the cells in which its effects were produced [9].

PDE5 inhibitors are the most widely used treatment for ED and their efficacy have been rigorously evaluated in numerous clinical trials [8]. Subjects receiving a PDE5 inhibitor report erections adequate for sexual intercourse [8, 15]. However, PDE5 inhibitors seem to be less effective in studies where male subjects have comorbid diseases such as diabetes [16]. Nevertheless, PDE5 inhibitors remain the primary line of oral treatment, and the most common reported side effects include headaches, dyspepsia, and nasal congestion [17-19]. In regard to cardiovascular (CV) safety, PDE5 inhibitors have proven to be safe in patients with CV disease; however, due to their mechanisms of action, PDE5 inhibitors are contraindicated in ED patients taking nitrates due to unpredictable hypotension [8]. On the other hand, it should be noted that the interaction between organic nitrates and PDE5 inhibitors varies according to the PDE5 inhibitor and the nitrate used [7].

2.1.1 Sildenafil

Since the launch of sildenafil as an effective basis for the treatment of ED in 1998, similar agents have undergone clinical trials and have been subsequently introduced into clinical practice [14]. There is clear evidence that sildenafil is efficacious in the treatment of ED for the broad population of men [20]. As a result, sildenafil has proven effective in cases when ED has arisen as a consequence of comorbid diseases such as diabetes, depression, cardiovascular disease, hypertension and lower urinary tract infections [9].

Sildenafil has shown efficacy when taken at doses of 25, 50, or 100 mg and has an onset of action usually within 25–60 minutes; however, absorption of the drug is slowed with food [9, 14, 21]. Minor side effects do occur with the use of sildenafil; the most reported side effects were headaches, flushing, indigestion, and visual changes [9, 19, 22]. Sildenafil will most likely continue to be the drug of choice for physicians, since there have not been any reports that have cast uncertainty on its safety for men with ED.

2.1.2 Udenafil (DA-8159)

Udenafil (DA-8159) is a PDE5 inhibitor; it is a long-acting drug with a half-time ($t1/2$) of 11–13 hours, and it has a relatively fast absorption with the plasma concentration after ingestion reaching its tmax, that is, its peak drug level, in 1–1.5 hours [4]. Phase II clinical trial data revealed that in men with mild-to-severe ED, udenafil produced a considerable improvement in erectile function after 12 weeks of treatment [8]. A phase III study in Korea evaluated the efficacy and safety of udenafil in ED patients. All responses to udenafil were significantly greater than the placebo ($p < 0.0001$) and patients receiving either udenafil doses of 100 mg or 200 mg were significantly ($p < 0.0001$) more satisfied with their sex life compared with men taking the placebo [4]. In animal studies, the administration of DA-8159 (0.3 or 1 mg/kg) induced a dose-frequency dependent increase in intracavernosal pressure (ICP); chronic treatment with DA-8159 restored erectile responses induced by electric stimulation, improved endothelial function, and significantly decreased plasma levels of both endothelin, (a potent vasoconstrictor), and asymmetrical dimethyl arginine (ADMA), (an inhibitor of NO production) [8]. Udenafil has been reported to be a well tolerated, since most of the adverse side effects were flushing, upset stomach and headaches, which were generally mild to moderate [4, 8].

2.1.3 Avanafil

Avanafil is a pyrimidine derivative synthesized to be a highly selective PDE5 inhibitor for the treatment of ED [9]. Studies have shown that up to 84% of avanafil doses resulted in sufficient erections for sexual activity, as compared to placebo [8]. In clinical trials, avanafil showed a higher selectivity, almost 120-fold, against PDE6 than both sildenafil and vardenafil [4]. Additionally, when compared with sildenafil, vardenafil, and tadalafil (described later), avanafil's chemical structure is distinctive from the standard nucleic base/sugar/phosphate diester model; avanafil's molecular structure is a nitrogen derivative of a pyrimidine carboxamide where the nitrogen atom of the amide substituent is bound to a pyrimidinylmethyl group [8]. As a result of its unique chemical structure, theoretically, avanafil can bind to the catalytic site of PDE5 regardless of the spatial orientation of the molecule, significantly increasing the effectiveness and affinity of the inhibitor for PDE5 [8]. In the pharmacokinetic evaluation of this drug, studies reported rapid absorption with a tmax approximately 35 minutes and a short t1/2 of less than 1.5 hours without any unwanted accumulation of the drug [4]. Favorable data from a nitrate interaction study showed only a modest impact on blood pressure and heart rate [23-24].

2.1.4 Lodenafil

Lodenafil carbonate is a newer PDE5 inhibitor; it is a dimer formed by two lodenafil molecules linked by a carbonate bridge [11]. After ingestion, the carbonate bridge is broken delivering the active lodenafil compound [8, 25]. The effects of lodenafil have been extensively investigated in vitro; the drug was noted to cause concentration-dependent relaxation of both rabbit and human corpus cavernosum tissue by amplifying the NO-dependent relaxation of the penile tissue in response to acetylcholine or transmural electrical field stimulation (EFS) [8]. In comparison lodenafil was shown to be approximately twofold more potent than sildenafil for inhibition of the breakdown of cGMP [26]. Its efficacy and safety at doses of 20 mg, 40 mg and 80 mg was also tested and shown to significantly improve erectile International Index of Erectile Function domain scores (IIEF domain scores: a widely used, multi-dimensional self-reporting instrument for the evaluation of male sexual function), with only mild to moderate adverse reactions such as headache, flushing, visual disorders, and dyspepsia [9, 26]. Lodenafil is an attractive pharmacotherapy agent for the treatment of ED [25-26].

2.1.5 Tadalafil

Tadalafil has proven to be efficacious in a number of special populations of men in which ED is due to a variety of conditions including diabetes, radiation therapy for prostatic cancer, spinal cord injury, and lower urinary tract infection [9, 27]. When taken at doses of 10 and 20 mg, tadalafil significantly improved erectile function and was well-tolerated, as the only reported side effects were headache, flushing, indigestion, nasal congestion, and back or girdle pain [9, 27-28]. At present there is no convincing evidence of any significant safety issues regarding cardiovascular contraindications with the use of tadalafil when taking the recommended doses of 2.5 mg and 5 mg per day [7, 28].

2.1.6 Vardenafil

Vardenafil is an effective vasoactive agent for the treatment of ED in a broad population at doses of 10 mg and 20 mg [9, 29]. Vardenafil was even able to cause adequate erections for sexual activity in special populations, where ED was a result of diabetes, chemotherapy, depression, hypertension, and spinal cord injury [9, 29]. Vardenafil has a mechanism of action similar to other PDE5 inhibitors, thus its side effects are similar to those reported by other PDE5 inhibitors such as headache, flushing, indigestion, and nasal congestion [4, 9]. Overall, vardenafil remains a highly recommended vasoactive agent, since it has been proven beneficial for a wide variety of patients with ED, and at present, there is no convincing evidence of any significant safety issues, regarding cardiovascular contraindications, with its use [7, 9, 29].

2.2 Trazodone

Trazodone is an "atypical" antidepressive agent and it selectively inhibits central 5-hydroxytryptamine (5-HT) uptake by increasing the turnover of brain dopamines [30]. Trazodone has alpha-adrenergic blocking effects (α-AR) and, together with its meta-chlorophenylpiperazine (*m*-CCP) metabolite, trazodone is known to induce erections in animal studies by selectively blocking the α-AR receptors and by increasing the spontaneous firing rate of cavernosal tissue nerves [31]. Despite its promising mode of actions within the cavernosum tissue, trazodone is not an effective treatment for most men with ED, since orally administered trazodone has been associated with high frequencies of priapism [32]. Furthermore, in a double-blind, placebo trial trazodone was not effective even at high doses of 150 to 200 mg per day [30, 33-34]. However, trazodone is still a viable option for men with psychogenic ED, resulting from anxiety or depression [33-34].

2.3 Melanocortin receptor agonists (PT-141)

PT-141 was initially produced as a tanning agent; however it was discovered, when it was injected subcutaneously, to initiate potent erections in men with nonorganic ED [35-36]. PT-141 is a synthetic cyclic nonselective melanocortin receptor agonist, with a high affinity to MC receptors 1, 3, and 4, and it is believed to be a metabolite of melanotan-II (MT-II) [36]. Theoretically, MC receptor agonists may have beneficial effects in patients with ED based on the results from a double-blind, placebo-controlled study in which PT-141, at doses ranging from 4 to 20 mg, was administered to 32 healthy subjects [37]. Results from this study showed that PT-141 significantly increased erectile activity even without visual sexual stimulation, compared with placebo-treated subjects. Additionally, in a placebo-controlled crossover trial, men with mild to moderate ED, treated with PT-141 together with visual sexual stimulation, experienced a threefold increase in erectile activity when compared to the placebo [37]. Co-administration of PT-141 with sildenafil 25 mg significantly increased penile rigidity when compared with sildenafil alone [7, 37]. It was also noted that, when patients took the two drugs in combination, there were no significant increase in the side effects, compared to those experienced, when taking either sildenafil or PT-141 alone [7].

2.4 Potassium-channel Openers

Potassium channel openers such as pinacidil, cromakalim, lemakalim, and nicorandil have all been shown as efficacious in achieving erections in men with ED [7]. Potassium channel openers work by hyperpolarizing the cell membrane, which increases the cell membrane permeability to potassium ions causing relaxation and subsequent erection [7]. Presently, clinical experience with these potassium channel openers for treatment of ED is limited; therefore, potassium channel agonist drugs have not been approved in controlled clinical trials as an alternative treatment for men with ED [7].

2.5 Rho-kinase inhibitors

Smooth muscle contraction and relaxation is related to the level of free cytosolic calcium, which is partly regulated by the accumulation of intracellular secondary messengers such as inositol triphosphate (IP_3) and diacylglycerol (DAG) via phospholipase C (PLC) activation [3]. PLC activation facilitates the release of and the increase of intracellular Ca^{2+}

concentration, resulting in calcium binding to calmodulin and subsequent activation of myosin light chain kinase [3]. When intracellular calcium levels decrease, RhoA, a small monomeric G protein, activates Rho-kinase; in turn, Rho-kinase phosphorylates and simultaneously inhibits the regulatory subunit of myosin light chain phosphatase [3, 38-39]. Thus, Rho-kinase is considered essential to the cell calcium sensitization system as its activation creates a cascade whereby the phosphorylation of myosin light chains triggers cycling of myosin cross-bridges along actin filaments, generating a contractile force that is maintained, unless inhibited, within the corpus cavernosum tissue [38]. It was first shown by Chitaley, K., et al. that Rho-kinase contributes to smooth muscle tone in the corpus cavernosum [40]. Injection of the Rho-kinase inhibitor Y-27632 into cavernosal sinuses increased intracavernosal pressure within minutes in a dose-dependent manner, without significantly decreasing systemic blood pressure [40]. Furthermore, the increase in intracavernosal pressure with Rho-inhibition was independent of the relaxing effects of N.O. and of guanylate cyclase, indicating that the Rho-kinase pathway may be an alternative therapeutic target for treating ED [38, 40]. In animal studies the Rho-kinase inhibitor fasudil, was effective against vasculogenic ED, in addition it was capable of reducing levels of pelvic atherosclerosis [41]. In a recent study involving diabetic-associated ED in rats, it was shown that chronic administration of fasudil was more effective, than other popular ED treatments, at reversing the damaging biochemical changes invoked by high insulin levels [42].

Human clinical trials have recently reported that low-dose atorvastatin (*Lipitor*), (a drug which works by inhibiting HMG-CoA reductase, an enzyme found in liver tissue, that plays a key role in production of cholesterol in the body), normalizes the diabetic response to sildenafil in streptozotocin (STZ) treated diabetic rats [43]. This result suggests that statins may also have inhibitory actions in the RhoA/Rho-kinase mechanism [42-43].

2.6 Alternative treatments for ED

2.6.1 HERBAL treatment for ED (Yohimbine)

Though herbal medicines are not a prescribed option of choice for patients in the United States, in other parts of the world like Asia, Africa and the Middle East, it is a widely used form of therapy for men with ED [44]. However, although there are a myriad of herbal treatments that are very appealing for patients with ED, caution must be warranted, since some herbal medicines may cause deleterious drug interactions, especially in men with comorbid diseases such as CV and diabetes. On the other hand, the herbal or traditional therapeutic approach may be more culturally acceptable with some patients, who may prefer this holistic option because of religious, social, monetary or other personal preferences. As a result, there is a growing interest among the population for alternative holistic treatment options, which has increased demand for such therapies in the United States [44]. Though there are many herbal remedies available at present for ED, this review will focus on the efficacy of yohimbine.

Yohimbine is an alkaloid derived from the African yohimbe tree (*Pausinystalia yohimbe*) [44]. Yohimbine has been well characterized as an alpha-2 adrenergic receptor (α_2-AR) antagonist [44]. It specifically inhibits the pre-synaptic α-2 adrenergic receptors in the brain; as a result there is a reduction of sympathetic tone since the brain and spinal cord noradrenaline levels are diminished [45]. The plasma half-life of yohimbine was found to be 0.6 hours, whereas the plasma noradrenergic effects of the drug lasted for more than 12 hours [46]. Theoretically, yohimbine should be a very effective treatment for ED; nevertheless, in several controlled trials on patients with different types of ED, yohimbine only produced modest effects [7]. However, a comprehensive systematic review demonstrated the advantage of yohimbine over a placebo in the treatment of ED [44, 47]. In combination with other drugs, oral yohimbine (15 mg daily) with trazodone (50 mg daily) was found to be a safe and effective treatment for psychogenic ED [44]. Despite its growing popularity, yohimbine is not currently recommended in most guidelines for management of ED, due to conflicting clinical reports concerning its efficacy [7].

2.6.2 Antioxidant therapy (Quercetin)

Oxidative stress occurs when there is an imbalance between pro-oxidants and antioxidants' ability to scavenge reactive oxygen species (ROS) [48]. ROS rapidly inactivate NO, thereby limiting its ability to relax smooth muscle [49]. Studies have also demonstrated that ROS have a central role in inducing apoptosis in cavernosum tissues [49-50]. Thus, there is overwhelming evidence implicating the role of oxidative stress in the pathophysiology of ED [48]. As a result, antioxidant treatment to regulate ROS is being explored as a potential therapeutic treatment for ED [49].

Quercetin (pentahydroxyflavone) is the most abundant flavonoid in the human diet, and it is available without a prescription as a dietary supplement [51]. Flavonoids are plant phenolic compounds with strong antioxidant properties, and they are found in various dietary sources, such as tea, onion, and broccoli. Quercetin is a potent anti-oxidant, and its mechanism of action involves the direct scavenging of free radicals such as hydrogen peroxide and superoxide, the inhibition of the pro-oxidant enzyme xanthine oxidase, the inhibition of lipid peroxidation, the chelating of iron and the altering of the anti-oxidant defense pathways in the cell [51-52]. Given its beneficial effects against oxidative damage, quercetin was hypothesized to be effective in the treatment of ED, in particular ED as a result of diabetes mellitus [51-52]. Animal studies have revealed that quercetin treatment effectively improved intracavernosal pressure of diabetic rats by preserving superoxide dismutase (SOD) activity, (an antioxidant enzyme), while simultaneously increasing endothelial nitric oxide synthase (eNOS) expression. The results clearly demonstrate that eNOS expression and NO levels in corpus cavernosum were significantly increased in diabetic rats, in response to quercetin treatment [52]. Though these studies show a promising potential for quercetin, more investigations are needed to establish its efficacy in human penile tissue.

3. Second-line treatment: Intracavernosal pharmacotherapy

Intracavernosal injection (ICI) is a second-line therapy that is mainly considered for patients who fail to respond to first-line therapy or those who cannot use the least invasive forms of currently available pharmacotherapy [53]. The ideal candidates for ICI therapy are those who use nitrates or could potentially use nitrates, have neural injury from pelvic surgery, trauma, diabetic patients, and patients who desire rapid onset of erection, greater rigidity and or duration of erection [54]. Contraindications for ICI therapy include patients with a history of priapism with vasoactive drug use, and those with severe penile fibrosis with the use of monoamine oxidase inhibitors (MAOIs); in addition, a nonresponse to ICI occurs mostly as a result of an inadequate dose, misdirected injection into the subcutaneous or

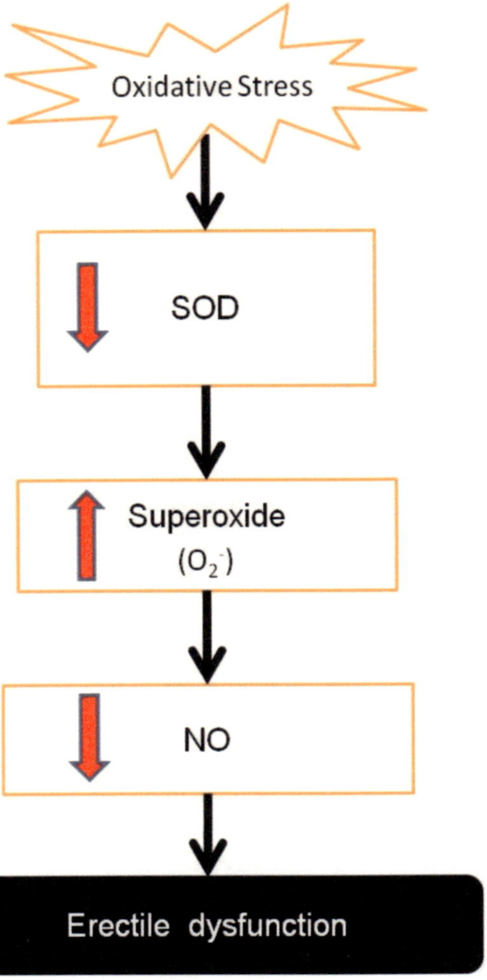

Fig. 1. **SOD in the Pathophysiology of Erectile Dysfunction**: During oxidative stress, SOD expression decreases causing an increase in superoxide (O_2^-). As O_2^- rises within the cell, NO production is attenuated leading to ED.

trabecular regions of the penis, leakage of vasoactive agent prior to ICI and insufficient sexual stimulation, or premature ejaculation [54].

Following an ICI and sexual stimulation, penile rigidity is achieved usually within 5-10 minutes, as a rapid increase in cavernosal artery blood flow leads to compression of subtunical venules located between the smooth muscle of the *corpora cavernosa* and the inner *tunica albuginea* (3). With venous outflow blocked, intracavernosal pressures can be greater than 100 mmHg. Vasoconstriction and the loss of penile rigidity occur as a result of an increase in sympathetic tone coincident with ejaculation (3). For ICI therapy, the most commonly prescribed vasoactive agents are prostaglandin E-1 (PGE-1), phentolamine, and papaverine (1, 3). However, with advances in medical research, other effective treatments are currently available, such as vasoactive intestinal polypeptide, calcitonin gene-related peptide, and guanylate cyclase activators.

3.1 Papaverine

Papaverine was discovered by Merck in 1848, it is an opium alkaloid originating from the poppy *Papaver somniferum*. In the treatment of ED, intracavernosal papaverine injection was the first pharmacological agent proven to be a clinically effective therapy for ED (1). Papaverine induces relaxation of the corpus cavernosal smooth muscle tissue and pudendal artery leading to penile erection via nonspecific inhibition of phosphodiesterase, leading to increased intracellular levels of cGMP and cyclic adenosine monophosphate (cAMP) (1). In *in vitro* studies, papaverine was shown to increase relaxation not only in isolated corpus cavernosum smooth muscle strips, but also in penile arteries and penile veins; in addition, these studies have also shown that papaverine was able to attenuate contractions induced by stimulation of adrenergic nerves and exogenous noradrenaline [9]. Papaverine may also regulate corpus cavernosum smooth muscle tone via a cAMP independent pathway by the inhibition of voltage-dependent L-type calcium channels [9, 55].

Although papaverine is an effective and inexpensive treatment for ED, compiled reports have implicated the use of papaverine with an increased rate of priapism and fibrosis [20, 56-57]. Penile pain is also very common following administration of papaverine [57-58]. Papaverine may cause other side effects such as flushing, sweating, upset stomach, loss of appetite, diarrhea, constipation, and irregular heartbeat [9, 59]

3.2 Alpha-adrenoreceptor antagonist (*Phentolamine*)

Although the beneficial vasoactive effects of phentolamine were discovered in the 1970s, the current clinical use of this drug is limited to use as a component of other vasoactive drug combinations [20, 60]. In the penile corpus cavernosum, there are at least three important alpha-adrenoreceptor iso-forms: α1A, α1B, and α1D. All three subtypes have been detected and the α1A and α1D proteins have been identified as the predominant subtypes in the *corpus cavernosa* [61-62]. However, the distinction and role of each individual receptor subtype to cell signaling pathways in erectile function remains mostly undetermined [63].

Alpha-1 and α2-adrenoreceptors are classified as G-protein coupled receptors which initiate several complex downstream processes [61]. It has been suggested that alpha 1 receptors preserve the penile contractile tone by increasing intracellular calcium levels followed by extracellular calcium influx [61]. It should also be noted that the α-adrenergic receptor system plays a critical role in the modulation of penile flaccidity (8). Contraction induced by post-junctional α2-receptors is caused by increased intracellular calcium but also involves the recruitment of ion channels, activation of phosphodiesterases and attenuation of adenylate cyclase activity [60, 64].

Phentolamine mesylate produces an α-adrenergic blockade; it is a nonselective α-adrenoreceptor antagonist with a similar affinity for α1 and α2-adrenoreceptors; it also has direct, positive inotropic and chronotropic effects on cardiac muscle, as well as vasodilator effects on vascular smooth muscle [20]. Although ICI of phentolamine increases corporal blood flow, a concurrent increase in noradrenaline prevents sinusoidal relaxation [65]. Studies have also shown that phentolamine induces the relaxation of corpus cavernosum erectile tissue independently of α1 and α2-adrenoreceptors blockades, via a noradrenergic, endothelium-mediated mechanism suggesting NO synthase activation (68, 77).

3.3 Prostaglandin E1

Prostaglandins were first characterized by Bergstrom, S., Bengt, S. and Vane, J. however, it was not until 1986 that the vasoactive effects of prostaglandin E1s (PGE-1) were described for intracavernosal use by Ishii, N. and Adaikan, PG. [20]. In 1996, PGE-1 became the first FDA-approved vasoactive intracavernosal drug for the treatment of ED, and its efficacy has been confirmed in three multi-centered, randomized prospective clinical trials with a six-month open-label extension [66]. Since then, a vast body of knowledge has described the efficacy and mechanism of this drug. Presently, PGE-1 is one of the most popular vasoactive agents for ICI therapy [67].

PGE-1 induces relaxation of human corpus cavernosum smooth muscle by regulating adenylate cyclase activity, upregulating the production of cAMP in the penis via activation of EP prostaglandin receptors, and subsequently leading to a decrease in intracellular calcium concentration, resulting in cavernosal smooth muscle relaxation [9, 20, 68-69]. PGE-1 mediated vaso-dilation occurs via gap junctions within the penis; additionally PGE-1 inhibits sympathetic activity by acting upon the presynaptic neurons, blocking the release of noradrenaline [70-72]. PGE-1 is metabolized by 15-hydroxydehydrogenase and has a blood plasma half-life of less than 1 minute, as liver, kidney, and penile enzymes all contribute to the conversion of PGE-1 to its inactive form [67]. Rates of priapism, a potentially devastating adverse effect, are low with the use of PGE-1, which makes it the most utilized injectable vasoactive agent [20].

3.4 Vasoactive Intestinal Polypeptide

Vasoactive intestinal peptide (VIP) is a naturally occurring neurotransmitter and a potent smooth muscle relaxing agent. VIP, which was isolated from the small intestine, was also first described as a specific neurotransmitter for inducing penile erection in 1986 [73]. While VIPergic nerves are most densely concentrated in the penis around the pudendal arteries, preliminary intracavernosal studies using VIP produced unsatisfactory results; however, when VIPs were used in combination with drugs such as papaverine and phentolamine, adequate penile erections were observed [9, 74]. As a result, current VIP therapy for ED is predominantly used in combination with phentolamine mesylate [20].

The effects of VIP are mediated via a specific G protein-coupled receptor (GPCR) which is linked to adenylate cyclase [9]. VIP co-localizes with nitric oxide synthase (NOS) within the perivascular and trabecular nerve fibers innervating the penis, thus regulating penile blood flow, and smooth muscle tone in the male genitalia [75]. Most of the NO and VIPergic nerves are cholinergic in nature, as they contain a vesicular acetylcholine transporter [76]. Given that the actions of VIP have been directly linked to adenylate cyclase, VIP can elevate cAMP concentrations in cavernosal tissues without affecting cGMP levels [77]. VIP has commonly observed side effects, such as facial flushing and headaches, which are frequent events characteristic of most vasoactive therapies [78].

3.5 Linsidomine chlorhydrate

Nitric oxide donors such as sodium nitroprusside (SNP) and linsidomine (SIN-1) can be used for the treatment of ED [79]. *In vivo* studies have shown that SNP and linsidomine (SIN-1) upregulates cGMP production, which increases NO release in a dose-dependent manner [80]. NO release causes the relaxation of vascular smooth muscle as well as cavernosum smooth muscle. Even though SIN-1 has a short half-life of only 1–2 min, there is a potential to cause systemic hypotension with use of this drug [81-82]. SNP and SIN-1 have positive hemodynamic effects promoting erectile function and show long-term promise as intracavernosal vasoactive agents compared to other forms of intracavernosal treatment [83].

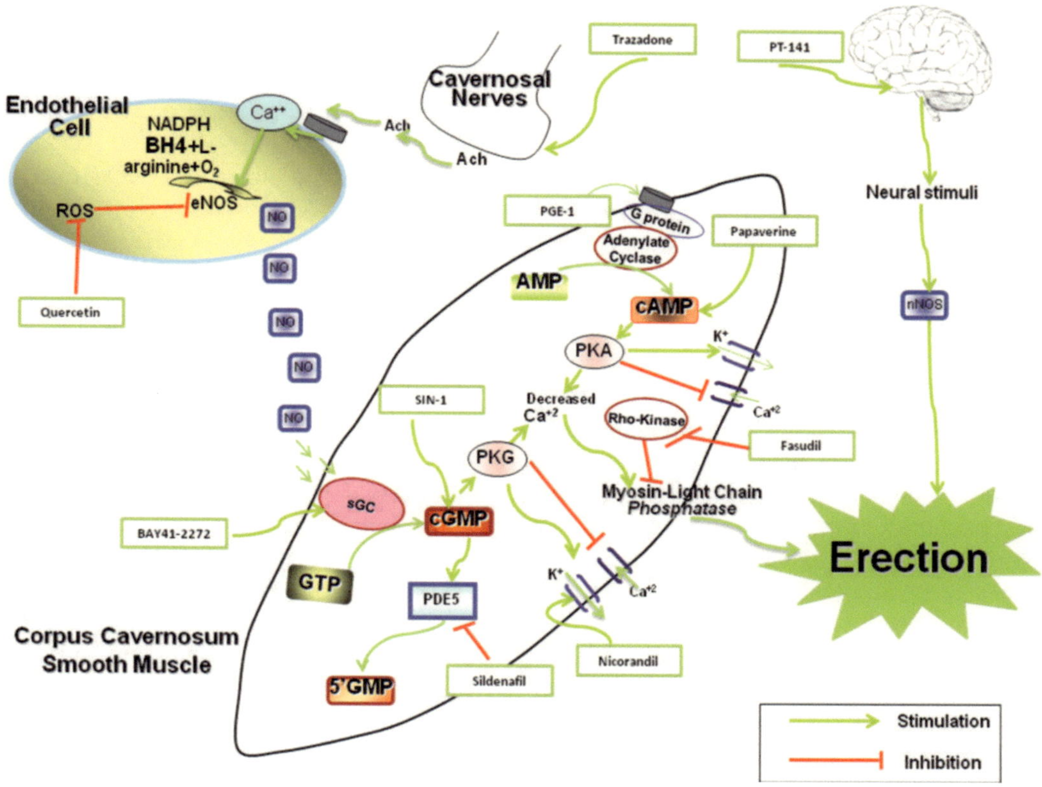

Fig. 2. **Pharmacotherapy treatments for ED**: Cavernosal nerves contribute to smooth muscle relaxation by releasing Acetylcholine (Ach). Trazadone increases cavernosal nerve firing, which increases Ach release, which stimulates eNOS, causing the release of NO. ROS causes eNOS uncoupling, which reduces its activity, however Quercetin has potent antioxidant effects and effectively reduces ROS generation. Once NO is released, it activates sGC, increasing the cGMP levels. SIN-1 and PDE5 inhibitors, such as sildenafil, also elevates cGMP levels resulting in the activation of PKG. On the other hand, PGE-1 and Papaverine elevates cAMP, causing the activation of PKA. PKG and PKA activation causes a cell signaling cascade which hyperpolarizes the cell membrane. Nicorandil also has similar hyperpolarizing effects by opening the potassium channels. Overall activation of PKG and PKA reduces intracellular calcium levels, resulting in increased activity of myosin-light chain phosphatase resulting in smooth muscle relaxation and subsequent erection. Fasudil also increases myosin-light chain phosphatase leading to smooth muscle relaxation by inhibition of Rho-kinase. Erections are also caused by neural stimulation, through the release of neuronal NO.

3.6 Calcitonin Gene-Related Peptide

Calcitonin-gene-related peptide (CGRP) causes an increase in penile arterial inflow, cavernosal smooth muscle relaxation and cavernosal outflow occlusion [84]. As a potent vasodilator, CGRP has also been shown to induce dose-related increases in penile blood flow with CGRP-specific receptor agonists [84-85]. For the treatment of ED, CGRP is usually co-administered with PGE-1, and this combined therapy has been proven successful in improving erectile function [86].

3.7 Guanylate Cyclase activator

Soluble guanylate cyclase (sGC) activators have been shown to increase intracavernosal pressure in corpus cavernosum tissue (23-24). BAY41-2272 is a sGC activator that has been shown to relax the human corpus cavernosum with or without the presence of NO (16). The sGC enzyme converts GTP to cGMP, which is activated when NO is released from erectile-autonomic nerves, resulting in smooth muscle relaxation. In the penis, cGMP is a down-stream cell-signal messenger that relaxes cavernosal smooth muscle, causing adequate blood flow for penile erection (23).

4. Conclusion

ED will continue to be a problem affecting many individuals. Though there are advances in the treatment of ED, there is still a need for more effective therapy for men with complex ED caused by comorbid diseases such as diabetes. In addition, there are an increasing number of patients with cardiovascular disease for whom first-line and second-line pharmacotherapy are contra-indicated. For first-line therapy, the major drawback is severe hypotension and bothersome side effects including headaches, dizziness, vision and hearing changes, which sometimes occur during sexual activity. For second-line therapy, even though it is an effective alternative for men who cannot tolerate or respond to first-line therapy, the chief drawback of such an approach is a high attrition rate. However, although this chapter did not focus on the option of combination therapy, (the combined used of various oral vasoactive drugs and or intracavernosal therapies), this form of therapy is becoming an increasingly popular option for patients and may represent the most promising alternative for men with complex ED. At present it is very common, especially for second-line ED treatment algorithms to include combination therapy. Therefore, as we move ahead into the future, we can better understand and provide more appealing options for the management of ED, through continued combined efforts of researchers and clinicians.

5. References

[1] Jackson, G., et al., *Cardiovascular aspects of sexual medicine.* J Sex Med, 2010. 7(4 Pt 2): p. 1608-26.

[2] Heidelbaugh, J.J., *Management of erectile dysfunction.* Am Fam Physician, 2010. 81(3): p. 305-12.

[3] Lasker, G.F., J.H. Maley, and P.J. Kadowitz, *A Review of the Pathophysiology and Novel Treatments for Erectile Dysfunction.* Adv Pharmacol Sci, 2010. 2010.

[4] Hatzimouratidis, K. and D.G. Hatzichristou, *Looking to the future for erectile dysfunction therapies.* Drugs, 2008. 68(2): p. 231-50.
[5] Virag, R., *Intracavernous injection of papaverine for erectile failure. 1982.* J Urol, 2002. 167(2 Pt 2): p. 1196.
[6] Dhir, R.R., et al., *Combination therapy for erectile dysfunction: an update review.* Asian J Androl, 2011. 13(3): p. 382-90.
[7] Andersson, K.E., *Mechanisms of penile erection and basis for pharmacological treatment of erectile dysfunction.* Pharmacol Rev, 2011. 63(4): p. 811-59.
[8] Uckert, S. and C.G. Stief, *Treatment of erectile dysfunction and lower urinary tract symptoms by phosphodiesterase inhibitors.* Handb Exp Pharmacol, 2011(204): p. 307-22.
[9] Eardley, I., et al., *Pharmacotherapy for erectile dysfunction.* J Sex Med, 2010. 7(1 Pt 2): p. 524-40.
[10] Truss, M.C., et al., *Role of the nitric oxide donor linsidomine chlorhydrate (SIN-1) in the diagnosis and treatment of erectile dysfunction.* Urology, 1994. 44(4): p. 553-6.
[11] Uckert, S., et al., *Phosphodiesterase isoenzymes as pharmacological targets in the treatment of male erectile dysfunction.* World J Urol, 2001. 19(1): p. 14-22.
[12] D'Amours, M.R., et al., *Potency and mechanism of action of E4021, a type 5 phosphodiesterase isozyme-selective inhibitor, on the photoreceptor phosphodiesterase depend on the state of activation of the enzyme.* Mol Pharmacol, 1999. 55(3): p. 508-14.
[13] Duan, H., et al., *2-Phenylquinazolin-4(3H)-one, a class of potent PDE5 inhibitors with high selectivity versus PDE6.* Bioorg Med Chem Lett, 2009. 19(10): p. 2777-9.
[14] Basu, A. and R.E. Ryder, *New treatment options for erectile dysfunction in patients with diabetes mellitus.* Drugs, 2004. 64(23): p. 2667-88.
[15] Stief, C., et al., *Sustained efficacy and tolerability with vardenafil over 2 years of treatment in men with erectile dysfunction.* Int J Clin Pract, 2004. 58(3): p. 230-9.
[16] Agarwal, A., et al., *Role of oxidative stress in the pathophysiological mechanism of erectile dysfunction.* J Androl, 2006. 27(3): p. 335-47.
[17] Kuthe, A., et al., *Gene expression of the phosphodiesterases 3A and 5A in human corpus cavernosum penis.* Eur Urol, 2000. 38(1): p. 108-14.
[18] Hatzimouratidis, K., *Can we cure erectile dysfunction?* Eur Urol, 2010. 58(2): p. 249-50.
[19] Hatzimouratidis, K., et al., *Guidelines on male sexual dysfunction: erectile dysfunction and premature ejaculation.* Eur Urol, 2010. 57(5): p. 804-14.
[20] Bella, A.J. and G.B. Brock, *Intracavernous pharmacotherapy for erectile dysfunction.* Endocrine, 2004. 23(2-3): p. 149-55.
[21] Hatzimouratidis, K., *Sildenafil in the treatment of erectile dysfunction: an overview of the clinical evidence.* Clin Interv Aging, 2006. 1(4): p. 403-14.
[22] Tsertsvadze, A., et al., *Oral sildenafil citrate (viagra) for erectile dysfunction: a systematic review and meta-analysis of harms.* Urology, 2009. 74(4): p. 831-836 e8.
[23] Gur, S., S.C. Sikka, and W.J. Hellstrom, *Novel phosphodiesterase-5 (PDE5) inhibitors in the alleviation of erectile dysfunction due to diabetes and ageing-induced oxidative stress.* Expert Opin Investig Drugs, 2008. 17(6): p. 855-64.
[24] Hatzimouratidis, K., et al., *Phosphodiesterase type 5 inhibitors in postprostatectomy erectile dysfunction: a critical analysis of the basic science rationale and clinical application.* Eur Urol, 2009. 55(2): p. 334-47.
[25] Glina, S., et al., *Efficacy and tolerability of lodenafil carbonate for oral therapy in erectile dysfunction: a phase II clinical trial.* J Sex Med, 2009. 6(2): p. 553-7.

[26] Toque, H.A., et al., *Pharmacological characterization of a novel phosphodiesterase type 5 (PDE5) inhibitor lodenafil carbonate on human and rabbit corpus cavernosum.* Eur J Pharmacol, 2008. 591(1-3): p. 189-95.
[27] Coward, R.M. and C.C. Carson, *Tadalafil in the treatment of erectile dysfunction.* Ther Clin Risk Manag, 2008. 4(6): p. 1315-30.
[28] Porst, H., et al., *Evaluation of the efficacy and safety of once-a-day dosing of tadalafil 5mg and 10mg in the treatment of erectile dysfunction: results of a multicenter, randomized, double-blind, placebo-controlled trial.* Eur Urol, 2006. 50(2): p. 351-9.
[29] Morales, A.M., et al., *Vardenafil for the treatment of erectile dysfunction: an overview of the clinical evidence.* Clin Interv Aging, 2009. 4: p. 463-72.
[30] Georgotas, A., et al., *Trazodone hydrochloride: a wide spectrum antidepressant with a unique pharmacological profile. A review of its neurochemical effects, pharmacology, clinical efficacy, and toxicology.* Pharmacotherapy, 1982. 2(5): p. 255-65.
[31] Steers, W.D. and W.C. de Groat, *Effects of m-chlorophenylpiperazine on penile and bladder function in rats.* Am J Physiol, 1989. 257(6 Pt 2): p. R1441-9.
[32] Sood, S., W. James, and M.J. Bailon, *Priapism associated with atypical antipsychotic medications: a review.* Int Clin Psychopharmacol, 2008. 23(1): p. 9-17.
[33] Azadzoi, K.M., et al., *Effects of intracavernosal trazodone hydrochloride: animal and human studies.* J Urol, 1990. 144(5): p. 1277-82.
[34] Meinhardt, W., et al., *Trazodone, a double blind trial for treatment of erectile dysfunction.* Int J Impot Res, 1997. 9(3): p. 163-5.
[35] Wessells, H., et al., *Synthetic melanotropic peptide initiates erections in men with psychogenic erectile dysfunction: double-blind, placebo controlled crossover study.* J Urol, 1998. 160(2): p. 389-93.
[36] King, S.H., et al., *Melanocortin receptors, melanotropic peptides and penile erection.* Curr Top Med Chem, 2007. 7(11): p. 1098-1106.
[37] Diamond, L.E., et al., *Double-blind, placebo-controlled evaluation of the safety, pharmacokinetic properties and pharmacodynamic effects of intranasal PT-141, a melanocortin receptor agonist, in healthy males and patients with mild-to-moderate erectile dysfunction.* Int J Impot Res, 2004. 16(1): p. 51-9.
[38] Walsh, M.P., *The Ayerst Award Lecture 1990. Calcium-dependent mechanisms of regulation of smooth muscle contraction.* Biochem Cell Biol, 1991. 69(12): p. 771-800.
[39] Somlyo, A.P. and A.V. Somlyo, *Signal transduction by G-proteins, rho-kinase and protein phosphatase to smooth muscle and non-muscle myosin II.* J Physiol, 2000. 522 Pt 2: p. 177-85.
[40] Chitaley, K., et al., *Decreased penile erection in DOCA-salt and stroke prone-spontaneously hypertensive rats.* Int J Impot Res, 2001. 13 Suppl 5: p. S16-20.
[41] Park, K., et al., *Chronic administration of an oral Rho kinase inhibitor prevents the development of vasculogenic erectile dysfunction in a rat model.* J Sex Med, 2006. 3(6): p. 996-1003.
[42] Li, W.J., et al., *Chronic treatment with an oral rho-kinase inhibitor restores erectile function by suppressing corporal apoptosis in diabetic rats.* J Sex Med, 2011. 8(2): p. 400-10.
[43] Morelli, A., et al., *Atorvastatin ameliorates sildenafil-induced penile erections in experimental diabetes by inhibiting diabetes-induced RhoA/Rho-kinase signaling hyperactivation.* J Sex Med, 2009. 6(1): p. 91-106.
[44] Ho, C.C. and H.M. Tan, *Rise of Herbal and Traditional Medicine in Erectile Dysfunction Management.* Curr Urol Rep, 2011.

[45] Simonsen, U., et al., *Prejunctional alpha 2-adrenoceptors inhibit nitrergic neurotransmission in horse penile resistance arteries.* J Urol, 1997. 157(6): p. 2356-60.

[46] Galitzky, J., et al., *Pharmacodynamic effects of chronic yohimbine treatment in healthy volunteers.* Eur J Clin Pharmacol, 1990. 39(5): p. 447-51.

[47] Ernst, E. and M.H. Pittler, *Yohimbine for erectile dysfunction: a systematic review and meta-analysis of randomized clinical trials.* J Urol, 1998. 159(2): p. 433-6.

[48] Zhang, W., et al., *Antioxidant treatment with quercetin ameliorates erectile dysfunction in streptozotocin-induced diabetic rats.* J Biosci Bioeng, 2011. 112(3): p. 215-8.

[49] Shukla, N., et al., *Effect of hydrogen sulphide-donating sildenafil (ACS6) on erectile function and oxidative stress in rabbit isolated corpus cavernosum and in hypertensive rats.* BJU Int, 2009. 103(11): p. 1522-9.

[50] Valente, E.G., et al., *L-arginine and phosphodiesterase (PDE) inhibitors counteract fibrosis in the Peyronie's fibrotic plaque and related fibroblast cultures.* Nitric Oxide, 2003. 9(4): p. 229-44.

[51] Bischoff, S.C., *Quercetin: potentials in the prevention and therapy of disease.* Curr Opin Clin Nutr Metab Care, 2008. 11(6): p. 733-40.

[52] Anjaneyulu, M. and K. Chopra, *Quercetin, an anti-oxidant bioflavonoid, attenuates diabetic nephropathy in rats.* Clin Exp Pharmacol Physiol, 2004. 31(4): p. 244-8.

[53] Montorsi, F., et al., *Pharmacological management of erectile dysfunction.* BJU Int, 2003. 91(5): p. 446-54.

[54] Pinsky, M.R., A. Chawla, and W.J. Hellstrom, *Intracavernosal therapy and vacuum devices to treat erectile dysfunction.* Arch Esp Urol, 2010. 63(8): p. 717-25.

[55] Iguchi, M., et al., *On the mechanism of papaverine inhibition of the voltage-dependent Ca++ current in isolated smooth muscle cells from the guinea pig trachea.* J Pharmacol Exp Ther, 1992. 263(1): p. 194-200.

[56] Kattan, S.A., *Maternal urological injuries associated with vaginal deliveries: change of pattern.* Int Urol Nephrol, 1997. 29(2): p. 155-61.

[57] Sahin, M., et al., *Short-term histopathologic effects of different intracavernosal agents on corpus cavernosum and antifibrotic activity of intracavernosal verapamil: an experimental study.* Urology, 2001. 58(3): p. 487-92.

[58] Salonia, A., et al., *Pathophysiology of erectile dysfunction.* Int J Androl, 2003. 26(3): p. 129-36.

[59] Virag, R., *Intracavernous injection of papaverine for erectile failure.* Lancet, 1982. 2(8304): p. 938.

[60] Domer, F.R., et al., *Involvement of the sympathetic nervous system in the urinary bladder internal sphincter and in penile erection in the anesthetized cat.* Invest Urol, 1978. 15(5): p. 404-7.

[61] Traish, A.M., et al., *Identification of alpha 1-adrenergic receptor subtypes in human corpus cavernosum tissue and in cultured trabecular smooth muscle cells.* Receptor, 1995. 5(3): p. 145-57.

[62] Goepel, M., et al., *Characterization of alpha-adrenoceptor subtypes in the corpus cavernosum of patients undergoing sex change surgery.* J Urol, 1999. 162(5): p. 1793-9.

[63] Yassin, A., et al., *Alpha-adrenoceptors are a common denominator in the pathophysiology of erectile function and BPH/LUTS--implications for clinical practice.* Andrologia, 2006. 38(1): p. 1-12.

[64] Hedlund, H., S. Fasth, and L. Hulten, *Efferent sympathetic nervous control of rectal motility in the cat.* Acta Physiol Scand, 1984. 121(4): p. 317-24.

[65] Juenemann, K.P., et al., *Hemodynamics of papaverine- and phentolamine-induced penile erection.* J Urol, 1986. 136(1): p. 158-61.

[66] Linet, O.I. and F.G. Ogrinc, *Efficacy and safety of intracavernosal alprostadil in men with erectile dysfunction. The Alprostadil Study Group.* N Engl J Med, 1996. 334(14): p. 873-7.

[67] Porst, H., *The rationale for prostaglandin E1 in erectile failure: a survey of worldwide experience.* J Urol, 1996. 155(3): p. 802-15.

[68] Paoletti, R., et al., *Calcium, calcium antagonists and experimental atherosclerosis.* Blood Press Suppl, 1996. 4: p. 12-5.

[69] Lin, J.S., et al., *Role of cyclic adenosine monophosphate in prostaglandin E1-induced penile erection in rabbits.* Eur Urol, 1995. 28(3): p. 259-65.

[70] Italiano, G., A. Calabro, and F. Pagano, *A simplified in vitro preparation of the corpus cavernosum as a tool for investigating erectile pharmacology in the rat.* Pharmacol Res, 1994. 30(4): p. 325-34.

[71] Molderings, G.J., et al., *Inhibition of noradrenaline release from the sympathetic nerves of the human saphenous vein by presynaptic histamine H3 receptors.* Naunyn Schmiedebergs Arch Pharmacol, 1992. 346(1): p. 46-50.

[72] Kifor, I., et al., *Tissue angiotensin II as a modulator of erectile function. I. Angiotensin peptide content, secretion and effects in the corpus cavernosum.* J Urol, 1997. 157(5): p. 1920-5.

[73] Adaikan, P.G., S.R. Kottegoda, and S.S. Ratnam, *Is vasoactive intestinal polypeptide the principal transmitter involved in human penile erection?* J Urol, 1986. 135(3): p. 638-40.

[74] Kiely, E.A., S.R. Bloom, and G. Williams, *Penile response to intracavernosal vasoactive intestinal polypeptide alone and in combination with other vasoactive agents.* Br J Urol, 1989. 64(2): p. 191-4.

[75] Polak, J.M., et al., *Vipergic nerves in the penis.* Lancet, 1981. 2(8240): p. 217-9.

[76] Hedlund, P., et al., *Cholinergic nerves in human corpus cavernosum and spongiosum contain nitric oxide synthase and heme oxygenase.* J Urol, 2000. 164(3 Pt 1): p. 868-75.

[77] Hedlund, P., et al., *Pituitary adenylate cyclase-activating polypeptide, helospectin, and vasoactive intestinal polypeptide in human corpus cavernosum.* Br J Pharmacol, 1995. 116(4): p. 2258-66.

[78] Simonsen, U., A. Garcia-Sacristan, and D. Prieto, *Penile arteries and erection.* J Vasc Res, 2002. 39(4): p. 283-303.

[79] Segarra, G., et al., *Comparative effects of dilator drugs on human penile dorsal artery and deep dorsal vein.* Clin Sci (Lond), 1999. 96(1): p. 59-65.

[80] Trigo-Rocha, F., et al., *Sodium nitroprusside: physiologic effects as a nitric oxide donor in three species.* Int J Impot Res, 1995. 7(1): p. 49-56.

[81] Brock, G., J. Breza, and T.F. Lue, *Intracavernous sodium nitroprusside: inappropriate impotence treatment.* J Urol, 1993. 150(3): p. 864-7.

[82] Martinez-Pineiro, L., et al., *Prospective comparative study with intracavernous sodium nitroprusside and prostaglandin E1 in patients with erectile dysfunction.* Eur Urol, 1998. 34(4): p. 350-4.

[83] von Heyden, B., et al., *Intracavernous injection of linsidomine chlorhydrate in monkeys: lack of toxic effect with long-term use.* Eur Urol, 1996. 30(4): p. 502-5.

[84] Stief, C.G., et al., *Calcitonin-gene-related peptide: a possible role in human penile erection and its therapeutic application in impotent patients.* J Urol, 1991. 146(4): p. 1010-4.

[85] Bivalacqua, T.J., et al., *Analysis of vasodilator responses to novel nitric oxide donors in the hindquarters vascular bed of the cat.* J Cardiovasc Pharmacol, 2001. 38(1): p. 120-9.

[86] Truss, M.C., et al., *Intracavernous calcitonin gene-related peptide plus prostaglandin E1: possible alternative to penile implants in selected patients.* Eur Urol, 1994. 26(1): p. 40-5.

9

Surgical Treatment of Erectile Dysfunction

Faruk Kucukdurmaz and Ates Kadioglu
Istanbul University, Istanbul Medical Faculty, Urology Department, Istanbul Turkey

1. Introduction

Erectile dysfunction (ED) is defined as the consistent or recurrent inability of a man to attain and/or maintain penile erection sufficient for sexual activity. According to current guidelines, a 3-month symptom duration is accepted to establish the diagnosis except for some cases of trauma or surgically induced ED (Lewis R 2010). ED affects physical and psychosocial health and has a significant impact on the quality of life (QoL) of sufferers and their partners and families. Epidemiologic studies for ED estimate the prevalence of ED ranging between 20-30 % among men aged between 40-80 years (Laumannn et al 2005, Lewis R 2010). These differences in reported incidences are probably due to variations in the methodology and the age and socioeconomic status of the study populations.

ED is a disorder in which subjective perception of patients is very important, therefore, the aim of the treatment should not only be organ focused but also be patient-outcome oriented. Patient satisfaction with sexual intercourse, their overall sex lives and ED treatments may represent reliable predictors of key patient-related treatment outcomes, in addition to pharmacological efficacy and safety (Carson C, et al. 2004)

The basic diagnostic work-up for patients who presented with ED should include a thorough medical and psychosexual history to identify common causes and risk factors of ED and assess psychological status of patients by using validated instruments (Hatzimouratidis K, et al. 2010). A focused physical examination should be the next step to evaluate possible penile deformities, prostatic diseases, signs of hypogonadism, cardiovascular and neurological status of the patients. Evaluation of serum glucose, lipid and testosterone levels is also an essential part of the initial evaluation of ED patients.

Patients suffering from ED should be treated with a structured strategy which may be influenced by efficacy, safety, invasiveness, cost effectivity and satisfaction of both the patient and his partner. These parameters should also be considered for the selection of the treatment option for each particular patient and his partner.

Although newer medical treatment alternatives such as PDE-5 inhibitors, vacuum erection devices and intracavernosal applications are considered first and second lines of ED therapy, respectively; surgical treatment, especially penile prosthesis implantation, is the standard of care in cases of medication-resistant ED. Surgical treatment options in order to correct ED are divided into three categories. These categories are:

1. Penile prosthesis implantation
2. Penile revascularization
3. Surgery for corporal veno-occlusive dysfunction

2. Penile prosthesis implantation

From the historical point of view, the wooden sticks that were either placed under the skin of the penis or into the urethra are known as the earliest implanted materials designed to improve erectile function (Henry GD, 2009). With increased knowledge of human anatomy, autologous materials were started to be implanted. The first real attempt to create an internal penile support and provide penile rigidity was described in 1936 by Bogoras who used a piece of cartilage as a penile stiffener in a total phallic reconstruction (Bogoras 1936). This is followed by Beheri who first documented successful intracavernosal placement of polyethylene rods in 700 patients in 1966 (Beheri 1966). The successful implantation of a new semirigid silicone cylinder that fulfills the whole corpora was described in 1973 which lead to the development of new implants that are currently used(Scott 1973).

2.1 Indications of surgery

There are many types of penile prosthesis designs that are currently available for implantation, but it should be kept in mind that not all patients with ED are candidates for penile prosthesis implantation. Implantation of penile prosthesis is indicated for the treatment of organic ED in men who fail or reject more conservative measures, such as oral PDE5 inhibitors, vacuum erection devices (VED), urethral alprostadil suppositories, and intracavernosal injection therapy. Additionally, implants are appropriate when medical therapy is contraindicated, cause severe side effects, vacuum erection therapy has proven unsatisfactory or unacceptable, and/or in men with end organ failure (e.g. diabetes mellitus), severe structural abnormalities (e.g. Peyronie's disease), cavernosal fibrosis (e.g. after prolonged priapism or infection). Patients who experience ED after radical prostatectomy or pelvic organ transplantation may also serve as the candidates for penile prosthesis implantation. Careful counseling before penile implant procedures will reduce the probability of problems that may result in postoperative dissatisfaction. The type of the prosthesis for each particular patient should be selected according to the patients' needs and expectations (Carson CC 2005). Patients at younger age with normal manual dexterity or who wear firm clothing often choose a three-piece inflatable penile prosthesis because appearance in the flaccid position is better than other designs (Hellstrom WG, et al. 2010). In addition, inflatable penile prosthesis should be the preferred option in patients with Peyronie's disease, history of previous implantation procedures or neurological disorders where considering interior tissue pressures are declined between uses and the risk of extrusion is diminished (Zermann DH, 2006). For some patients such as paraplegics, malleable prostheses can be chosen since inflatable ones have much higher malfunction rates. Malleable penile prosthesis can be better served in those patients who lack adequate manual dexterity, or those with significant obesity (Hellstrom WG, et al. 2010).

2.2 Types of implants

There are three classes of penile implants including hydraulic, semi-rigid and soft silicone. The hydraulic implants consist of two types, the three-piece inflatable and the two-piece inflatable. The only two-piece device currently available is AMS Ambicor(Fig.1). When this nondistensible device is deflated, the cylinders collapse and the penis, unlike that with a malleable prosthesis, is not rigid. When the scrotal pump is cycled, a small volume of fluid is transferred from the rear tips of the cylinders into the distal nondistensible chambers filling and then pressurizing them. Different from 3-piece inflatable prosthesis, Ambicor does not increase in size with inflation. Flaccidity and erection are more compromised with this model when compared with 3-piece device due to low, restricted reservoir volume. Also the device is not available with antibiotic impregnated forms as of yet, but has an acceptable short-term mechanical reliability (Levine LA 2001).

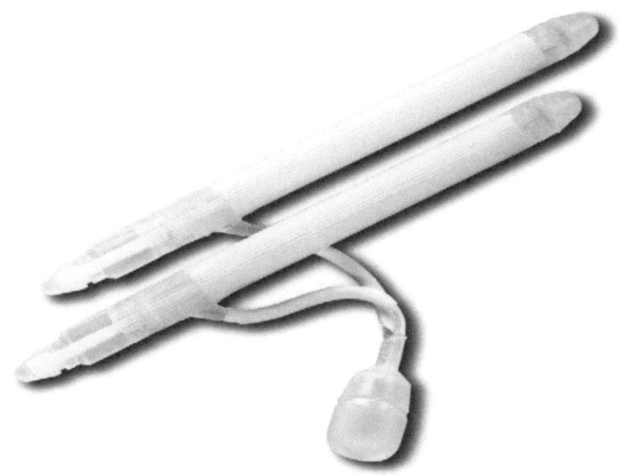

Fig. 1. AMS Ambicor two-piece inflatable penile prosthesis

The ideal penile prosthesis would produce flaccidity and erection that mimics natural condition. Three-piece inflatable prostheses provide these conditions by transferring fluid into and out of cylinders. These devices consist of a pair of cylinders, reservoir and a pump. AMS and Coloplast are the two main companies that manufacture 3-piece inflatable prostheses. Coloplast manufactures the Titan Inflatable Penile Prosthesis (Fig. 2) and the Titan Narrowbase Inflatable Penile Prosthesis. The Narrowbase implant is developed for patients with small penises or for cases in which dilation is limited because of scarring from corporal fibrosis or previous surgery. All of these cylinders expand in girth, but not in length. AMS manufactures the AMS 700 CX Inflatable Penile Prosthesis (Fig. 3), the AMS 700 LGX Inflatable Penile Prosthesis, and the AMS 700 CXR Inflatable Penile Prosthesis. The CXR device, like the Titan Narrow-base prosthesis, has smaller diameter cylinders and is used in revision cases and less commonly in men with small penises.

Apart from other devices, AMS LGX cylinder has a unique property that it expands both in girth and length (Fig 4). The CX and CXR have a unidirectional weave that allows only girth expansion, whereas the LGX has a bidirectional weave permitting expansion both in length and girth. In patients with organic ED and penile deformity or curvature, girth only expanding devices may provide better cosmetic outcome. In men with small penises or men with scarring due to ischemic priapism or previous penile surgery where corporeal dilation is limited, smaller diameter CXR cylinders often serve as a better alternative.

Infections are known to be the most significant and unwanted complications in IPP surgery, especially for revision/replacement, which may develop due to decreased host resistance,

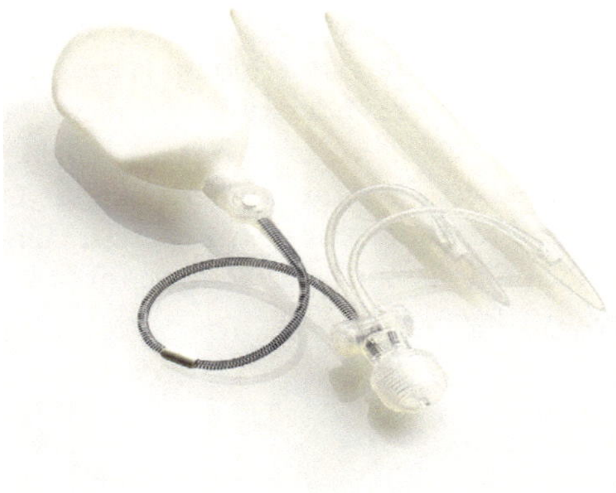

Fig. 2. Hydrophilic-coated Coloplast Titan™ threepiece prosthesis with reservoir lock-out valve to minimize autoinflation

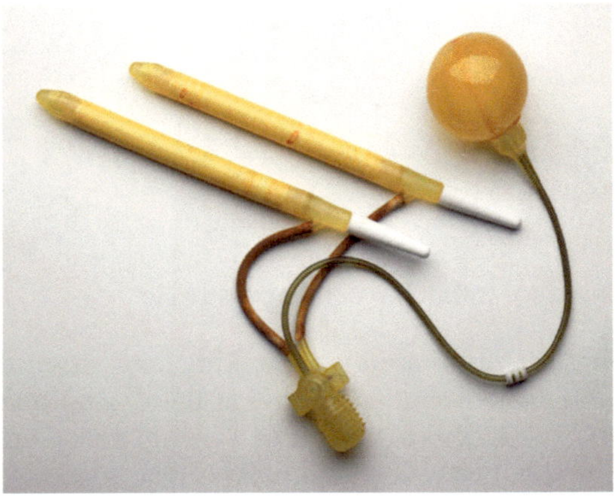

Fig. 3. AMS 700 CX inflatable penile prosthesis

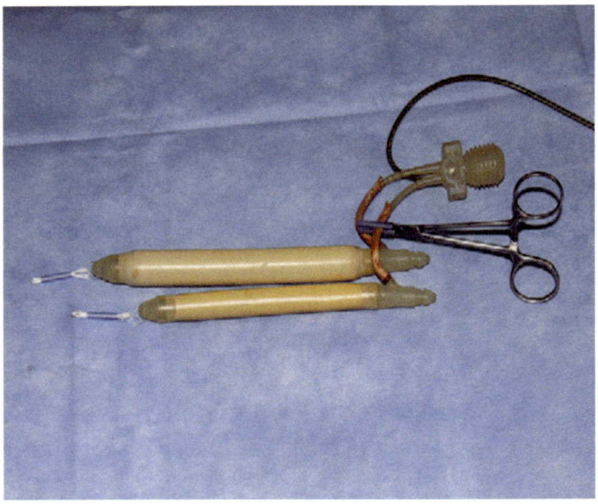

Fig. 4. AMS LGX inflatable penile prosthesis

impaired antibiotic penetration due to capsule formation, and decreased wound healing related to scarring. Most bacteria produce a mucin coat or biofilm that is the bacterial colonisation over the device and resistant to systemic antibiotic treatment due to decreased metabolic needs (Silverstein A, et al 2003). Antibiotics or the body's defense mechanisms can not eradicate the bacteria inside the biofilm without removing all prosthetic components and irrigation of the implant spaces (Stewart et al 2001). Both manufacturers developed advances in the designs of prosthesis in order to decrease the incidence of infections by applying coatings to the prosthesis designed to retard bacterial growth. In 2001, AMS introduced InhibiZone™ (Fig. 5) which is a patented antibiotic surface treatment that impregnates minocycline and rifampin into the external silicone surfaces of all the components, except the RTE, giving the orange-like color.

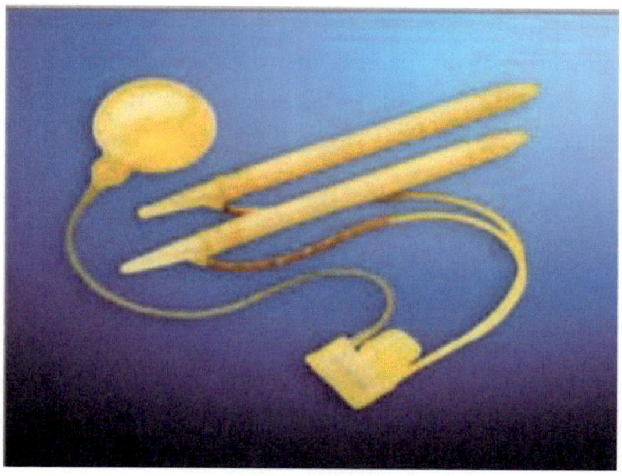

Fig. 5. AMS 700 MS™ series cylinder with Inhibizone® antibiotic surface treatment. AMS = American Medical Systems.

The antibiotics reach into the implant space within 10 days. They seem effective in the prevention of bacterial colonization and development of biofilm layer (Nickel JC, et al.1998). Minocycline and rifampin may help decrease the probability of developing bacterial resistance by inhibition of protein synthesis and inhibition of DNA-dependent RNA polymerase, respectively (Darouiche RO, et al 1999). In-vitro and in-vivo studies have demonstrated the effectiveness of minocycline in retarding the emergence of staphylococcal strains that are resistant to rifampin (Raad et al 1995). Short-term follow-up for this prosthesis enhancement shows statistical improvement in infection reduction for first time implant patients by a single surgeon (Wilson SK, et al 2002). Coloplast also produced antibiotic-coated devices named as Titan and Titan NB. The hydrophilic coating absorbs much more water and the idea is the adherence of antibiotics to the surface of prosthesis when soaked into antibiotic solutions.

It should be remembered that pumping systems of inflatable devices require some manual dexterity and patients who lack this ability may experience difficulties in order to make these devices work. AMS developed Momentary Squeeze Pump (MSP) that contains a much smaller pump with the inflation part in the most dependent site and deflation part in the upper portion of pump. It delivers more volume per squeeze and is easier to find deflation button. The main difference with the previous pump is that the MSP deflates completely after pressing the deflation button for a few moments. It also has a lock-out valve precluding auto-inflation of the implant. Early clinical studies reported significant reduction in time spent instructing the patient in use of this device (Henry GD, et al 2004).

Semi-rigid rod prostheses are constructed of two solid prostheses that are independently placed in each corpus cavernosum(Sadeghi-Nejad H 2007). They are divided into two types as the malleable and the mechanical. Coloplast's Genesis is a malleable device that consists of a braided silver wire surrounded by a silicone hydrophilic coat. The AMS 650 and 600 implants have similar construction of silicone surrounding a stainless steel woven core. Soft silicone rods were originally manufactured in France by Subrini (Subrini L 1982). They are ideal for patients in whom the cosmetic advantages of the inflatable devices are not as important as the ease of use and the lower chances of mechanical failure in semirigid implants. Pelvic organ transplant recipients may be well served by the semirigid devices rather than a three-piece inflatable device due to the results of a study addressing the higher incidence of reservoir complications in the retroperitoneal space (Cuellar DC, 2001). The narrow cylinders are appropriate for thin penises and for the penises with scar tissue where dilation to a large caliber corporal body is not easily performed.

Implantation of three-piece inflatable prostheses is a complex issue since they require a reservoir which has a large volume to be placed in the abdominal cavity. Since reservoir has a high capacity, complications such as stretching of pliant tunica and compression of erectile tissue that cause deterioration of the erectile tissue with time which are observed with the use of self-contained or two-piece devices with no reserve fluid volume are not seen in three-piece inflatable implants (Wilson SK, et al 1996). The three-piece inflatable also gives the best flaccidity, as all fluid can be drained out of the cylinders into the reservoir when the non-erect state is desired. Satisfaction rates of 70–87% are reported from patients after appropriate consultation.

2.3 Patient selection

The surgeon has three choices when selecting a prosthesis for a particular patient which include semirigid, two-piece inflatable, and three-piece inflatable prosthesis. Generally, the decision of the type of the prosthesis to be used depends on the physician's comfort with the surgical approach, assessment of body habitus, penile size, previous abdominal surgery and manual dexterity of the patient. Recently, the 3-piece inflatable prosthesis is accepted as the gold standard option in industrialized countries.

The semi-rigid rods are easy to implant and manipulate since they are bendable and can easily be maneuvered (Hellstrom WG et al, 2010). This kind of implants may have tendency to be eroded through glans because of cylinder pressure and loss of sensation in patients with spinal cord injury. Implantation of inflatable prostheses in this patient population can be recommended even if the implant is used only to make condom catheter urinary drainage easier (Rossier 1984).

Two-piece inflatable devices have the advantage of avoiding intra-abdominal reservoir placement. They provide better functional outcomes than rod implants in terms of rigidity and flaccidity.

Although three-piece inflatable devices provide the best rigidity, it should be beneficial to use these devices in patients with a larger penis. Similarly, patients with shorter penises mostly prefer three-piece devices because of the difficulty to hide semi-rigid rods and two-piece implants. Semi-rigid rods are generally selected in patients with limited manual dexterity or those who experience problems with the use of hydraulic devices. A motivated partner who may manipulate the device will be an exception to this issue.

Penile prosthesis implantation restores penetrative ability, however, it has no effect on recovery of sexual drive, glandular sensitivity and ejaculatory functions. If the removal of implants occurs at a later date, the capsule remains and the empty space will partially fill with proliferating scar tissue which makes it difficult for the patient to respond sufficiently to other medical treatment alternatives. Therefore, it is important that the patient should be aware of his expectations about the penile prosthesis. Also, a detailed discussion between surgeon and patient about the outcomes and potential complications of the procedure such as infection which may necessiate reoperation with a rate of 1-4% and mechanical dysfunction should be performed (Govier et al 1998, Wilson et al 1999).

2.4 Preoperative preparation and postoperative care

Preoperative preparation of patient aims to reduce the risk of infection (AUA Guidelines 2005). Lower urinary tract should be investigated before prosthetic surgery to find out some abnormalities such as urinary tract infection and urethral stricture. A urinalysis, determination of post-void residual urine, and cystoscopy in indicated cases should be performed in order to rule out these abnormalities. If infection is detected, it should be treated or the patient should be placed on prophylactic antibiotic treatment before the surgery. Any obstruction that may be due to prostatic hypertrophy or bladder neck contracture should be treated prior to prosthetic surgery. Simultaneous insertion of penile prosthesis and artificial urinary sphincter may be recommended in patients who suffer from urinary incontinence after radical prostatectomy. Although there are some studies which reported that a better control of blood sugar in patients with diabetes mellitus is associated with a lower risk of infection, larger studies detected no difference in infection rates in normal or elevated blood glucose level (Wilson SK, et al 1998). More recently, Mulcahy et al reported the results of 6071 diabetic patients who underwent penile prosthesis implantation with antibiotic (minocycline and rifampin) impregnated and 624 patients implanted with non-antibiotic impregnated implants with initial revision rates of 1.47% and 4.17%, respectively(Mulcahy et al 2011). At the end of 7 year-follow-up, authors found out the rate of infection related revisions significantly lower for antibiotic impregnated implant (1.62%) than for nonimpregnated implants (4.24%). It is also determined that diabetic men had a significantly higher rate of revisions due to infection at 7 yr (1.88%) than men without diabetes (1.53%). Finally, authors concluded that this long-term evidence obtained from the largest patient population establishes that the use of an antibiotic-impregnated IPP can decrease revisions due to infection and this decline may represent a significant medical advance in erectile restoration for diabetic patient population. There are a few measures to decrease the risk of infection such as showering with antibacterial soap, shaving operation area and use of broad-spectrum antibiotics one hour prior to surgery. Insertion of a catheter may facilitate urethral dissection and provide space for reservoir placement by emptying the bladder if a scrotal incision is carried out. The catheter may remain until the following morning. Some surgeons have tendency to use drains at the end of the surgery to reduce edema and provide an exit for bleeding. Such a drain is removed the following morning and has not demonstrated an increased incidence of prosthesis infection (Wilson SK, et al 1996).

Most patients need oral pain medication following the surgery. Heavy exercise and other activities which may cause displacement of the reservoir into the inguinal canal are proscribed for 4 weeks. Patients are instructed to use the device and return the sexual activity at the postoperative period of 4 to 6 weeks (Montague DK. 2011). Since initial inflation of the prosthesis may be difficult to perform; it will be beneficial to instruct the patients to inflate and deflate the device twice daily for the first month after surgery.

2.5 Operative technique

There are a variety of approaches for the implantation of penile prostheses described in the literature. These are distal penile, infrapubic and penoscrotal approaches. The distal penile approach is generally preferred for insertion of a semirigid or malleable penile prosthesis. Better visualization for the reservoir placement is the advantage of infrapubic approach. However, neurovascular injury which may result in decreased distal penile sensation is more likely due to close relationship with neurovascular bundle. Two-piece devices, due to the absence of a separate reservoir, are best implanted through a penoscrotal incision. Infrapubic approach may be preferred in patients with the history of previous abdominal surgeries where reservoir placement is complicated, however, penoscrotal approach provides ease in massive obese patients. In conclusion, the approach chosen for each particular patient should be based upon the type of prosthesis available, anatomy and surgical history of patient and preference of the surgeon.

2.5.1 Distal penile approach

This approach is generally accepted as the best approach for insertion of a semirigid or malleable penile prosthesis. It provides some advantages such as well incision healing, allowing corporeal dilation, and facilitation of rod placement.

After placement of a foley catheter, a circumcoronal incision is carried out and dissection is performed down to the layer of Buck's fascia with special consideration to prevent harm to dorsal penile nerves, which course within Buck's fascia. After identification of Buck's fascia, stay sutures are placed in the two corpora through the tunica albuginea lateral to the penile nerves. Dilation of corpora is performed by large scissors to establish a track in the corporal tissue. Dilation then follows with Hegar or Brooks dilators from 9 to 14 depending upon required cylinder girth. Once the corpora are measured by using a Furlow or other dilator, the cylinders can be placed. The corporotomy is then closed with 2-0 absorbable, synthetic sutures. With noninflatable cylinders, a penile block can be performed and a noncompression dressing is applied.

2.5.2 Infrapubic approach

The infrapubic approach is carried out by a horizontal or vertical incision approximately one finger below the symphysis pubis. After performing incision, subcutaneous tissue is dissected down to the rectus fascia. The rectus fascia is then incised and dissected for approximately 2 to 3 cm. A midline separation of the rectus muscles is achieved by sharp and blunt dissection to create a pouch beneath the rectus muscles in order to insert the reservoir without any discomfort. Dissection is then carried out over the corpora cavernosa. Sharp and blunt dissection is performed on either side of the fundiform ligament, identifying the dorsal neurovascular bundle. At this point, it should be remembered that the dorsal nerves of the penis lie approximately 2 to 3 mm lateral to the deep dorsal vein. Once Buck's fascia has been dissected free from the tunica albuginea, the shiny white tunica albuginea is fixed with longitudinal traction sutures. Then, a corporotomy incision is performed between the traction sutures. Following corporotomy, scissors are used to initiate the tunneling of the corpora cavernosa. Hegar dilators from size 9 to 14 can also be used. If corporeal fibrosis is encountered, Rossillo cavernotomes can be used to dilate to size 12. After performing dilation bilaterally, Furlow introducer can be used to measure corporal length by using the traction suture as the reference point.

Proximal and distal measurements are added to give total corporal length and choose appropriately sized inflatable cylinders. A length slightly less than the total measurement is usually used to permit comfortable positioning of the cylinders. Rear tip extenders of size 0.5, 1, 2, 3 cm, or combinations thereof are placed on the proximal cylinder end to adjust length.

Following measurement, interrupted sutures can be placed for subsequent corporotomy closure. When the corporotomy sutures are placed, cylinders are positioned in the dilated corpora cavernosa using the Furlow inserting tool with distal needle to pull the cylinders into position. It is important to ensure that adequate positioning of proximal and distal ends of cylinders has been performed. The corporal incision should be placed proximal enough to allow easy exit of the input tube and minimize cylinder/input tube contact. Closure of the corpora cavernosa is carried out with traction on the cylinder placement suture to maintain it in a flat, nonkinking position and ensure adequate seating. Following placement of cylinders and closure of the corporotomy incision, cylinder inflation can be tested by pumping fluid to identify any abnormalities in position, curvature, or related problems. A finger is placed beneath Scarpa's fascia down into the scrotum on one side to develop a sub dartos pouch for the pump. The pump is then positioned in the most dependent portion of the scrotum. The reservoir is then placed into the previously prepared area and filled with saline. Before connection, it is important to release pressure on the filling syringe and determine if any backfilling is observed. This backfilling or backpressure may predict an autoinflation problem in the future. Tubing connection is then carried out using quick connectors or suture tie plastic connectors. The tubing is tailored to eliminate excessive length but to allow for adequate pump positioning. Shodded clamps are used to compress the ends of tubes. Following tailoring, tubes are irrigated to eliminate small particles or blood clots. After the tubing is connected, the adequacy of the connection is tested by gently pulling on the connectors. All shodded clamps are removed and the device is inflated and deflated on multiple occasions to ensure adequate location, placement, and erection.

After that, thorough irrigation with antibiotic solution and then closure of rectus fascia with interrupted sutures are carried out. The wound then is closed in the standard fashion with two layers of subcutaneous tissue and a subcuticular skin suture leaving the cylinders partially inflated for 24 hours to improve haemostasis. A dry, sterile dressing is applied and a foley catheter is placed at the end of the procedure. Suction drains may be used according to surgeon's preference. The catheter is usually removed in the first postoperative day. The cylinders are deflated and patient discharged after the removal of drain. At discharge, patients are prescribed with a one-week antibiotic regimen and instructed to start cycling the device. Sexual activity can usually be resumed 6 weeks postoperatively (Garaffa G, et al 2010).

2.5.3 Penoscrotal approach

Three-piece inflatable penile prostheses, as well as semirigid and two-piece prostheses can be implanted by a transverse or vertical penoscrotal incision. This approach has distinct advantages in obese patients and is the most common approach for routine penile prosthesis implantation. Since differentiation of corpus spongiosum and corpus cavernosum is mandatory during dissection in this approach, initial insertion of a foley catheter is generally recommended. The incision is placed in the upper portion of the scrotum one finger below the penoscrotal junction. Once the skin incision has been carried out, dissection is continued lateral to the corpus spongiosum and urethra to expose the corpora cavernosa. Incision, dilation, and closure of the corpora cavernosa are similar to that described previously for the infrapubic incision, but synthetic absorbable sutures should be used with this approach because the suture line may be palpable postoperatively. Cylinder sizing and placement are as described above. Pump placement is likewise in the most dependent portion of the scrotum just below the dartos fascia. Dissection for reservoir placements can be carried out with a second separate infrapubic incision, but is more commonly performed through the penoscrotal incision. The scrotal skin incision is retracted to the area of the external inguinal ring and dissection is carried out medial to the spermatic cord. It is important to drain the bladder completely at this point. The transversalis fascia is then identified and incised sharply using large scissors pushed firmly through the medial aspect of the external inguinal ring. Dilation is carried out with the index finger after incision of the transversalis fascia. The reservoir balloon is then positioned over the index finger and placed in the perivesical space. Inflation of the reservoir is carried out with care that no backpressure is observed. Pocket enlargement should be performed to prevent autoinflation in case of syringe refilling. Once the reservoir is placed, inflated, and tubing connected as previously described, the device is tested in inflation and deflation modes. Closure is carried out with a subcuticular suture in the standard fashion.

2.6 Complications of penile prosthesis implantation

Complications of penile prosthesis can be divided into two categories as intraoperative and postoperative complications. Intraoperative complications include corporal cross-over and corporal/urethral perforation. Corporal cross-over can be subdivided into proximal and distal and might be encountered during corporal dilatation or cylinder placement (Garaffa et al 2010). This complication may be easily detected and corrected during the procedure. Testing for cross over is performed by side by side placement of dilators in each corpus cavernosum with special consideration to symmetry and proper positioning. If a crossover is detected, the dilator may be simply redirected with the contralateral dilator left in situ to prevent repeat crossover. Corporal perforation may also be recognized and easily repaired during the procedure, however, if urethral perforation is suspected, the procedure should be abandoned to allow for spontaneous recovery of the tear or a direct repair through a separate incision should be performed while the cylinder is in place.

Postoperative complications include infection, mechanical failure, auto-inflation, glans tumescence or coolness, reservoir displacement, cylinder erosion or extrusion and cavernosal fibrosis.

The two main complications of penile prosthesis implantation are mechanical failure and infection. Mechanical failure of penile prosthesis can include leakage from the cylinders, tubing fracture, reservoir malfunction, connector disruption, tube kinking and cylinder aneurysm. Historically, mechanical failure rates have been known to be low with many studies reporting rates of failure between 5-15% (Milbank et al 2002, Deuk et al 2001, Daitch et al 2001). Although, mechanical failure rates are low, manufacturers provided some improvements in the design of prostheses to achieve more successful outcomes. Five year freedom from mechanical failure rates reached over 90% after these improvements. More recently, Dhar et al. reported the long-term results of 455 patients who underwent penile prosthesis implantation with AMS 700 CX and found out that the overall freedom from reoperation was 74.9% and from mechanical failure was 81.3% after ten years (Dhar NB, et al 2006). A large-scale study performed with 2384 patients who had undergone penile prosthesis implantation with four different implant types reported revision-free survivals for all reasons to be 68.5% at 10 years and 59.7% at 15 years. For freedom from mechanical failure, the results were 79.4% at 10 years and 71.2% at 15 years (Wilson SK, et al. 2007). In another recently published, long-term study, Kim et al. reported the mechanical reliability results of AMS 700CX/CXM in 397 men with mean age of 63.1 years and follow-up duration of 113 months (Kim et al 2010). Mechanical survival rates of the prostheses were 97.6%, 93.2% and 78.2% at 3, 5, and 10 years after implantation, respectively. It is also reported that the overall survival of implants were significantly lower in patients with neurogenic ED when compared to non-neurogenic ones which may be due to decreased glandular sensation and difficulty in having natural position during sexual intercourse.

Infection is the bane of penile prosthesis surgery because, if it occurs in the space around the implant, total removal of all prosthetic material will be needed. Penile prosthesis reimplantation is more difficult due to corporal fibrosis in these patients.

A number of measures have been taken to decrease the risk of infection in prosthesis implanted patients. The most popular approach to reduce the rate of infection is the impregnation of antibiotics to the surface of prosthetic devices. Initial research suggests these newer interventions decrease the rate of prosthetic infection. With antibiotic prophylaxis, the infection rate is 2–3% and may be further reduced by using an antibiotic impregnated or hydrophilic-coated implant. Recently, Carson et al. reported the results of the retrospective comparison of the initial revision events due to infection in patients who underwent antibiotic impregnated or non-impregnated implantation with a follow-up of 7.7 years. At the end of follow-up, it is determined that initial revision rates due to infection were significantly lower in the impregnated group (Carson CC 2011). In another study, the antimicrobial activity of InhibiZone-coated IPPs produced by AMS was compared with the Titan hydrophilic-coated implants (produced by Coloplast) dipped in vancomycin, in both in-vivo and in-vitro animal models (Mansouri MD, et al 2009). The antimicrobial activity of the two implants was also compared against a control. In-vivo zones of inhibition were compared for each group against methicillin-resistant Staphylococcus aureus (MRSA), methicillin-resistant S. epidermidis (MRSE), vancomycin-resistant Enterococcus (VRE), and Escherichia coli. It is found that the InhibiZone-treated implants produced a larger zone of inhibition against MRSA, VRE, and E. Coli when compared with the vancomycin-dipped Titan implant and control and zones of inhibition were equivalent for MRSE in both implants. Similar results were obtained in animal models. Authors concluded that InhibiZone prostheses have a broader spectrum in vitro and a more durable antimicrobial activity in vitro and in an animal model than implants dipped in vancomycin. Therefore, the use of InhibiZone implants may help reduce the incidence of penile implant infection.

The use of prophylactic broad spectrum antibiotics is widespread in penile prosthetic surgery; however, the timing of the administration of these antibiotics varies among different studies. According to the guidelines "infusion of the first antimicrobial dose should begin within 60 minutes before surgical incision and that prophylactic antimicrobials should be discontinued within 24 hours after the end of surgery". It is well-known that infection rates in revision penile prosthetic surgery have been higher than primary implant surgery. During the revision surgery, the entire device is removed and the implant spaces are lavaged with multiple antiseptic solutions before implantation of a new device, the infection rate is similar to that with first time (primary) penile prosthesis implantation (Henry GD, et al 2005). Mulcahy et al. reported an 82% success rate achieved by using salvage therapy which involves removal and reimplantation immediately following thorough irrigation of the corpora with a multiantibiotic solution (Mulcahy et al 1996). More recently, the success rate increased to 84% in 101 patients who had infected implants (Mulcahy et al 2003). The salvage protocol described by Mulcahy should be performed in a stepwise fashion which consists of the removal of all prosthetic parts and foreign material, irrigation of wound and all compartments with 7 antiseptic solutions, changing operative equipment such as gloves, drapes and implantation of new prosthesis, closing the wound primarily without any drain and prescribe oral antibiotics according to culture for one month. The 7 antiseptic solution contains kanamycin and bacitracin, half strength hydrogen peroxide, half strength povidone iodine, water pic pressure irrigation with 1 gm vancomycin and 80 mg gentamicin in 5 liters, half strength povidone iodine, half strength hydrogen peroxide, kanamycin and bacitracin.

Autoinflation of a three-piece device may cause discomfort for the patient. In a study, the rate of autoinflation was reported between 3-5% (Hollenbeck BK et al 2002).

In order to prevent auto-inflation, Mentor developed a lockout valve mechanism that is added to prosthetic reservoir stem. This mechanism decreased the risk of autoinflation by transferring the fluid from reservoir in response to negative pressure from the pump (Wilson SK, et al 2002). Autoinflation risk decreased to the rate of 1.3% after this modification.

Coloplast developed Coloplast Titan One-Touch Release (OTR) pump to make device deflation easier for the patient. The new OTR pump allows cylinder deflation with one firm squeeze to the release pads. One firm squeeze of these pads causes the deflate valve to shift into the open position, providing a new pathway for fluid flow from the cylinders to the reservoir. In a recent study, Shaw et al assessed the functionality and surgeon experience with 100 consecutive patients implanted with a Titan OTR pump, compared with 100 prior consecutive patients implanted with a Titan Genesis pump (Shaw et al.2011). At the end of a mean length of follow-up of 20.8 months in the Genesis group and 8.4 months in the OTR group, the average number of postoperative teaching sessions needed to teach the patient how to operate the device was significantly lower in the OTR group (1.87 vs. 1.19). It is also reported that no pump malfunctions were seen in either group and the OTR pump was subjectively easier for the surgeon and the patient to deflate when compared with the Genesis pump.

Reservoir complications are not commonly encountered, however, they include herniation into inguinal canal and upper scrotum or erosion into adjacent viscera. Reservoir herniation is a rare complication that occurs in approximately 0.7% of three-piece inflatable prosthesis surgery cases (Sadeghi-Nejad et al. 2001). This complication is exclusively limited to cases when the penoscrotal approach is used. It may be caused by vigorous postoperative coughing or failure of proper initial reservoir placement under the transversalis fascia. Reservoir protrusion through an unrecognized existing hernia or a large tranversalis defect created intraoperatively are other possible contributory factors. Decreased spontaneous autoinflation of the cylinders in the immediate postoperative period may result in a lower incidence of this adverse event. Correction of this complication is by revision through an inguinal incision with placement of the reservoir in its proper position and repairing the defect (Hellstrom WG, et al.2010).

Some patients may suffer from poor support of the glans by the tips of the prosthesis. This angulation of the glans penis is called as the supersonic transport (SST) deformity because of the similarity of its appearance to the supersonic transport of aircraft. This deformity may develop secondary to small-size prosthesis or incomplete distal dilation of the corpora. If the problem occurs during the operation, following the achievement of adequate distal dilation, a larger rear-tip extender may be placed to lengthen the cylinder and see whether the defect is corrected. If the problem is noted in the immediate postoperative period, it is wise to wait a few weeks and allow for complete healing and scar formation, which may result in glans fixation and resolution of the SST deformity (Carson C. 1999)

Device extrusion may develop as an isolated finding or may be a sign of the device infection. Semirigid prosthesis are more prone to erosion, as the rate was reported as 18.1% for semirigid prostheses, 2.4% for self contained inflatable and 0% for 3-piece inflatable ones (Zermann et al 2006). Distal cylinder extrusion can be corrected by preparing a new cavity for the distal cylinder behind the back wall of the fibrotic sheath containing it (Mulcahy JJ. 1999). An alternative technique is to perform distal corporoplasty using synthetic material. Proximal perforation of the crura during the implant procedure can be repaired by the constructing wind sock of vascular prosthetic material and anchoring this to the prosthesis. More recently, Shindel et al described a novel technique of transglanular repair of the impending distal erosion of penile prostheses and reported successful outcomes in 4 of 6 patients during the follow-up (Shindel et al. 2010).

2.7 Outcomes of penile prosthesis surgery

Different from other treatments of ED, inflatable prostheses allow men to achieve a rigid erection on demand and as often as desired and also allow them to maintain the erection for a long period of time. Men with ED may develop performance anxiety and loss of confidence in their sexual capabilities, however, implantation of penile prosthesis may restore both erectile capacity and men's sexual confidence and provides the best results among all ED treatment modalities in terms of satisfaction.

In a study performed with 138 ED patients, the satisfaction rates were found to be significantly higher in patients treated with penile prosthesis implantation when compared with patients treated with sildenafil and intracavernous prostoglandin E1(Rajpurkar et al 2003). There are various studies that reported high satisfaction rates for both patients and partners after penile prosthesis implantation for the treatment of ED. Montorsi et al reported the results of 200 consecutive patients who underwent prosthetic surgery with 3-piece inflatable implants and reported a 98% patient and 96% partner satisfaction rate. Authors noted that the major factors that contribute to these high satisfaction rates are the rapid ability of the implants to produce an erection and consistent excellent rigidity (Montorsi et al 2000). However, loss of penile length which is likely to occur in revision surgeries after infection or penile shortening in Peyronie's disease may result in much lower satisfaction rates (Montorsi et al 1996).

There are many factors that may influence the patient satisfaction, such as postoperative pain and edema, occurrence of postoperative complications, cosmetic outcome, functional integrity of the device, ability to use and partner acceptance. Apart from these factors, reduced sensitivity, diminished sexual drive, unnatural feeling and perception of having a diminished role in initiating erection by the partner may be accepted as the other reasons of dissatisfaction. In a study performed by Akin-Olugbade et al over 114 penile prosthesis recipients, all patients showed significant improvement in IIEF and EDITS scores, however, patients with Peyronie's disease, body mass index over 30 and who underwent radical prostatectomy had lower satisfaction rates than the overall group. It should be kept in mind that these men have shorter penile length and failure of the implants to restore this length loss may contribute to increased rate of dissatisfaction (Akin-Olugbade et al 2008). High complication rates and unrealistic expectations are the other reasons of this low satisfaction rate.

More recently, Natali et al reported the results of 200 patients who underwent penile prosthesis implantation with AMS 700 CX, AMS Ambicor and AMS 600-650 with a mean follow-up of 5 years and found out a patient satisfaction rate of 97%, 81% and 75%, respectively (Natali et al 2008). In the same study, partner satisfaction rate was reported as 92%,91% and 75%, respectively. In another case series, 41 of 42(97.6%) patients reported successful intersourse after penile prosthesis implantation (Xuan XJ et al 2007). Paranhos et al reported the outcomes of 139 patients who underwent penile prosthesis implantation with a mean follow-up of 40 months (Paranhos et al 2010). The overall satisfaction rate was 86.3% for patients and 83.4% for partners at the end of the follow-up. In a recently performed study, Bettocchi et al evaluated 80 patients who underwent prosthesis surgery and reported that seventy-six patients (97%) affirmed to use penile prostheses frequently. Fifty-four patients (69%) and 70 partners (90%) affirmed that they never had problems with the use of the prosthesis and they considered themselves satisfied. Outcomes of these studies of penile prosthesis implantation concerning patient and partner satisfaction are summarized in table-1.

3. Penile arterial revascularization

Penile microarterial bypass surgery which was first described by Michal, is considered as a milestone in the treatment of ED because it is accepted as the only treatment option that is capable of restoring normal erectile function without the need of using any external mechanical (vacuum erection) devices, vasoactive medications or surgical placement of

Author	Year of publication	No of pts	Patient satisfaction rate	Partner satisfaction rate	Implant type/Comment
Montorsi et al	2000	200	98%	91%	AMS 3-piece implant
Xuan et al	2007	42	97.6%	NA	Patients who achieve coitus
Natali et al	2008	62/98/40	97%/81%/75%	92%/91%/75%	AMS 700CX/ Ambicor/600-650
Knoll et al	2009	69	86%	NA	AMS 700 Momentary squeeze
Paranhos et al	2010	139	86.3%	83.4%	RP and DM as negative predictors of satisfaction
Bettocchi et al	2010	80	97%	90%	AMS 700 CX

Table 1. Outcomes of the penile prosthesis procedures

penile prosthesis (Michal 1973). The objective of the surgery is to bypass arterial lesions that cause obstruction in the hypogastric-cavernous arterial bed (Hellstrom WJ, et al. 2010). Specifically, this surgery aims to increase the cavernosal arterial perfusion pressure and blood inflow in patients with vasculogenic ED that is developed due to pure arterial insufficiency. Lack of standardization in patient selection, hemodynamic evaluation and surgical technique as well as limited long-term outcome data using validated instruments have resulted in this surgery being considered by many surgeons as an experimental procedure. However, guidelines recommended that this type of surgery is proposed only to men with recently acquired ED secondary to focal arterial lesions and with the evidence of no existing generalized vascular disease. Additionally long operation time and the requirement for microsurgical expertise resulted in less frequent use of penile revascularization procedures. The efficacy of this surgery is still controversial and not evidence-based, largely because the selection criteria, outcome measurements, and microsurgical techniques have not been objective or standardized. The patients who are candidates for MABS (microarterial by-pass surgery) should fulfill some criteria such as age younger than 55 years with recently acquired ED due to focal occlusive disease of the common penile or cavernosal arteries detected by penile Doppler ultrasound, cavernosometry and selective internal pudendal arteriography. The patients who have vascular risk factors (diabetes, hypertension, tobacco use, hypercholesterolemia), evidence of neurological ED (eg multiple sclerosis, pelvic surgery, lumbosacral radiculopathies etc), nontreated hormonal abnormalities, psychiatric disorders (severe depression, bipolar disease, schizophrenia), Peyronie's disease, premature ejaculation and any evidence of corporo-occlusive dysfunction should not be considered as a candidate for this type of surgery. Young men who have sustained traumatic arterial lesions appear to have better outcomes compared to elderly patients.

Historically, Michal et al who reported the first MABS, performed a direct anastomosis between the inferior epigastric artery (IEA) and the corpus cavernosum (Michal I) which provided a sufficient flow rate and intraoperative erection. However, this procedure resulted in anastomotic stenosis in all patients and unsatisfactory success rates. Consequently, they performed the anastomosis between the IEA (end-to-side) and the dorsal penile artery (DPA) and achieved a success rate of 56% (Michal II)(Michal et al 1980).

Virag et al. performed the anastomosis between the IEA to the deep dorsal vein in order to increase penile perfusion in a retrograde fashion and reported a 49% success rate and an additional 20% improvement (Virag et al 1981). Furlow et al. also performed arterialization procedures of the dorsal vein with ligation of the circumflex branches to avoid glanular hyperemia, with success rates of 62% (Furlow et al 1988). Hauri reported a complicated side-to-side anastomosis between the dorsal artery and vein covered by a spatulated IEA that resulted in success rates of 80% (Hauri 1984)

MABS techniques that are currently defined include an anastomosis between the IEA to the dorsal vein (arterialization) or artery (revascularization). Artery-to-vein procedures are easier to perform than artery-to-artery, however, the failure rates are higher due to some reasons such as that the dorsal vein has valves that most likely impair penile reperfusion and may be associated with anastomotic thrombosis. Also, the use of a valvulotome may improve retrograde reperfusion to the corpora, but may also cause endothelial injury, which may activate the intrinsic pathway of the clotting system, leading to early thrombosis and failures. Finally, artery-to-artery MABS eliminates the possibility of penile hyperemia. Munarriz et al reported the long-term results of the patients who underwent MABS and although not supported by their data, they favor a MABS with the anostomosis between IEA- and the dorsal artery(Munarriz et al 2009).

MABS has three steps which include dorsal artery dissection, IEA harvesting, and microsurgical anastomosis (Munarriz et al 2004).

1. Dorsal artery dissection is performed via a 5-cm semilunar incision 2 cm below the penoscrotal junction. While the penis is stretched, blunt dissection is carried out along Buck's fascia towards the glans to invert the penis. The fundiform ligament is identified and preserved to minimize penile shortening. The selected dorsal artery is isolated and mobilized proximally, avoiding injury of the dorsal nerves. Temporary scrotal closure is performed.

2. Harvesting of IEA begins with a 5-cm transverse incision between umbilicus and pubis. Dissection is carried down through Scarpa's fascia, the rectus fascia is divided vertically, and the rectus muscle mobilized medially. The IEA is identified and mobilized from its origin at the level of the common external iliac artery to the umbilicus. If arterial branches are found, they are controlled with bipolar cautery and divided. During the mobilization of the IEA, papaverine is utilized to prevent vasospasm. The distal end of the IEA is clipped near the umbilicus and divided. Subsequently, the scrotal staples are removed and a clamp is utilized to transfer the IEA to the dorsal aspect of the penis through the external inguinal ring. The abdomen is closed in a multilayer fashion using a running technique with 0 polyglycolic acid suture for the rectus fascia, 2-0 for Scarpa's, and a 4-0 monocryl for the skin.

3. *Microvascular Anastomosis:* The dorsal artery is mobilized and divided in a proximal location on the penile shaft. The proximal end is cauterized using the bipolar cautery.

Aneurismal clips are placed on the dorsal artery and IEA. The adventitia of the distal end of the IEA and proximal dorsal artery is sharply excised with microscissors to prevent thrombosis of the anastomosis. A microsurgical anastomosis is performed using a simple interrupted technique with 10-0 Nylon stitches. The dorsal aneurismal clip is removed and back blood flow is observed, documenting anastomotic patency. The IEA aneurismal clip is removed and if there is no anastomotic leak, the penis is placed back on its normal anatomical position, the Dartos closed with a running 2-0 polyglycolic acid suture, and the skin with a 4-0 polyglycolic acid suture. Patency of the anastomosis is further confirmed by Doppler ultrasound.

3.1 Complications of the penile revascularization surgery

Penile shortening and decreased penile sensitivity may be observed in up to 25% of the patients after the procedure (Munarriz 2010). It is thought that penile shortening is the result of fibrosis/scarring of the fundiform ligament and its incidence may be minimized by the preservation of this ligament during the procedure. Decreased penile sensation is mostly seen due to a denervation injury during surgery, however, patients who underwent this operation may still report improvement in their orgasmic function. Glans hyperemia is another commonly observed complication with a rate of 13% in some series (Manning M, et al 1998). Other less common complications are wound infection and inguinal hernia.

3.2 Outcomes of penile revascularization surgery

Generally, the studies reporting the results of penile revascularization surgery are retrospective, had small numbers of patients, short term follow-up, variable patient selection criteria and type of surgery. To make a standardization and proper evaluation of these studies published, however, AUA guidelines recommend some inclusion criteria such as presence of a normal serum testosterone level, failure of pharmacologic erection test, abnormal nocturnal penile tumescence or penile duplex Doppler ultrasonography, abnormal penile arteriogram, artery to artery or artery to dorsal vein anastomosis employed in surgical technique, objective follow-up data reported by either duplex Doppler ultrasonography, penile arteriogram, or validated outcome questionnaire in the absence of diabetes mellitus and history of smoking. Also the follow-up period of studies to be included should at least have a period of 12 months. There are only four studies fulfilling these criteria which report variable success rates with different surgical techniques (Table-2).

Author	Type of surgery	No of pts	Months of follow-up: overall (mean)	Success Rate% (N) Success	Criteria
Ang (1997)	Dorsal vein	6	8-37(20)	66 (4)	NPT,Doppler
De Palma (1995)	Dorsal artery	11	12 to 48	60% (7)	Doppler
Grasso (1992)	Dorsal artery	22	12 months for all	68 (15) 36 (8)	NPT, Doppler
Jarow (1996)	Mixed	11	12 to 84 (50)	91 (10)	Doppler
Munarriz (2010)	Dorsal artery	71	NA(34.5)	88.7% (63)	IIEF

Table 2. Outcomes of the penile revascularization procedures

Apart from these studies, Kawanishi et al. reported the results of 51 men with arteriogenic ED who had objective outcome data reported by color Doppler duplex studies and a longer follow up period (Kawenishi et al 2004). The patency of the neoarterial blood flow either by the Hauri or Furlow-Fischer procedure was assessed objectively by color flow duplex Doppler. The authors reported the objective estimated efficacy rate as 84.9 % at 3 and 65.5% after 5 years of follow-up.

Although guidelines do not recommend this kind of procedures in elderly people, Kayigil et al reported the results of deep dorsal vein arterialization (DDVA) in 43 carefully selected healthy elderly patients with a mean follow-up of 22 months(Kayıgil et al 2008). All patients underwent DDVA using the Furlow-Fisher technique. Surgical outcome was tested postoperatively by IIEF score. The success rate of the operation was 60.5% at the end of follow-up. More recently, Kayıgil et al reported the long-term results (73.2 months) of 110 men who underwent revascularization surgery and reported an overall success rate of 72%(Kayıgil et al 2011). The success rates were 81.8% at 3 months, 77.2% at 1 year, 70% at 2 years, 66.3% at 3 years, and 63.6% at 5-year after surgery in the patients who achieved a no-ED threshold score of more than 26 in the IIEF-15. Authors concluded that this procedure may serve as a better alternative to prosthesis surgery by using a physiological restoration mechanism further studies are needed to compare the outcomes of different treatment modalities.

Recently, Babei reported a systematic review and metaanalysis to determine the results of patients with arteriogenic ED who underwent penile revascularization surgery. Characteristics of participants, study qualities, types of interventions, cure rates and adverse events were analyzed. Outcomes of procedures were found to be better in men younger than 30 years old and in men with the absence of venous leakage and history of smoking. In conclusion, the authors noted that inconsistent measurements of outcomes limited the findings, and none of the studies were randomized controlled trials. Authors also concluded that this kind of procedures may be beneficial in highly selected patients, however, randomized-controlled trials examining penile revascularization techniques are needed to recommend one technique over another (Babei et al 2009).

Robot-assisted vessel harvesting for penile revascularization is a new surgical approach in patients who suffered pelvic crush injuries resulting in post-traumatic ED. Raynor et al. reported five patients that underwent penile revascularization using a modified Virag-V technique (Raynor et al.2010). The epigastric artery was harvested robotically and transposed through a 3 cm incision at the base of the penis. Microscopic revascularization was performed by anastomosing the epigastric artery to the deep dorsal vein. Distal dorsal vein ligation of the subcoronal plexus was performed to prevent glans hyperemia. The procedure was successful in 4 patients. Authors concluded that this procedure is an ideal minimally invasive complement to penile revascularization which may shorten operation time and offer a novel option for the use of minimally-invasive technology.

4. Surgical treatment of Corporal Veno-Occlusive Dysfunction (CVOD)

Cavernous veno-occlusive dysfunction is another type of ED which may result from congenital reasons or trauma in young men, and acquired factors such as Peyronie's disease, diabetes mellitus and late onset hypogonadism in older men.

Pathophysiology of venogenic ED (VED) consists of formation of large venous channels draining the corpora cavernosa, degenerative changes to the tunica albuginea, structural alterations of the cavernous smooth muscle and endothelium (Ghanem et al 2008). Whatever the cause is, the objective of the treatment is to obstruct this leakage. It is found out that the deep dorsal vein is the major site of venous leakage in more than 75% of cases (Fuchs et al.1989).

Surgical treatment for VED should be considered when medical treatment fails to provide sufficient erection. Selection criteria for surgery include the patients with erections of short duration or tumescence only with sexual stimulation; younger than 50 years; normal cavernous arterial inflow in response to an intracavernous injection agent; and who are more likely to have venous leakage after performing Doppler ultrasound or penile cavernosography in the absence of chronic systemic diseases (Manning M et al 1998).

Surgery for penile venous leakage is not recommended in older men because penile venous leakage often results from atrophy of the intracorporeal muscles or the tunica albuginea (Lue TF 1999, Montague DK, et al 1996). However, when venous leakage is congenital, the deficiency is usually in the large, ectopic, superficial and deep dorsal veins or the large crural veins (Lue TF, 1999, Ebbehoj et al. 1979). Currently, there is no evidence from randomized controlled trials to recommend a standardized approach for the diagnosis and effective treatment of veno-occlusive ED. Since it is generally accepted that venous leakage is an effect rather than a cause, and newer pathophysiologic mechanisms that cause CVOD and therapeutic possibilities that might address these causes, are being examined. Research continues to detect an effective surgical treatment alternative.

Although there is no standard evidence-based surgical option, ligation of superficial dorsal vein, deep dorsal vein, crural vein, crural plication/ ligation, arterialization of deep dorsal or cavernosal veins or extraperitoneal laparoscopic penile vein ligation are some of the intervention types used in CVOD surgery.

Recently, Cayan et al reported the results of a study including 26 men with a mean age of 34, who underwent penile venous surgery for primary venous leakage with a mean follow-up of 42 months (Cayan 2008). Surgical procedure consists of resection of the superficial and deep dorsal veins, ligation of the cavernous vein and 2 crura proximal to the entrance of the cavernous artery with umbilical tapes, and preservation of the dorsal artery and nerve on each side. In the follow-up, erectile function improved in 19 men and remained unchanged in 7 men. Patient satisfaction with no additional treatment or with phosphodiesterase-5 inhibitors was 88.4% and only 3 patients were unsatisfied with the surgery. It is concluded that penile venous surgery with crural ligation for venous leakage has excellent long-term results, high patient satisfaction rate and should be offered to young men with primary cavernous ED. Additionally, young patients who have normal penile arterial system and no risk factors such as diabetes are the best candidates for the improved postoperative outcome. Since the surgery of ligation or resection for venous leakage has not been very successful and unsatisfactory long-term results have reduced the indications for venous surgery, a new technique which is the embedding of dorsal vein for dorsal venous leakage is reported to improve the long-term outcomes (Zhang et al 2009). The procedure is performed through a curved incision made over the root of the penis. Following the dissection of deep dorsal vein, a whole thickness tunica albuginea excision of about 0.8 cm was performed and the dissected vein is embedded to this newly formed groove. At the end of 42 months of average follow-up, 14 of 17 patients reported satisfactory intercourse and three had sufficient erection after oral treatment. Besides, it was also noted that there were significant improvements in terms of IIEF-5 scores and some Doppler USG parameters in all patients. According to these results, authors concluded that this new surgical technique is a simple operation which seems to provide promising results with the need of future studies in the treatment of penile deep dorsal venous leakage of ED.

Possible complications that may be encountered in the post-operative period include wound infection, skin necrosis, glandular hyperemia or hypoesthesia, inguinal hernia, penile curvature, shortening or edema.

If CVOD surgery is going to be performed, a long-term follow-up of at least 48 months is recommended with the use of pre and postoperative validated scales (e.g. IIEF). Post-operative follow-up should include objective evaluation of the penile vascular and erectile status. Penile color duplex ultrasound after complete cavernosal smooth muscle relaxation is the gold standard investigation of choice for both pre-op and post-op objective assessment.

The type of operation offered to the patient should be determined depending on the experience and preference of the surgeon and the basis of the site, nature, and size of the leak.

5. Conclusion

Penile prosthesis implantation is currently the most effective treatment option in terms of both patient and partner satisfaction in the management of ED. Satisfaction rates and prosthesis survival significantly increased with the improvements in both prosthesis design and surgical techniques. Among prosthesis types, inflatable 3-piece prosthesis have the best outcomes and recommended for younger patients with normal manual dexterity, patients with Peyronie's disease, neurological disorders, patients who underwent radical prostatectomy and in revision procedures. Preoperative preparation and use of antibiotic impregnated devices during surgery are the essential points to reduce the risk of prosthesis infection. The ideal prosthesis aims to mimic natural erection and flaccidity as well as possible and research to find the ideal prosthesis still continues. Further technological improvements may provide additional significant increases in satisfaction and survival rates and decrease the number of infected implants. Penile revascularization is not a commonly performed procedure and its use is limited only to selected cases because of the variabilities in inclusion and exclusion criteria, short length of follow-up, and lack of objective follow-up data. However, patients who are younger than the age of 55, non-smoker, non-diabetic with the absence of venous leakage may have a better outcome after the procedure. Penile venous surgery is not a recommended surgical treatment modality due to absence of a standardized surgical technique and follow-up data. This operation may only be recommended for young patients with site-specific congenital, posttraumatic or post-inflammatory venous leaks with informed consent. The type of the operation for each particular patient should be decided according to experience of surgeon, site, size and nature of the venous leak.

6. References

Akin-Olugbade O, Parker M, Guhring P, Mulhall J.(2006) Determinants of patient satisfaction following penile prosthesis surgery. J Sex Med Jul: 3:743-8

Ang LP, Lim PH. Penile revascularisation for vascular impotence. (1997) Singapore Med J. Jul: 38:285-8

AUA Guidelines. Management of Erectile Dysfunction (2005)

Babei AR, Safarinejad MR, Kolahi AA. (2009)Penile revascularization for erectile dysfunction: a systematic review and meta-analysis of effectiveness and complications. Urol J. Winter: 6:1-7

Bettocchi C, Palumbo F, Spilotros M, Lucarelli G, Palazzo S, Battaglia M, Selvaggi FP, Ditonno P.(2010) Patient and partner satisfaction after AMS inflatable penile prosthesis implant. J Sex Med.Jan;7(1 Pt 1):304-9.

Bogoraz.(1936) On complete Plastic reconstruction of a penis sufficient for Coitus (in Russian). Soviet Surgery (Sovetskaya). 8:303-9

Carson C, Giuliano F, Goldstein I, Hatzichristou D, Hellstrom W, Lue T et al. (2004) The 'effectiveness' scale—therapeutic outcome of pharmacologic therapies for ED: an international consensus panel report. Int J Impot Res 16: 207–213.

Carson C. (1999) Complications of penile prostheses and complex implantations. In: Carson C, Kirby R, Goldstein I, eds. Textbook of male erectile dysfunction. Oxford, UK: Isis Medical Media. 435–50.

Carson CC, Mulcahy JJ (2011) J Urol. Long-term infection outcomes after original antibiotic impregnated inflatable penile prosthesis implants: up to 7.7 years of followup.

Carson CC, Noh CH. (2002) Distal penile prosthesis extrusion: treatment with distal corporoplasty or Gortex windsock reinforcement. Int J Impot Res.Apr: 14:81-4

Carson CC. (2005) Penile prosthesis implantation: surgical implants in the era of oral medication. Urol Clin North Am. Nov: 32:503-9, vii

Cayan S. (2008) Primary Penile Venous Leakage Surgery With Crural Ligation in Men With Erectile Dysfunction. J Urol. 180, 1056-1059.

Cuellar DC, Sklar GN. (2001) Penile prosthesis in the organ transplant recipient. Urology 57:138–41.

Daitch JA, Angermeier KW, Lakin MM, Ingleright BJ, Montague DK. (1997) Long-term mechanical reliability of AMS 700 series inflatable penile prostheses: comparison of CX/CXM and Ultrex cylinders. J Urol. Oct: 158:1400-2

Darouiche RO, Smith JA, Jr., Hanna H, et al. (1999) Efficacy of antimicrobial-impregnated bladder catheters in reducing catheter-associated bacteriuria: a prospective, randomized, multicenter clinical trial. Urology. Dec: 54:976-81

DePalma RG, Olding M, Yu GW, et al. (1995) Vascular interventions for impotence: lessons learned. J Vasc Surg. Apr: 21:576-84; discussion 84-5

Deuk Choi Y, Jin Choi Y, Hwan Kim J, Ki Choi H. (2001) Mechanical reliability of the AMS 700CXM inflatable penile prosthesis for the treatment of male erectile dysfunction. J Urol. Mar: 165:822-4

Dhar NB, Angermeier KW, Montague DK. (2006)Long-term mechanical reliability of AMS 700CX/CXM inflatable penile prosthesis. J Urol. Dec: 176:2599-601; discussion 601

Ebbehoj J and Wagner G. (1979) Insufficient penile erection due to abnormal drainage of cavernous bodies. Urology 13:507.

Fuchs AM, Mehringer CM, Rajfer J. (1989) Anatomy of penile venous drainage in potent and impotent men during cavernosography. J Urol 141:1353–6.

Furlow, W.L. and Fisher, J. (1988) Deep dorsal vein arterialization: clinical experience with a new technique for penile revascularization. *J. Urol.* 139, 298A, Abstr. 543

Garaffa G, Moncada I, Ralph DJ. (2010) Surgical management of erectile dysfunction. Arch Esp Urol.63;8: 728-738.

GE B. (1964) Surgical Treatment of Impotence. Plast Reconst Surg. 34:71-3

Ghanem H, Shamloul R. (2008) An evidence-based perspective to commonly performed erectile dysfunction investigations. J Sex Med. 5:1582–9.

Govier FE, Gibbons RP, Correa RJ, Pritchett TR, Kramer-Levien D.(1998) Mechanical reliability, surgical complications, and patient and partner satisfaction of the modern three-piece inflatable penile prosthesis. Urology. Aug: 52:282-6

Grasso M, Lania C, Castelli M, Deiana G, Francesca F, Rigatti P. (1992) Deep dorsal vein arterialization in vasculogenic impotence: our experience. Arch Ital Urol Nefrol Androl. Dec: 64:309-12

Hatzimouratidis K, et al. (2010) Guidelines on Male Sexual Dysfunction: Erectile Dysfunction and Premature Ejaculation. Eur Urol 57:804-814.

Hauri, D. (1984) Therapiemoglichkeitem bei der vascular bedingten erectilein impotenz. *Akt. Urol.* 15, 350

Hellstrom WJ, Montague DK, Moncada I, Carson C, Minhas S, Faria G, Krishnamurti S. (2010) J Sex Med. Jan;7(1 Pt 2):501-23.

Henry GD WS, Delk JR. (2004) Early results with new ribs and pads AMS 700 pump: Device instruction easier. J Sex Med. 1:81

Henry GD, Wilson SK, Delk JR, 2nd, et al. (2005) Revision washout decreases penile prosthesis infection in revision surgery: a multicenter study. J Urol. Jan: 173:89-92

Hollenbeck BK, Miller DC, Ohl DA. (2002)The utility of lockout valve reservoirs in preventing autoinflation in penile prostheses. Int Urol Nephrol.34:379-83

Jarow JP, Defranzo AJ. (1996) Long-term results of arterial bypass surgery for impotence secondary to segmental vascular disease. J Urol. 156:982-5.

Kawanishi Y, Kimura K, Nakanishi R, Kojima K, Numata A. (2004) Penile revascularization surgery for arteriogenic erectile dysfunction: the long-term efficacy rate calculated by survival analysis. BJU Int. Aug: 94:361-8.

Kayigil O, Agras K, Okulu E. (2008)Is deep dorsal vein arterialization effective in elderly patients? Int Urol Nephrol. 40:125-31

Kayıgil O, Okulu E, Aldemir M, Onen F. (2011)Penile revascularization in vasculogenic erectile dysfunction (ED): long-term follow-up. BJU Int.

Kim DS, Yang KM, Chung HJ, Choi HM, Choi YD, and Choi HK. (2010) AMS 700CX/CXM inflatable penile prosthesis has high mechanical reliability at long-term follow-up. J Sex Med 7:2602–2607

Laumann EO, Nicolosi A, Glasser DB, Paik A, Gingell C, Moreira E et al. (2005) Sexual problems among women and men aged 40–80 y: prevalence and correlates identified in the Global Study of Sexual Attitudes and Behaviors. Int J Impot Res;17: 39–57.

Levine LA, Estrada CR, Morgentaler A. (2001) Mechanical reliability and safety of, and patient satisfaction with the Ambicor inflatable penile prosthesis: results of a 2 center study. J Urol. Sep: 166:932-7

Lewis RW, Fugl-Meyer KS, Corona G, Hayes RD, Laumann EO, Moreira ED Jr, Rellini AH, Segraves T. (2010) Definitions/Epidemiology/Risk factors for sexual dysfunction. J Sex Med. Apr;7(4 Pt 2):1598-607

Lue TF: Surgery for crural venous leakage. Urology 1999; 54: 739.

Manning M, Junemann KP, Scheepe JR, Braun P, Krautschick A, Alken P. (1998) Long-term followup and selection criteria for penile revascularization in erectile failure. J Urol. Nov: 160:1680-4

Mansouri MD, Boone TB, Darouiche RO.(2009) Comparative assessment of antimicrobial activities of antibiotic-treated penile prostheses. Eur Urol Dec;56(6):1039-45.

Michal V, Kramar R, Pospichal J et al. (1973) Direct arterial anastomosis on corpora cavernosa penis in the therapy of erective impotence. Rozhl Chir 52: 587.

Michal, V., Kramer, R., and Hejhal, L. (1980) Revascularization procedures of the cavernous bodies. In *Vasculogenic Impotence: Proceedings of the First International Conference on Corpus Cavernosum Revascularization*. Zorgniotti, A.W. and Ross, G., Eds. Charles C Thomas, Springfield, IL. pp. 239–255

Milbank AJ, Montague DK, Angermeier KW, Lakin MM, Worley SE. (2002) Mechanical failure of the American Medical Systems Ultrex inflatable penile prosthesis: before and after 1993 structural modification. J Urol. Jun: 167:2502-6

Montague DK, Barada JH, Belker AM, Levine LA, Nadig PW, Roehrborn CG et al (1996) Clinical guidelines panel on erectile dysfunction: summary report on the treatment of organic erectile dysfunction. J Urol 1996; 156: 2007.

Montorsi F, Guazzoni G, Barbieri L, et al. (1996)AMS 700 CX inflatable penile implants for Peyronie's disease: functional results, morbidity and patient-partner satisfaction. Int J Impot Res. Jun: 8:81-5; discussion 5-6

Montorsi F, Rigatti P, Carmignani G, et al.(2000) AMS three-piece inflatable implants for erectile dysfunction: a long-term multi-institutional study in 200 consecutive patients. Eur Urol. Jan: 37:50-5

Mulcahy JJ. (1999) Distal corporoplasty for lateral extrusion of penile prosthesis cylinders. J Urol. Jan: 161:193-5

Mulcahy JJ. (2003) Treatment alternatives for the infected penile implant. Int J Impot Res. Oct: 15 Suppl 5:S147-9

Munarriz R, Uberoi J, Fantini G, Martinez D, Lee C. (2009) J Urol. Microvascular Arterial Bypass Surgery: Long-Term Outcomes Using Validated Instruments Vol. 182, 643-648

Munarriz, R., Mulhall, J., and Goldstein, I. (2004) Penile arterial reconstruction. In *Glenn's Urologic Surgery*. 6th ed. Lippincott Williams & Wilkins, Philadelphia. pp. 573–581.

Natali A, Olianas R, Fisch M.(2008) Penile implantation in Europe: successes and complications with 253 implants in Italy and Germany. J Sex Med. Jun: 5:1503-12

Nickel JC, Heaton J, Morales A, Costerton JW. (1986)Bacterial biofilm in persistent penile prosthesis-associated infection.J Urol. Mar: 135:586-8

Paranhos M, Andrade E, Antunes AA, Barbieri ALN, Claro JA, Srougi M.(2010) Penile Prosthesis Implantation in an Academic Institution in Latin America. Int Braz J Urol 36 (5): 591-601

Raad I, Darouiche R, Hachem R, Sacilowski M, Bodey GP. (1995)Antibiotics and prevention of microbial colonization of catheters. Antimicrob Agents Chemother. Nov:39:2397-400

Rajpurkar A, Dhabuwala CB. (2003) Comparison of satisfaction rates and erectile function in patients treated with sildenafil, intracavernous prostoglandin E1 and penile implant surgery for erectile dysfunction in urology practice. J Urol 170(1):159-163.

Rossier AB, Fam BA. (1984) Indication and results of semirigid penile prostheses in spinal cord injury patients: long-term followup. J Urol. Jan: 131:59-62

Sadeghi-Nejad H, Sharma A, Irwin RJ, Wilson SK, Delk JR.(2001) Reservoir herniation as a complication of three-piece penile prosthesis insertion. Urology. Jan: 57:142-5

Sadeghi-Nejad H. (2007)Penile prosthesis surgery: A review of prosthetic devices and associated complications. J Sex Med 4:296–309

Scott FB BW, Timm GW. (1973) Management of erectile impotence. Use of implantable inflatable prosthesis. Urology. 2:80-2

Shaw T and Garber BB. (2011) Coloplast Titan inflatable penile prosthesis with one-touch release pump: Review of 100 cases and comparison with genesis pump. J Sex Med 8:310–314.

Shindel AW, Brant WO, Mwamukonda K, Bella AJ, Lue TF. (2010) Transglanular repair of impending penile prosthetic cylinder extrusion. J Sex Med. Aug;7(8):2884-90

Stewart PS, Costerton JW. (2001)Antibiotic resistance of bacteria in biofilms. Lancet;358:135–8.

Subrini L. (1982) Subrini penile implants: surgical, sexual and psychological results. Eur Urol. 8:222-6

Virag, R., Zwang, G., Dermange, H., and Legman, M. (1981) Vasculogenic impotence: a review of 92 cases with 54 surgical operations. *Vasc. Surg*. 15, 9–16.

Wilson SK DJ, Henry GO. (2002) Short-term Follow-up for Enhanced American Medical Systems CX Prosthesis. J Urol. 169:1333A

Wilson SK DJ. (1996) Scrotal hematoma prevention following penile prothesis implantation; to drain or not to drain. J Urol. 155:634A

Wilson SK, Cleves M, Delk JR, 2nd.(1996) Long-term results with Hydroflex and Dynaflex penile prostheses: device survival comparison to multicomponent inflatables. J Urol. May: 155:1621-3

Wilson SK, Cleves MA, Delk JR, 2nd.(1999) Comparison of mechanical reliability of original and enhanced Mentor Alpha I penile prosthesis. J Urol. Sep: 162:715-8

Wilson SK, Delk JR, Salem EA, et al. (2007)Long-term survival of inflatable penile prostheses: single surgical group experience with 2,384 first-time implants spanning two decades. J Sex Med 4:1074–9

Wilson SK, Henry GD, Delk JR, Cleves MA. (2002)The Mentor Alpha I penile prosthesis with reservoir lock-out valve: effective prevention of auto-inflation with improved capability for ectopic reservoir placement. J Urol.168:1475-8.

Xuan XJ, Wang DH, Sun P, Mei H.(2007) Outcome of implanting penile prosthesis for treating erectile dysfunction: experience with 42 cases. Asian J Androl. Sep: 9:716-9

Zermann DH, Kutzenberger J, Sauerwein D, Schubert J, Loeffler U. (2006) Penile prosthetic surgery in neurologically impaired patients: long-term followup. J Urol. Mar: 175:1041-4; discussion 4

10

Gene and Stem Cell Therapy in Erectile Dysfunction

Trevor Hardigan, R. Clinton Webb and Kenia Pedrosa Nunes
Georgia Health Sciences University, Augusta, Georgia
USA

1. Introduction

Erectile dysfunction (ED) is a complex, multifactorial issue commonly affecting men of all ages. ED is currently defined as "the inability to achieve and/or maintain penile erection sufficient to permit satisfactory sexual intercourse", and has been associated with such risk factors as hypertension, diabetes, alcoholism, smoking, and pelvic surgery [1]. This condition has seriously impacted the men's quality of life. Even though nowadays there are a large number of options to treat ED, a considerable number of patients do not answer adequately the conventional therapies available. Penile erection is achieved through a neurovascular response exhibiting an increase in arterial inflow, relaxation of corporal smooth muscle, and restriction of the venous outflow. Relatively recent pharmacological advances, namely oral phosphodiesterase-5 (PDE5) inhibitors, have become the first line of treatment in ED. PDE5 inhibitors allow the patient to achieve a penile erection via the effects on the nitric oxide (NO) signaling pathway, which is the principal mediator of corporal smooth muscle relaxation. The inhibition of the degradative actions of PDE5 on 3',5'-cyclic guanosine monophosphate (cGMP), the second messenger molecule of NO signaling, lead to an increased bioavailability of NO in the corporal smooth muscle thus promoting vasodilation and penile erection. However, despite the widespread efficacy of these medications, there are still men for which oral PDE5 inhibitors are ineffective. ED in men with diabetes, for example, is typically more severe, exhibiting a less effective response to PDE5 inhibitors when compared to non-diabetic patients. The vascular injuries that accompanies diabetes is often too damaging to endothelial physiology to allow adequate penile erections [4] and thus complicates use of the oral medications as treatment for ED. Due to the vast array of potential causes of ED ranging from neurogenic and vasculogenic to hormonal issues, there exists a continuing need to address these deficiencies in patient management of ED and pursue new treatments. Two avenues showing a great deal of promise in ED treatment are gene therapy and stem cell therapy, both of which could possibly provide methods to prevent or even cure ED. This chapter will focus on recent studies in both gene and stem cell therapies in ED research, with the objective to establish that continued scientific exploration into these fields will yield clinically applicable approaches to combat this condition.

2. Gene therapy and ED

Gene therapy is the introduction of exogenous genetic material into cells that either restores or enhances normal cellular function that is defective, or essentially attenuates the functional effects of the mutant genetic phenotypic expression. This is accomplished through the use of vectors, which are designed to deliver or transfect a given gene into an organism allowing the organism to subsequently reproduce the gene and its protein product. Many different types of vectors have been characterized; viral vectors such as retroviruses and adenoviruses, cell-based vectors such as myoblasts and endothelial cells, as well as non-viral vectors such as plasmid DNA and naked DNA. Viral vectors are commonly used due to their high cellular transfection efficiency; however they have been shown to trigger immune and inflammatory responses which can reduce their effects [5]. The host's immune response can generate antibodies to the virus being used as vector, prompting destruction of the delivery system before it generates a therapeutic effect [1]. Additionally, many of the viruses used as vectors do not exhibit tissue specificity, contributing to issues associated with viral migration through the systemic circulation to other unwanted tissues or organ systems [1].

Several molecules have been examined as potential gene therapeutic approaches for ED, including vascular endothelial growth factor (VEGF), NO synthase, precalcitonin gene-related peptide, brain derived neurotrophic factor, and the calcium sensitive potassium (maxi-K) channel [5]. The penis is considered to be a well suited structure for gene therapy due to its limited blood supply, which would decrease the risks associated with non-target infection via the systemic circulation. Its external positioning allows for an ease of accessibility for genetic manipulation, and the intracellular transference of the erectile tissue response to the delivery by gap junctions of corporal smooth muscle further make gene therapy a useful approach as only a proportion of cells are required to be transfected [5]. The relatively low turnover rate of vascular smooth muscle cells indicates the potential for long term expression of introduced genes and thus would yield an improvement over the short term effects of current pharmacological therapies [4]. The role of NO in regulating corporal smooth muscle relaxation is a primary area of concern in ED, and consequently a great deal of the research examining potential gene therapeutic treatments focuses on ways to repair deficient endothelial NO production. [4]

2.1 eNOS gene therapy

eNOS, or nitric oxide synthase 3, is an enzyme found in endothelial cells that produces the NO required for relaxation of the surrounding smooth muscle. It has been shown in patients with ED that a lack of eNOS expression potentiates the difficulties in achieving and maintaining adequate penile erection through low bioavailability of NO and subsequent increase in vascular tone [4]. There have been several studies examining the role of eNOS gene therapy to treat many of the underlying vascular pathologies leading to ED. Champion et al. studied the effects of using adenoviral gene transfer of eNOS in an age-related rat model of ED. Through the increase in production of eNOS mRNA and subsequent increase in protein expression, it was observed that there was a notable increased erectile response to cavernous nerve stimulation, PDE5 inibitors, and also acetylcholine post-treatment. Within the aged-penis there was also an increase in the presence of cGMP noted. In diabetic rat models, intracavernosal pressure recorded during cavernosal nerve stimulation is markedly lower when compared to the control animals [1]. Bivalacqua et al. have shown that the use of intracavernous eNOS transfection is also a viable therapy, improving both the erectile response to cavernous nerve stimulation and the levels of corporal NO in diabetic rat model of ED. These findings were assessed in conjunction with the use of a PDE5 inhibitor in the diabetic rat model, and it was observed that when combined with intracavernous eNOS transfection the erectile response to the pharmacologic treatment was increased along with levels of cGMP in the penis.

2.2 VEGF gene therapy

Vascular endothelial growth factor (VEGF) is a multifunctional protein and a critical mediator of endothelial and smooth muscle physiology. It stimulates angiogenesis and increases vascular permeability as well inhibits apoptosis, and as such it provides a potential therapeutic approach for the treatment of ED by increasing NO levels through the expansion of penile vasculature [1]. The increase in vasculature would bring about an accompanying increase in endothelial cells, thus creating an increase of NO production in the target organ. Both VEGF and its receptor flk-1 have been shown to be downregulated in certain types of ED [4], suggesting a possible pathological association. There have been several studies indicating the potential benefits of VEGF treatment for ED. Intracavernous injection of VEGF has been shown to provide a protective effect against hypercholesteremia in penile corporal endothelium from an atherosclerotic rabbit model of ED. This protective effect of VEGF has also been shown in other models of ED such as those accompanying diabetes or in traumatic arteriogenic ED. Additionally, endothelial hypertrophy and hyperplasia were observed following intracavernous VEGF protein delivery in another hypercholesteremic ED model [4]. It is believed that the anti-apoptotic effects of VEGF are associated with this hyperplasia and hypertrophy of endothelial cells, potentially by directly inducing anti-apoptotic pathways in the endothelium. Other potentially therapeutic effects of VEGF in connection with ED are an increase in the expression of eNOS and a stimulatory effect on eNOS phosphorylation.

Further studies have utilized the data supporting the benefits of VEGF protein introduction as a foundation for designing VEGF gene therapy treatments. The goal was that introducing VEGF DNA would increase long-term expression of VEGF and ameliorate any deficiencies in protein amount, essentially acting as a curative treatment for ED [4]. In a study by Rogers et al., an adeno-associated virus was used to transfect VEGF DNA into a model of venogenic ED, with resulting active angiogenesis indicated by endothelial cell hypertrophy and hyperplasia. A similar study examining VEGF DNA delivery in a venogenic model of ED using an adenovirus was shown to increase phosphorylation of eNOS leading to a concurrent increase in the bioavailability of NO and recovery of erectile function [10]. VEGF introduction has also been examined using a combined gene therapy approach with angiopoetin-1, an angiogenic growth factor that promotes the creation of new blood vessels from pre-existing vessels. Using an adenovirus for both VEGF and angiopoetin-1 in a hypercholesteremic rat model of ED, it was found that the ratio of phosphorylated eNOS to total eNOS was markedly higher in animals receiving the gene therapy versus the control animals. The combined gene therapy approach was found to increase factor VIII-positive endothelial density with a subsequent increase in erectile response to electrical stimulation, suggesting the importance of functional endothelium in management of ED.

2.3 SOD gene therapy

Another potential target for gene therapy in ED is utilizing superoxide dismutase (SOD) to decrease the levels of reactive oxygen species (ROS). Reactive oxygen species have been shown to play a critical role in endothelial cell dysfunction, primarily through the actions of superoxide scavenging of NO to form the toxic substance peroxynitrite [4]. Superoxide and peroxynitrite create a cascade of ROS formation by uncoupling eNOS within the endothelium, decreasing the production of NO and thus impairing erectile function. This creation of ROS is exacerbated by the expression of inducible nitric oxide synthase (iNOS) during oxidative stress conditions, leading to the production of even more ROS. Antioxidants are involved in attenuating the toxic effects of ROS. SOD, found in cells such as vascular endothelium, helps to decrease levels of superoxide by catalyzing the dismutation of the ROS into hydrogen peroxide and water [4].

In a study by Bivalacqua et al., intracavernous adenoviral gene transfer of extracellular SOD was performed in an age-related rat model of ED in an attempt to decrease the levels of ROS. In the rat model there was an observed increase in superoxide production, a decrease in cGMP production as well as a decrease in erectile response to cavernous nerve stimulation. Additionally, they used nitrotyrosine staining as a measure of oxidative stress and found elevated levels in the aged rats. Following transfection of extracellular SOD DNA, there was an increase in extracellular SOD mRNA, protein, and activity levels, along with an increase in cGMP production. Oxidative stress was again measured using nitrotyrosine staining and a decrease was observed post therapeutic treatment. Erectile response to cavernous nerve stimulation was also restored, suggesting that the introduction of extracellular SOD DNA holds potential a viable gene therapy treatment to combat ED resulting from ROS damage to penile endothelium. It has also been shown that ROS play a role in diabetes-related vascular dysfunction and also ED [4], prompting studies on the effects of extracellular SOD gene therapy in diabetic models of ED. Extracellular SOD expression was notably decreased in the diabetic penis, contributing to an increase in the levels of ROS present. Adenoviral transfection of extracellular SOD decreased levels of superoxide and increased cGMP production, which together improved erectile function in an endothelium dependent manner.

2.4 Anti-arginase gene therapy

Supplementation of the amino acid L-arginine, either through the diet or direct infusion, has been shown to cause an increase in NO and a subsequent enhancement of endothelium-related vasodilation in the penis [2]. L-Arginine is used as a substrate by both eNOS and arginase, the latter of which converts L-arginine to urea and L-ornithine. This creates a synergistic relationship between the two enzymes, as an increase in arginase activity leads to a downregulation of NO biosynthesis through competition with eNOS [2]. The enzyme arginase has two isoforms, arginase I and arginase II. Arginase I and II are commonly referred to as the hepatic type and extrahepatic type, respectively, though in a study by Bivalacqua et al. which showed an increase in arginase activity in human diabetic corpus cavernosum that both arginase isoforms were found. It was suggested that the impaired endothelium-derived NO bioactivity or signaling via an increased expression of arginase plays a role in the reduction of endothelium-dependant response in the penis of aged mice [2]. Utilizing adeno-associated viral gene transfer of anti-arginase, Bivalacqua et al. found that there was a decrease of arginase-1 protein and mRNA in the aged mouse penis accompanied by restoration of endothelial and erectile function in vivo [2]. The increase in erectile function was attributed to the increase in constitutive NOS activity and penile cGMP levels, suggesting that arginase can interfere with normal erectile function by decreasing production of endothelium-derived eNOS in the penis. Interestingly, it has been shown that in the aged rat penis there is an increase in eNOS protein expression in endothelial cells due to a reduction in caveolin-1, a protein that regulates eNOS. This increase in eNOS protein expression is accompanied by a significant decrease in eNOS activity, suggesting that the upregulated protein is not biologically active. This is supported by the restoration of endothelial vascular responses as a result of increased eNOS activity following adeno-associated viral gene transfer of anti-arginase [2]. While arginase inhibition was shown to improve erectile function, it was not shown to fully restore it, suggesting that there are likely multifactorial mechanisms of endothelial dependant erectile response impairment. Even still, the enhanced penile eNOS activity and cGMP levels resulting from arginase inhibition via anti-arginase gene therapy make it a potential molecular therapeutic treatment of age-associated vasculogenic ED [2].

When considering gene therapy as a treatment for ED, there are a number of potential issues that need to be taken into consideration. As mentioned previously, there is the risk that viral vectors could enter the systemic circulation and thus cause random transgene expression in unwanted tissues or organs. Increasing the specificity of viral vectors, such that they could target appropriate cells without damaging other cells, could allow for injection systemically rather than intracavernously. There are several methods that have been examined by which to increase the specificity of the viral vectors such as transcriptional and transductional targeting. Transcriptional targeting works through the selection of a cell specific promoter , whereas transductional targeting utilizes cell specific membrane markers to induce delivery of the genetic material. The risk of an immune response to the commonly studied viral vectors is also a concern, as this could hinder use of the therapy in both, acute or repeated clinical treatments. To limit the possibility of an unwanted immune and inflammatory response, it would be beneficial to lower the necessary load of virus required to transduce cells in the penis. Future studies exploring gene therapy for the treatment of ED should look to create as normal of an erectile response as possible by maximizing the specificity of the treatments as well as decreasing any potential unwanted side effects.

3. Stem cell therapy and ED

Stem cells have become increasingly popular as a potential treatment for a wide variety of diseases, including ED. Stem cells are defined by the capacity to self renew and differentiate into one or more distinct cell types. The stem cell's potential to differentiate can be extensive, being referred to as pluripotent when it can differentiate into any cell type in the organism. Other levels of differentiation ranging from multipotent to the more limited progenitor cells exist, providing numerous avenues from which potential therapies can be pursued. With the advent of induced pluripotential stem cells (iPS cells), scientists now have access to a line of pluripotent cells with which to work without many of the moral and ethical concerns revolving around the use of human embryonic stem cells. Adult-derived stem cells are also an area of current research, utilizing cell types such as mesenchymal stem cells and adipose-derived stem cells to replace lost or damaged cells in target tissues [2]. Stem cell treatment is attractive as a potential therapy for ED due to the underlying multifactorial pathologies responsible for the disease. The ability to replace whole cells could correct several of the associated specific molecular pathologies of ED with one type of treatment [2]. Stem cell replacement of penile endothelial cells may allow for recovery of normal erectile response, as endothelial dysfunction is one of the primary causes of ED.

3.1 MSC therapy

One of the more commonly used adult stem cells is mesenchymal stem cells (MSCs). There are produced in the bone marrow, as well as certain other tissues and organs, and they possess the ability to differentiate into a wide variety of cell types depending on the biological environment [2]. They are able to be isolated and expanded *ex vivo,* making them an advantageous choice for cell therapy [3]. It has been shown previously that MSCs are able to differentiate into endothelial and smooth muscle cells to repair vascular injury *in vivo,* making them a viable option for the treatment of vasculogenic ED. In a study by Bivalacuqa et al., MSCs were used to differentiate into endothelial cells, thereby improving endothelium-derived NO bioavailability and thus erectile physiology. The MSCs were injected intracavernously with or without simultaneous eNOS gene therapy, and in both groups there was a marked increase in erectile response, eNOS activity, and cGMP levels. The MSCS were found to still be present and expressing endothelial and smooth muscle cell markers not present before injection twenty-one days post injection, which suggests that the differentiated stem cells could provide long term replacement of damaged cells. Other studies have also examined the combined use of MSCs and gene therapy. In a recent study by Qiu et al., the efficacy of MSCs both alone and in combination with VEGF gene therapy for the treatment of ED in a type 1 diabetic rat model was observed. The survival of engrafted stem cells in the target tissue is always a concern during treatments, including in this study following intracavernous implantation. Survival of MSCs has been shown to increase when coupled with VEGF treatment, as noted by the accompanying increase in pro-survival factors phosphorylated Akt and Bcl-xL. Improved erectile function and an increase in the number of endothelial and smooth muscle cells were noted post injection, with the rats receiving the combined stem cell and VEGF gene therapy exhibiting the greatest increase compared to the animals treated with MSCs alone or the control group [3]. This suggests that the use of MSCs is a potential route for stem cell therapy of ED, especially when considered with concurrent gene therapeutic treatments.

3.2 ADSC therapy

Another type of adult stem cells that has been examined for the treatment of ED is adipose-derived stem cells (ADSCs). They are found in fat tissue and possess the qualities of stem cell, namely self-renewal and differentiation into multiple cell phenotypes, as well as the ability to provide functional repair of damaged tissue. In terms of differentiation and therapeutic potential, ADSCs are similar to MSCs but are easier and safer to harvest in large quantities as adipose tissue is a readily available biological source. ADSCs have been shown to be vascular precursor stem cells, making them an appropriate choice for stem cell therapy of ED [24]. In a study by Bella et al., the effects of ADSCs to repopulate endothelial and smooth muscle cells in erectile tissue following bilateral cavernous nerve crush injury were examined. Using intracavernosal pressure (ICP) as a measure of erectile function, the animals treated with ADSCs were observed to have higher ICP response and thus a better recovery of erectile function when compared with the control animals. The ability of ADSCs to help restore erectile function in this study was suggested to result from their differentiation into local penile cell types, as well through the secretion of growth factors that recruited local stem cells to differentiate, promoted IGF-1 mediated local functional cell growth, and exhibited a neurotrophic effect to promote nerve regeneration [26].

In another study using ADSCs, Garcia et al. tested the use of ADSCs for the treatment of ED in obese type 2 diabetic ZDF rats. These rats were shown previously to have an 85% prevalence of impotence (ICP≤60 cmH2O) among their population, making them an appropriate model to test the efficacy of ADSCs to survive in-vivo and subsequently restore erectile function. Three weeks after ADSCS injection into the rat penis, there was a noted functional improvement in erectile function when compared with untreated animals, as indicated by an improvement in ICP. It was determined that the effect of the treatment may be a result of an increase in the population of endothelial cells and a decrease in intracorporal tissue apoptosis among the treated rats. The survival of the ADSCs was assessed using BrdU labeling, which did not indicate the presence of many injected ADSCs after three weeks post injection. This suggests that the observed therapeutic effects likely result from elaboration of cytokines and growth factors from the ADSCs as opposed to direct differentiation in local cell types. An increase in nNOS (NOS type 1) was also seen, indicating that there may have been a restorative impact on nitrergic neuron axons and ganglia leading to improved erectile function. However, it is also possible that this increase

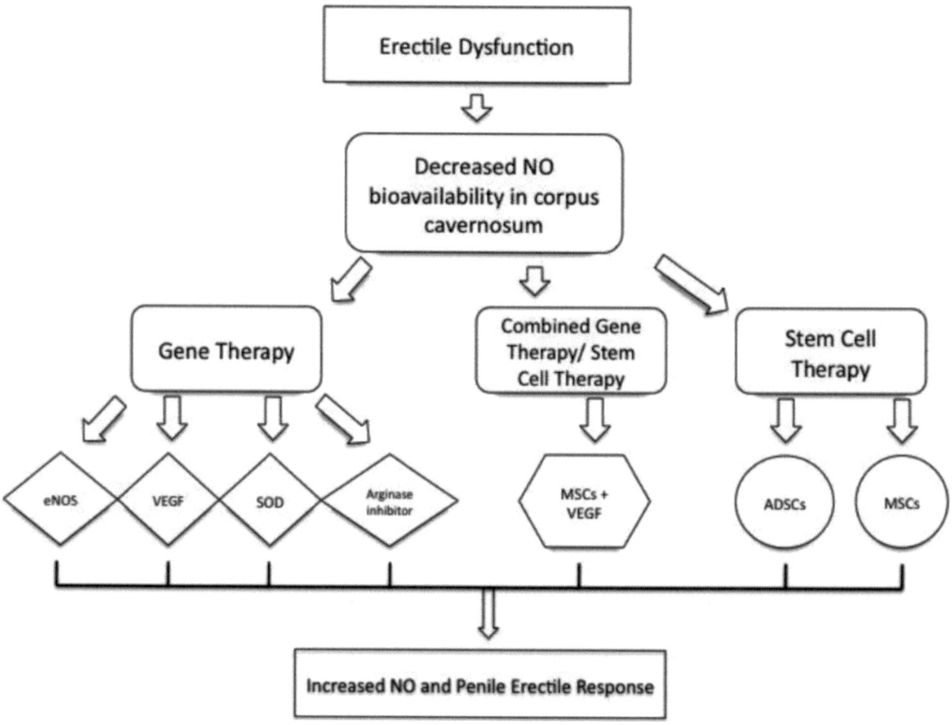

Fig. 1. Gene and stem cell therapies for the treatment of ED. Gene therapy treatments consist of eNOS, VEGF, SOD, and arginase inhibitor vectors. Stem cell therapy treatments include adipocyte-derived stem cell (ADSCs) and mesenchymal stem cell (MSCs) introduction into the cavernosal tissue. A combined gene therapy and stem cell therapy approach utilizing MSCs and VEGF has also been studied.

in nNOS was a result of increased oxygenated blood flow supplying more dorsal nerve nNOS following erectile function improvement. The use of ADSCs is an attractive therapeutic option in future studies, as the ease with which great numbers of cells can be harvested eliminates the need for ex vivo cell culture, thereby reducing the risk of contamination from a variety of organisms.

4. Conclusion

The advent of gene and stem cell therapy has unveiled new horizons for the future of medicine and clinical treatments. Among the many potential diseases able to be positively altered by these therapeutic treatments, ED has already been shown to be an appropriate pathological target. The use of gene and stem cell therapies alone or in combination with each other and other treatments such as pharmacological interventions holds great promise in the future care of patients afflicted with ED (Figure 1).

5. References

[1] Mills, J.N., et al., *The molecular basis of erectile dysfunction: from bench to bedside.* Reviews in urology, 2005. 7(3): p. 128-34.

[2] Bivalacqua, T.J., et al., *Overexpression of arginase in the aged mouse penis impairs erectile function and decreases eNOS activity: influence of in vivo gene therapy of anti-arginase.* American journal of physiology. Heart and circulatory physiology, 2007. 292(3): p. H1340-51.

[3] Qiu, X., et al., *Combined Strategy of Mesenchymal Stem Cells Injection with VEGF Gene Therapy for the Treatment of Diabetes Associated Erectile Dysfunction.* Journal of andrology, 2011.

[4] Strong, T.D., et al., *Endothelium-specific gene and stem cell-based therapy for erectile dysfunction.* Asian journal of andrology, 2008. 10(1): p. 14-22.

[5] Burnett, A.L., *Erectile dysfunction management for the future.* Journal of andrology, 2009. 30(4): p. 391-6.

[6] Champion, H.C., et al., *Gene transfer of endothelial nitric oxide synthase to the lung of the mouse in vivo. Effect on agonist-induced and flow-mediated vascular responses.* Circulation research, 1999. 84(12): p. 1422-32.

[7] Bivalacqua, T.J., et al., *Gene transfer of endothelial nitric oxide synthase partially restores nitric oxide synthesis and erectile function in streptozotocin diabetic rats.* The Journal of urology, 2003. 169(5): p. 1911-7.

[8] Bivalacqua, T.J., et al., *Effect of combination endothelial nitric oxide synthase gene therapy and sildenafil on erectile function in diabetic rats.* International journal of impotence research, 2004. 16(1): p. 21-9.

[9] Lin, C.S., et al., *Intracavernosal injection of vascular endothelial growth factor induces nitric oxide synthase isoforms.* BJU international, 2002. 89(9): p. 955-60.

[10] Musicki, B., et al., *Phosphorylated endothelial nitric oxide synthase mediates vascular endothelial growth factor-induced penile erection.* Biology of reproduction, 2004. 70(2): p. 282-9.

[11] Rogers, R.S., et al., *Intracavernosal vascular endothelial growth factor (VEGF) injection and adeno-associated virus-mediated VEGF gene therapy prevent and reverse venogenic erectile dysfunction in rats.* International journal of impotence research, 2003. 15(1): p. 26-37.

[12] Ryu, J.K., et al., *Combined angiopoietin-1 and vascular endothelial growth factor gene transfer restores cavernous angiogenesis and erectile function in a rat model of hypercholesterolemia.* Molecular therapy : the journal of the American Society of Gene Therapy, 2006. 13(4): p. 705-15.

[13] Xu, J., et al., *Oxygen-glucose deprivation induces inducible nitric oxide synthase and nitrotyrosine expression in cerebral endothelial cells.* Stroke; a journal of cerebral circulation, 2000. 31(7): p. 1744-51.

[14] Bivalacqua, T.J., et al., *Gene transfer of extracellular SOD to the penis reduces O2-* and improves erectile function in aged rats.* American journal of physiology. Heart and circulatory physiology, 2003. 284(4): p. H1408-21.

[15] Bivalacqua, T.J., et al., *Superoxide anion production in the rat penis impairs erectile function in diabetes: influence of in vivo extracellular superoxide dismutase gene therapy.* The journal of sexual medicine, 2005. 2(2): p. 187-97; discussion 197-8.

[16] Bivalacqua, T.J., et al., *Increased expression of arginase II in human diabetic corpus cavernosum: in diabetic-associated erectile dysfunction.* Biochemical and biophysical research communications, 2001. 283(4): p. 923-7.

[17] Bakircioglu, M.E., et al., *Decreased trabecular smooth muscle and caveolin-1 expression in the penile tissue of aged rats.* The Journal of urology, 2001. 166(2): p. 734-8.

[18] Sadeghi, H. and M.M. Hitt, *Transcriptionally targeted adenovirus vectors.* Current gene therapy, 2005. 5(4): p. 411-27.

[19] Waehler, R., S.J. Russell, and D.T. Curiel, *Engineering targeted viral vectors for gene therapy.* Nature reviews. Genetics, 2007. 8(8): p. 573-87.

[20] Wu, X., et al., *Mesenchymal stem cells participating in ex vivo endothelium repair and its effect on vascular smooth muscle cells growth.* International journal of cardiology, 2005. 105(3): p. 274-82.

[21] Wang, T., et al., *Cell-to-cell contact induces mesenchymal stem cell to differentiate into cardiomyocyte and smooth muscle cell.* International journal of cardiology, 2006. 109(1): p. 74-81.

[22] Bivalacqua, T.J., et al., *Mesenchymal stem cells alone or ex vivo gene modified with endothelial nitric oxide synthase reverse age-associated erectile dysfunction.* American journal of physiology. Heart and circulatory physiology, 2007. 292(3): p. H1278-90.

[23] Pons, J., et al., *VEGF improves survival of mesenchymal stem cells in infarcted hearts.* Biochemical and biophysical research communications, 2008. 376(2): p. 419-22.

[24] Lin, G., et al., *Potential of adipose-derived stem cells for treatment of erectile dysfunction.* The journal of sexual medicine, 2009. 6 Suppl 3: p. 320-7.

[25] Garcia, M.M., et al., *Treatment of erectile dysfunction in the obese type 2 diabetic ZDF rat with adipose tissue-derived stem cells.* The journal of sexual medicine, 2010. 7(1 Pt 1): p. 89-98.

[26] Bella, AJ., et al., *Non-cell line induced autologous adult adipose tissue derived stem cells enhance recovery of erectile function in the rat following bilateral cavernous nerve crush injury.* Sexual Medicine Society of North America Meeting, 2008. 68p.

11

The Assessment of Atherosclerosis in Erectile Dysfunction Subjects Using Photoplethysmography

Yousef Kamel Qawqzeh, Mamun Ibne Reaz and Mohd Aluadin Mohd Ali
Systems Design Lab, Department of Electrical, Electronic and Systems Engineering
National University of Malaysia
Malaysia

1. Introduction

Cardiovascular disease (CVD) is a major factor in mortality rates around the world and contributes to more than one-third of deaths in the United States [1]. The distribution of blood volume to different parts of the human vascular system can be seen in Figure 1. CVDs are the world's largest killers, claiming 17.1 million lives a year [1]. Tobacco use, an unhealthy diet, physical inactivity and harmful use of alcohol increase the risk of heart attacks and strokes [2]. Table 1 introduces the common risk factors of CVD. In addition, Table 1 shows some common types of CVD risk factors.

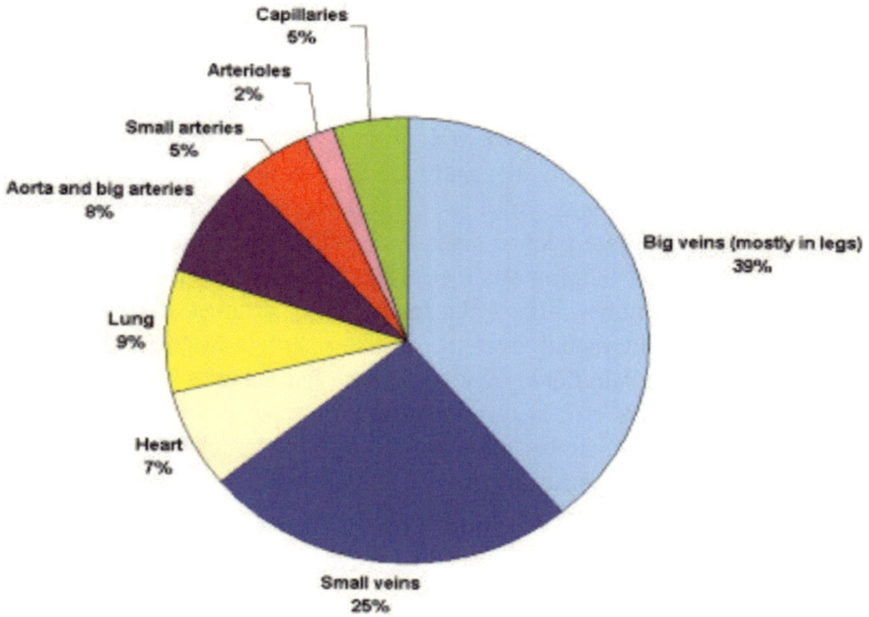

Fig. 1. Distribution of blood volume for the different parts of the human vascular system
Source: [3]

Risk factor	Risks can't be changed	Risks can be modified or treated	Factors contribute to heart disease risk
1	Increasing age	Tobacco smoke	Response to stress
2	Gender	High blood cholesterol	Drinking alcohol
3	Heredity	high blood pressure	Smoking
4	Family history	Physical inactivity	
5		Obesity	
6		Diabetes mellitus	

Table 1. Common types of CVD risk factors

The underlying cause of CV disease is atherosclerosis, a chronic inflammatory process that is clinically manifested as coronary artery disease, carotid artery disease, or peripheral artery disease [1; 4]. The frequency and prevalence of atherosclerosis are difficult to be assessed exactly. It has been predicted that atherosclerosis will be the primary cause of death in the world by 2020 [5]. Usually, atherosclerosis is an asymptomatic condition that might begin from childhood, whereas symptomatic organ-specific clinical manifestations often do not appear until 40 years of age or older when it is most commonly diagnosed [6]. Atherosclerosis can be characterized as a slow disease in which the arteries become hardened. In other words, it is characterized by the formation of arterial lesions or plaques as a result of an inflammatory response to endothelial injury [7]. Atherosclerosis eventually leads to artery enlargement, arterial stenosis, and may ultimately produce an arterial rupture [8]. The more commonly used subclinical vascular markers in the clinical setting are carotid intima media thickness (CIMT) and plaque measured by ultrasound, coronary artery calcium detected by cardiac computed tomography (CT), ankle–arm index pressure (AAI) measured by distal pressure Doppler measurement, and aortic pulse wave velocity (PWV) measured from carotid and femoral pressure wave recordings with a Doppler or mechanographic device [9-10]. Atherosclerosis can occur because of fatty deposits on the inner lining of arteries, calcification of the wall of the arteries, or thickening of the muscular wall of the arteries from chronically elevated blood pressure [11]. Atherosclerosis does not usually produce any symptoms until a CVD occurs. Therefore the prediction of atherosclerosis might contribute a lot to disease stratification and risk prevention. Figure 3 represents the process of developing atherosclerosis in the carotid intima-media arteries. It seems clearly that, inflammation affects the formation of arteries and the propagation of blood stream as well. Endothelial dysfunction is observed in the early stages of the atherogenic process, and it is initiated by injury to the arterial endothelium [1]. Such injury has been associated with CV risk factors including diabetes mellitus or impaired glucose metabolism, hypertension, cigarette smoking, dyslipidemia, obesity, and/or metabolic syndrome [12]. Endothelial dysfunction is the initial step of the atherosclerotic process involving many vascular districts, including penile and coronary circulation [13]. Endothelial dysfunction is associated with CVD risk factors [14-15]. Endothelial dysfunction has been proposed to be an early event of patho-physiologic importance in the atherosclerotic process [16-17] and provides an important link between diseases such as hypertension, chronic renal failure, or diabetes and the high risk of cardiovascular events in patients exhibiting these conditions [18].

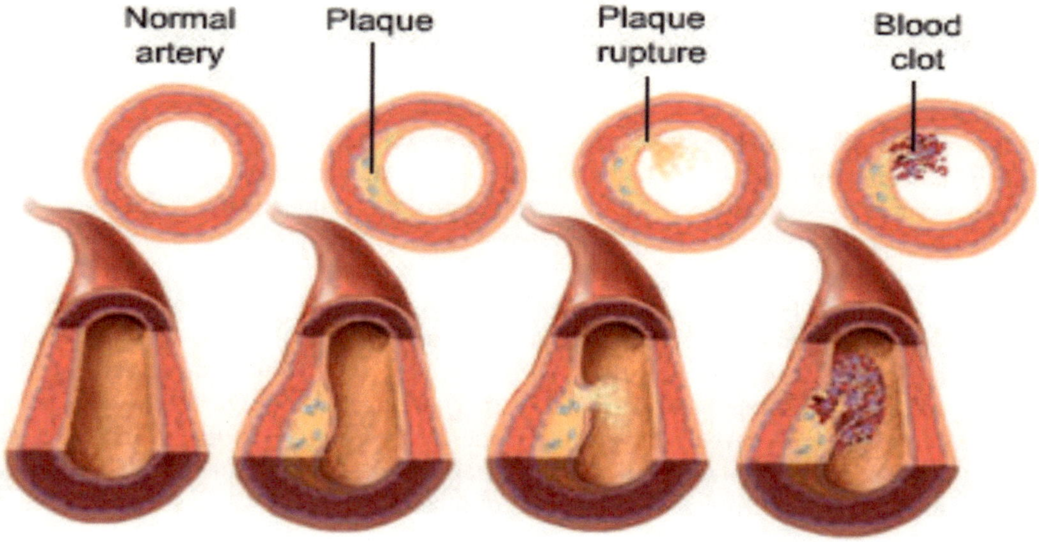

Fig. 2. The process of atherosclerosis development in general. Source: [38]

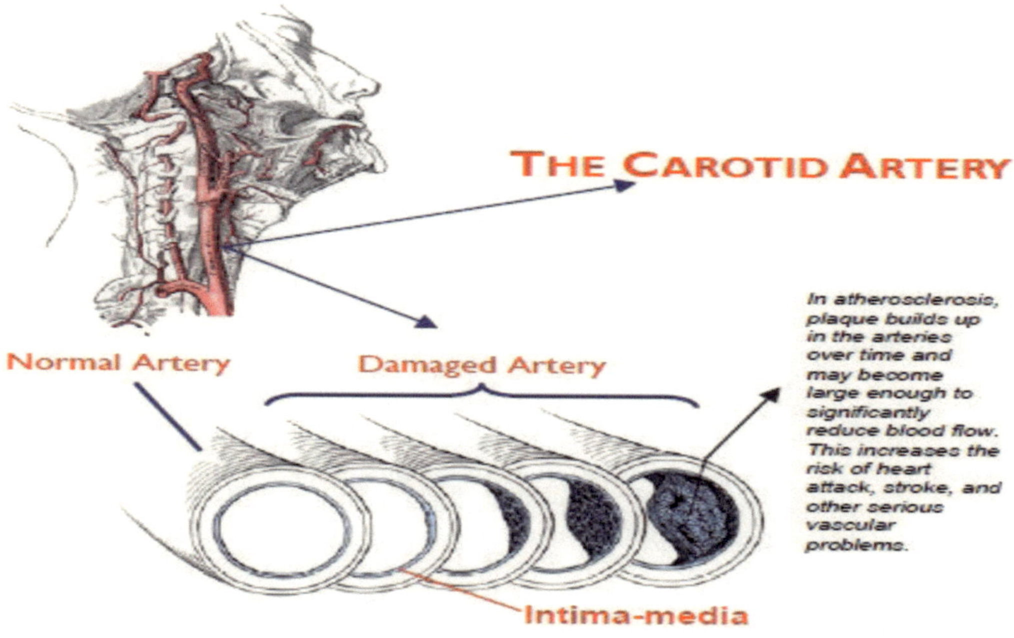

Fig. 3. Atherosclerosis risk at carotid intima-media arteries, Source: [39]

Elevated blood pressure reflects the existence of atherosclerosis. There is irresistible evidence that high blood cholesterol increases the risk of developing atherosclerosis; but cholesterol is not the damaging mechanism. In fact, the risk of atherosclerosis is more precisely assessed by measuring the proportional association between HDL cholesterol and LDL cholesterol [18]. Stiffening of large arteries predicts adverse cardiovascular outcomes [19-21]. Until now, measurements of arterial stiffness required the use of complex ultrasound equipment or explanation tonometry at the level of the peripheral arteries, with the subjects in the supine or sitting position [22-23]. Medically, atherosclerosis is considered the dominant pattern of arteriosclerosis which affects primarily the elastic and large- to medium-sized muscular arteries. Therefore, hypertension is an established risk factor for the development of atherosclerosis [24]. Atherosclerosis is the term applied to a focal condition of the intima of arteries associated with medial changes. In fact, atherosclerosis can involve many of the body's blood vessels with a variety of presentations [25]. Pathological and epidemiological data confirm that atherosclerosis begins in early childhood, and advances seamlessly and inexorably throughout life [26]. Risk factors in childhood are similar to those in adults, and track between stages of life. When diagnosed, aggressive treatment should begin at the earliest indication, and continue for years. For those patients at intermediate risk according to global risk scores, C-reactive protein (CRP), coronary artery calcium (CAC), and carotid intima-media thickness (CIMT) are available for further stratification. Atherosclerotic lesions develop slowly, but continuously leading to the main causes of mortality in diabetic patients such as coronary arterial disease, stroke, and renal failure [27]. In diabetic children, the presence of subclinical atherosclerotic disease as a precursor of macrovascular complications has been shown in several studies [28]. Also, impaired endothelial function preceding atherosclerotic changes has been observed [29]. As the measurement of the intima-media thickness of the carotid arteries is considered a surrogate marker of subclinical atherosclerosis, this method has been used widely in these patients to asses vascular health [28]. CIMT is a noninvasive and reproducible method to detect and quantify subclinical atherosclerosis [30]. Autopsy studies have demonstrated a direct histoligical relationship between carotid and coronary atherosclerosis [31-32]. CIMT measurements have been used to measure differences in the progression of atherosclerosis in clinical trials [33]. In observational trials, increased CIMT is associated with prevalent and incident cardiovascular disease [34-36]. Although ultrasound measurement of CIMT has been recommended as a clinical screening tool, its use has been limited to research studies or selected institutions, in part because of labor- and time-intensive measurement protocols [37].

Mainly, atherosclerosis starts with oxidation of LDL particles in the arterial wall [40-41]. Oxidative modified LDL (oxLDL) damages the endothelium of the artery - a pathophysiology similar to that of vascular erectile dysfunction (ED) [41-42]. As a result, the elasticity of the arteries deteriorates. Impaired arterial elasticity and increased levels of circulating oxLDL as well as elevated fibrinogen and resting heart rate associate with subclinical atherosclerosis and increased risk of cardiovascular disease (CVD) events [43-48]. Besides similar pathophysiology, ED and CVD share same risk factors [49]. In addition, a high prevalence of both silent and clinical CVD has been reported among ED patients [49-50]. ED has also been reported as an independent predictor of incident CVD [51-52]. Since ED often precedes CVD symptoms from other vascular beds, it is thought to be an early clinical manifestation of systemic atherosclerosis [49; 53]. There is increasing evidence of a strong link between ED and atherosclerosis [54-55]. ED and atherosclerosis share similar risk factors and both conditions are characterized by endothelial dysfunction and impaired nitric oxide bioavailability [56]. Peripheral artery disease (PAD) as similar to ED is associated with atherosclerotic risk factors [57].

With advanced age, men experience decreases in important health indicators (muscle amount, muscle power, physical activity, bone density, blood generation, and sexual drive)

[58]. Various research [57-59] on the decrease in blood testosterone with aging suggests that many clinical characteristics related to age, including ED, are closely related to lack of testosterones. Recent research results indicate that testosterone and ED are closely related to one other [60-61], which suggests that supplementary therapy with testosterone may be one useful method in the treatment of ED [62]. However, the link between ED and atherosclerosis is well known to doctors. Doctors thought of atherosclerosis to be the main cause of ED. The thought was driven from the hypothesis that small arteries will be clotted before the large or medium ones. Since erection depends mainly on the amount of delivered blood to the penis, normal arteries thought to have no problem in supporting the process of blood delivering. In contrast, if the arteries become stiffen due to the deposition of atherosclerosis (which in turn will reduce their compliance as a result of the increment in arteries walls resistance), the amount of delivered blood will be declined which affects the process of erection. Atherosclerosis as an indicator of endothelium dysfunction, thought to be the underlying cause of CVDs and ED. Once the arteries start losing their elastic properties, the atherosclerosis is proven to be existed. The development of atherosclerosis prevents endothelial cell from regulating blood flow. Moreover, the accumulation of atherosclerosis affects the propagation of blood which can be detected by the recording of Photoplethysmogram (PPG) signal. PPG is an optoelectronic technique that reflects blood volume changes in arteries [63]. It functions by illuminating the skin with a light by light-emitting diode (LED) and recording the scattered lights by a photodetector.

ED as a vasculogenic disorder may indicate that, blood vessels anywhere in the body are not in perfect health. ED still has no establish method for diagnosing subjects to be subject with ED or normal subject (normal erection). Therefore, linking ED to atherosclerosis is the most acceptable thought in this area. ED may be a sign that coronary artery disease is developing some risk factors. That's why; being under-risk of atherosclerosis raises the chance of experiencing ED at any age. The endothelium can be damaged by high cholesterol, high blood pressure, smoking, or diabetes. They also cause atherosclerosis. Once damaged, the endothelium can't expand arteries to increase blood flow as well. Less blood flow into the penis means a less tumescence and consequently no satisfactory erection. In this study, a sample of 68 ED patients were hired to run a research that aims to investigate and evaluate the associations between atherosclerosis and ED. The PPG signal was used to predict the high-risk of atherosclerosis. Its noteworthy that, CIMT test was used to evaluate the risk of atherosclerosis. Since the CIMT method continues to be a measure of atherosclerosis, the value of 0.7 was determined as the critical point. As a result, any value below or equal to 0.7 (CIMT=<0.7mm) represents a normal case, otherwise, it represents a case under risk. And since the diagnostic test is used to reveal the health status of the subject, a new index derived from CIMT which is called high-risk atherosclerosis (HRART) was used to discriminate between at-risk-of-the-disease and normal subjects based on the critical value of 0.7. Statistically, HRART was taken as the dependent variable. All subjects were from Urology clinic at the medical center of the National University of Malaysia (PPUKM).

Thinking of atherosclerosis as the main cause that might cause ED represents a big motivation for the development of a predictive model for high-risk atherosclerosis assessment. Once atherosclerosis has been predicted, ED can be examined and checked by means of atherosclerosis. The measurement of CIMT and PPG were done at the same time. We started our research by hypothesizing that PPG is willing to predict high-risk atherosclerosis by utilizing PPG's contour analysis technique. Since PPG reflects changes in blood volume, it will be affected clearly by aging and by atherosclerosis. Therefore, the aim was to extract some indices from PPG waveform morphology and relate these indices to atherosclerosis measured by CIMT test. Since the pulsatile components of PPG waveform are the important features due to their ability to reflect blood flow and blood volume changes in the arteries, we paid extra attention to PPG amplitude indices without neglecting PPG time indices. Atherosclerosis plays an important role in the process of blood propagation and blood volume changes. As we age, PPG amplitude is subject to reduction because of the accumulated atherosclerosis, which in turn increases the resistance of arteries and reduces arterial compliance. It is noteworthy that, atherosclerosis affects the elastic properties of the arterial wall, making it stiffen. As arteries become stiffer, blood propagation becomes faster and pulse amplitude becomes lower as well. In this research 12 main indices of PPG were extracted and evaluated Table 2 demonstrates the extracted parameters.

Index	B	S.E.	Wald	df	Sig.	Exp (B)
Age	.071	.028	6.198	1	.013**	1.07
BMI	-.025	.058	.179	1	.673	.976
SP	.04	.024	2.7	1	.1	1.04
DP	-.017	.034	.25	1	.614	.98
MAP	.016	.033	.23	1	.634	1.02
PP	.071	.032	4.8	1	.028**	1.07
H	-.114	.045	6.3	1	.012**	.89
PT	1.02	1.6	.4	1	.52	2.76
MET	52.8	32.5	2.6	1	.1	8.7E+22
ST	15.4	6	6.57	1	.01**	4732574
DT	4.96	6	.68	1	.41	143
PPT	-14.7	6.96	4.5	1	.034**	.00
SI	.04	.087	.23	1	.63	1.04
MEV	-552.3	1231	.2	1	.65	.00
PM	-1.08	10.2	.01	1	.92	.338
DM	1.76	15.2	.013	1	.9	5.8
RI	1.78	1.9	.88	1	.35	5.9
b/a	-5.43	1.88	8.3	1	.004**	72.6
c/a	-.073	3.75	.00	1	.98	.93

Note: Each index was tested separately to obtain any statistically significant against the dependent variable. The table represents their collection.

Table 2. Initial variables tested for model development

Given the importance of the medical data in pathogenesis of atherosclerosis, clinical interest has focused on the development of markers of risk. Therefore, blood pressure (SP, DP, PP, and MAP) in addition to body mass index were recorded as well. Among the medical data measurements mentioned, PP was found to be a significant factor contributing to the process of atherosclerosis. PP is an independent predictor of myocardial infarction (MI) [64]. The progression of atherosclerosis is accompanied by an increase in PP [65]. Our results supported such an observations by revealing a positively association between PP and atherosclerosis.

In addition, subject's height (H) was inversely correlated with atherosclerosis in our results. Height was inversely associated with risk of MI [66], and an inverse association between height and risk of coronary heart disease (CHD) has been reported in several analytic studies [67-68]. Therefore, H and PP were statistically significant in this research. Detail on H and PP characteristics in the follow sections.

Basically, the first attention was to utilize PPG technique only in the assessment of high-risk atherosclerosis. But, as a result from the final research, PP and H were contributable to the risk of atherosclerosis. Which in turn resulted in a predictive model represents the contribution of PPG (b/a ratio), PP and H to the development of atherosclerosis. Obviously, it is worthy to investigate the contribution of PPG (b/a ratio) alone to atherosclerosis and the contribution of PP, H and PPG (b/a ratio) together. To make these investigations achieved, we conducted the analysis of logistic regression (Backward: LR). Logistic regression (LR) is used normally to model the relationship between a binary response variable and one or more predictor variables, which may either be discrete or continuous. Binary outcome data is common in medical applications. In our work, the binary response variable might be whether or not a patient is at risk of atherosclerosis. In multiple regressions, we are concerned with finding an appropriate combination of predictor variables to help explain the binary outcome. However, a logistic regression model was developed to assist in the early prediction of high-risk atherosclerosis, and to be used as an alternative rapid measure for screening for atherosclerosis.

The developed model went through three main methods of logistic regression. The first method (ENTER: LR) was used to test the significance of each index separately against the dependent variable, Risk of atherosclerosis initiated from CIMT test. The second method (Forward: LR) was used to test the significance of the significant indices against the dependent variable. The final method (Backward: LR) was used to test the significance of the significant indices against the dependent variable as well. Both forward and backward methods were used for the same techniques and they were fed with the same significant indices; and the one with a higher performance in terms of (Nagelkerke R-square and likelihood ratio) was used to implement the final model. The results revealed that some indices (age, PP, H, PPT, ST, and b/a) were statistically significant and that they could be used to initiate the model. The six chosen indices were fed to forward: LR and backward: LR methods. Table 3 shows the associated Nagelkerke R-square for each variable.

Index	R-square	Likelihood-ratio
Age	.133	87.14
PP	.11	88.4
H	.138	86.8
PPT	.094	89.3
ST	.135	87
b/a	.184	84.2

Note: R-square represents the amount that this index contributes to the process of high-risk of atherosclerosis.

Table 3. Nagelkerke R-square for the selected indices

However, to investigate the effects of the multiple variables together in the model, the forward: LR method was used first. After feeding the model with all the chosen variables, forward: LR responded as follows:

- Two out of six indices remained in the model (b/a and H), therefore age, PP, PPT, and ST were excluded from the calculations. Table 4 illustrates the model summary of the forward: LR method.
- The model revealed a value of Nagelkerke R-square (.288) and a likelihood ratio of 77.69
- Step 2, forward: LR was chosen to represent the model based on this method.

Step	-2 Log likelihood	Cox & Snell R Square	Nagelkerke R Square
1	84.179	.138	.184
2	77.694	.216	.288

Note: Step 2 is used to represent the final decision about the model

Table 4. Model summary of forward: LR

On the other hand, backward: LR responded better than the forward: LR method. The model revealed a higher Nagelkerke R-square value (.372). A summary of the model is shown in Table 5. After feeding the model with all chosen variables, backward: LR responded as follows:

- Three out of six indices remained in the model (b/a, PP, and H); Therefore PPT, age and ST were excluded from the calculations. Table 5 illustrates the model summary of the backward: LR method.
- The model revealed a value of Nagelkerke R-square (.372) and a likelihood ratio of 74
- Step 4 backward: LR was chosen to represent the model based on this method.

Step	-2 Log likelihood	Cox & Snell R Square	Nagelkerke R Square
1	71	.287	.383
2	71	.287	.383
3	72	.279	.372
4	74	.258	.372

Note: Step 4 was used to represent the final decision about the model

Table 5. Model summary of backward: LR

Moreover, it is helpful to demonstrate the relationship between the predicted outcome and certain characteristics found in observations. Table 6 represents the final characteristics of the developed model.

Our chief interest was to use the logistic model to predict the outcome for a new subject. How good was this model for prediction? When we have a new subject, we can use the logistic model to predict his probability of having high-risk atherosclerosis. Let us say we have a black box where we input the b/a index, PP and H of a subject and the output is a number between 0 and 1 which denotes the probability of the subject having a high-risk of atherosclerosis (Figure 4).

	B	S.E.	Wald	Df	Sig.	Exp(B)	95% C.I.for EXP(B)	
							Lower	Upper
BA	-4.758	2.020	5.55	1	.019	.009	.000	.450
H	-.123	.052	5.62	1	.018	.884	.798	.979
PP	.066	.037	3.27	1	.047	1.07	.994	1.148
Constant	20.696	8.924	5.38	1	.020	973357650		

Note: Model's final selected factors and their characteristics

Table 6. The final factors included into the model and model characteristics

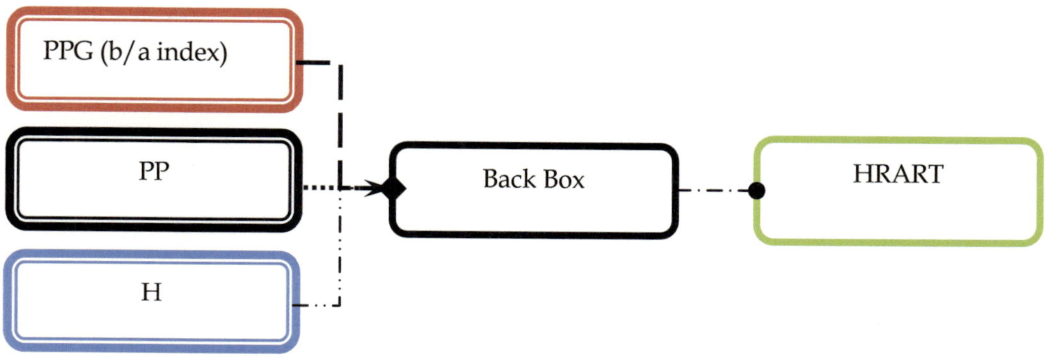

Fig. 4. The logistic regression predictive model

In the black box we have the equation for calculating the probability of having high-risk atherosclerosis, which is given by Y (Model's outcome) = 20.696 - 4.758*b/a + 0.066*PP - 0.123*H. Therefore, the probability of having high-risk atherosclerosis can be calculated as HRART = Exp (Y) / (1+Exp (Y)). This tells us that increasing the b/a value decreases the risk of atherosclerosis. Moreover, increasing PP increases the chance of being under high-risk of atherosclerosis. Finally, increasing height decreases the risk of atherosclerosis. The classification table of the predictive model is shown in Table 7.

Observed		Predictive HRART No-risk	High-risk	Percentage correct
Step 1	No-risk	24	10	70.6
	High-risk	9	25	73.5
Overall percentage				72.05
Step 2	No-risk	25	9	73.5
	High-risk	7	27	79.4
Overall percentage				76.5

Note: Classification table based on backward: LR

Table 7. Classification table of the predictive model

2. Agreement between the PPG and the CIMT

We often hope to have data on, for example, atherosclerosis or arteriosclerosis where direct measurement without adverse effects is difficult or impossible. The true values remain unknown. Therefore, indirect methods are used, and a new method has to be evaluated by comparison with an established method rather than with the true quantity. If the new method agrees adequately well with the old one, the new one may be used as an alternative measure, or the old one may be replaced. In this work, CIMT is an established method for the measurement of atherosclerosis. The PPG as a new method comes into this work to assist or replace CIMT. And since CIMT is the used method, the convention of assisting or interchanging use of the two methods was employed.

However, the Bland-Altman plot [69] is a graphical method to compare two measurement methods. In this graphical method the differences (or alternatively the ratios) between the two methods are plotted against the averages of the two methods. On the other hand [70] the differences can be plotted against one of the two methods, if this method is a reference or "gold standard" method. Horizontal lines are drawn at the mean difference, and at the limits of agreement, which are defined as the mean difference plus and minus 1.96 times the standard deviation of the differences. It is noteworthy that the agreement between the two methods must be done using the raw data (CIMT vs. b/a (PPG)).

A comparison between CIMT and PPG in the measurement of high-risk atherosclerosis is plotted in Figure 5. PPG is a new non-invasive method. Here the mean difference is 0.05 percentage points with a 95% confidence interval. The limits of agreement (-0.81 and 0.91) are small enough for us to be confident that the new method (PPG) can be used to assist CIMT for clinical purposes.

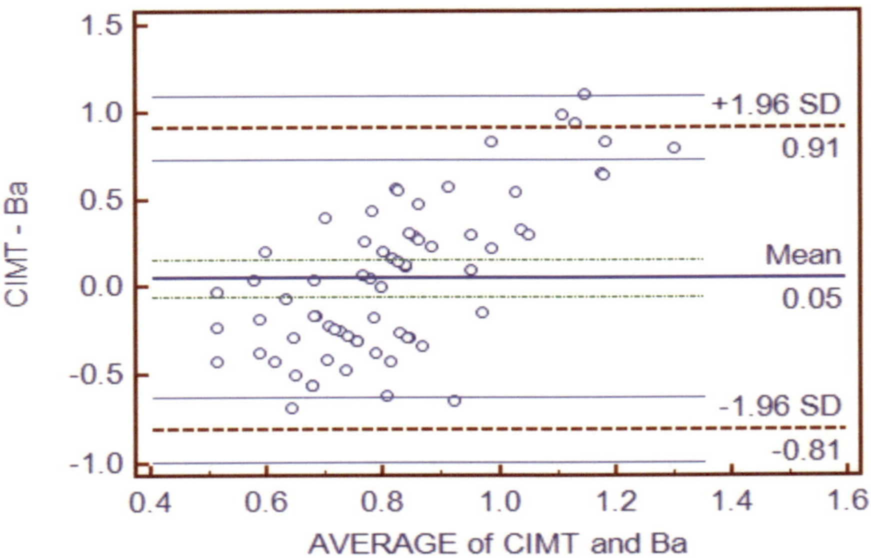

Fig. 5. Agreement of CIMT and PPG in the measurement of risk atherosclerosis

The plot reveals good agreement between the two methods, since the data are scattered around the mean. In addition, the mean value (0.05) is so close to zero that this strengthens the agreement between CIMT and PPG. Such agreement raises the possibility of using PPG as an alternative rapid measure of high-risk atherosclerosis.

3. Model performance

The new proposed measure of high-risk atherosclerosis, (PPG's b/a index), needs to be evaluated to be used in clinical settings. Basically, the performance of any established test or any newcomer test must be assessed. The diagnostic performance of a test or the accuracy of a test to discriminate risky cases from non risky cases is evaluated using Receiver Operating Characteristic (ROC) curve analysis [71-72]. ROC curves can also be used to compare the diagnostic performance of two or more laboratory or diagnostic tests [73]. Moreover, a measure of how well an index can distinguish between two diagnostic groups (risky/non risky) can be evaluated by the area under the ROC curve (AUC). Since the CIMT method continues to be a measure of atherosclerosis, the value of 0.7 was determined as the critical point. As a result, any value below or equal to 0.7 (CIMT=<0.7mm) represents a normal case, otherwise, it represents a case under risk. And since the diagnostic test is used to reveal the health status of the subject, a new index derived from CIMT which is called high-risk atherosclerosis (HRART) is used to discriminate between at-risk-of-the-disease and normal subjects based on the critical value of 0.7. HRART was taken as the dependent variable. Figure 6 demonstrates the error bar plot for b/a index based on HRART data.

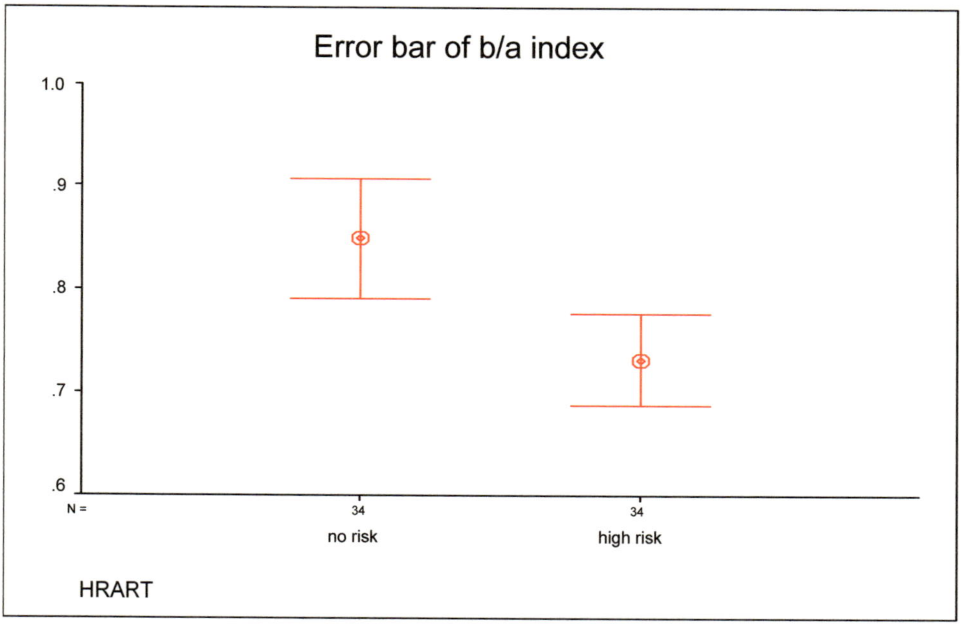

Fig. 6. Error bar of PPG (b/a index) based on HRART

Statistically, an ROC curve provides an objective measure of the discriminatory power of a screening test and also an idea of where to place the cut-off point. Therefore, a ROC test (HRART vs. b/a) was run to obtain the sensitivity (the true positive rate) and the 100-specificity (the false positive rate) for different cut-off points of the PPG (b/a ratio). MedCalc software (version 11.4.4) was used to obtain the ROC curve and the AUC. The ROC curve for (HRART vs. b/a index) is shown in Figure 7.

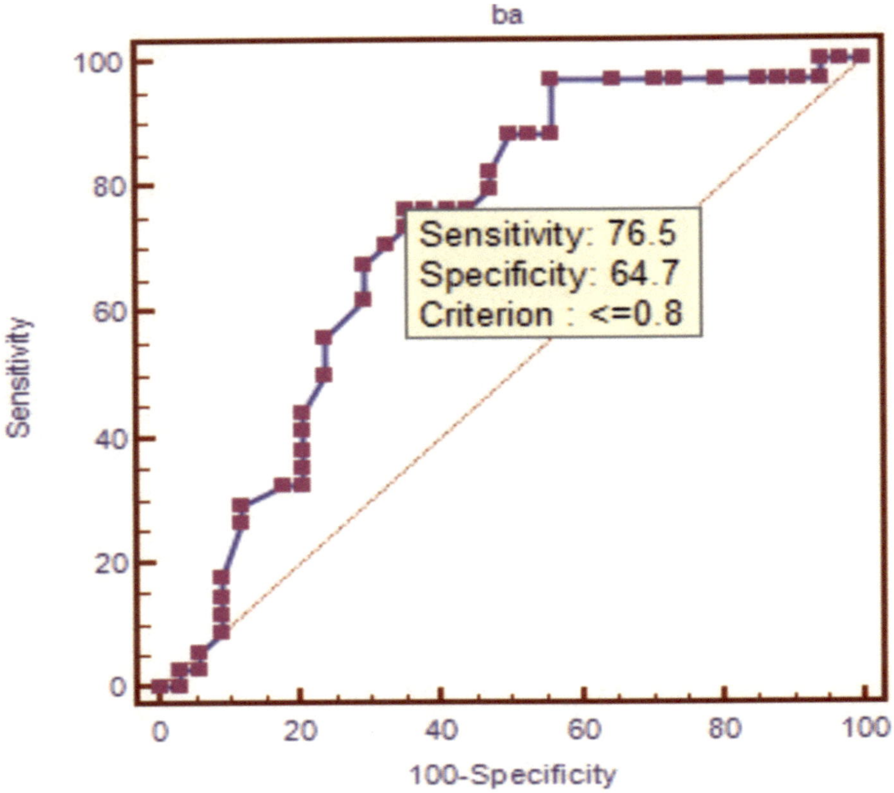

Fig. 7. ROC curve of HRART vs. PPG (b/a index)

As seen in Figure7, the ROC curve revealed a sensitivity of 76.5% and a specificity of 64.7% in the discrimination between risky and normal subjects. A sensitivity of 75% would be reasonable [74-76]. When the probability of disease and the sensitivity and specificity of the test are known, the predictive value positive (PVP) and the predictive value negative (PVN) can be calculated [77]. Moreover, the combination of ROC curves for all model factors can be obtained to reflect the relationship between each factor and the dependent variable. The three factors (b/a index, PP and H) contributed by some means to the process of atherosclerosis. Figure 8 represents the ROC curves for all the model's factors.

The combined ROC for the model's factors revealed the contribution of each factor to the development of atherosclerosis inside our arteries. As a result of that, each factor contributed separately to the atherosclerosis process, and all of them together contributed also to the process of atherosclerosis development partially. Partially means "not making a full contribution," in other words, there are some other untested factors that might be contributing to atherosclerosis. However, the model produced a highly satisfactory Nagelkerke R-square value (0.372) which makes it a good rapid measure for the prediction of atherosclerosis risk. The effectiveness of the diagnosis is measured by the AUC.

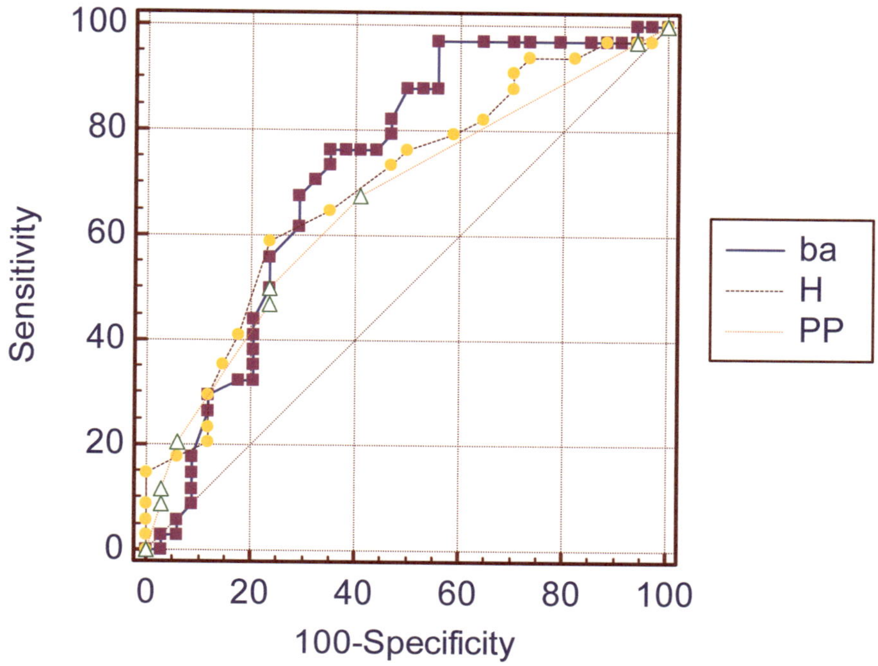

Fig. 8. The obtained ROC curves for b/a index, PP and H

3.1 Area Under the Curve (AUC)

The correctness of any medical test depends on how well the test separates the sample being tested into those with or without the disease. The area under the ROC curve (AUC) is frequently used as a measure for the effectiveness of diagnostic markers [78]. Moreover, AUC is an overall test for the performance of the test. Statistically, the area of 1 represents a perfect test which rarely appears in real empirical data. The analysis of our data produced an AUC of 0.724, which is fair enough to ensure that the test is reliable in discrimination between normal and risky specimens. The details of the AUC obtained can be seen in Table 8.

Variable **Classification variable**	**b/a index** **HRART**
Sample size	68
Positive group: HRART = 1	34
Negative group: HRART = 0	34
Disease prevalence (%)	50.0
Area under the ROC curve (AUC)	0.724
Standard error	0.06
95% Confidence interval	0.6 to 0.83
Z statistic	3.5
Significance level P (Area = 0.5)	0.0004

Table 8. The AUC obtained and its characteristics

Basically, AUC can be interpreted as the probability that the test result from a randomly selected diseased subject is more indicative of disease than that from a randomly selected non-diseased subject. Therefore, getting a value of AUC to be 0.724 can be an indicator of the good performance of the developed predictive model. The interactive dot diagram (Figure 9) illustrates a sensitivity of 76.5% and a specificity of 64.7%. During the present study we defined normal subjects (without risk of atherosclerosis) who had a value of b/a index to be greater than 0.8. Otherwise, the subject will be diagnosed as a subject at risk of atherosclerosis, which in turn will make the subject aggressive about his/ her health status.

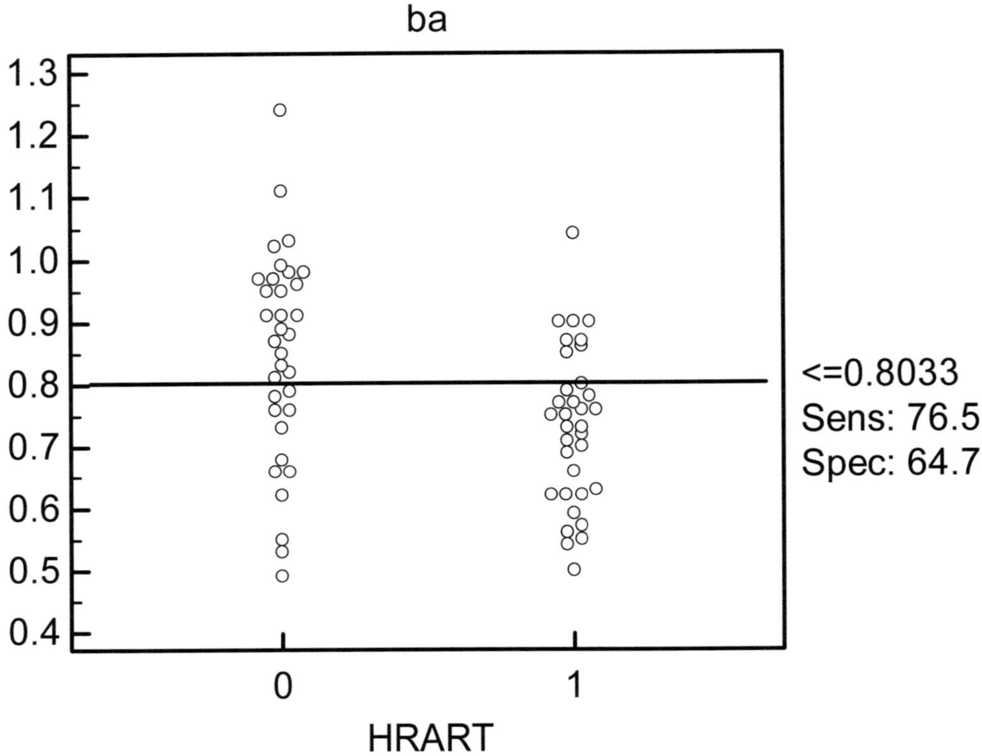

Fig. 9. Interactive dot diagram of b/a index based on HRART

In conclusion, this investigation introduced the acquired results based on our analysis. Moreover, a detailed discussion on the developed model and its characteristics were presented. The focus was completely on the association between atherosclerosis and the PPG signal indices. The developed model revealed a sensitivity of 76.5% and a specificity of 64.7% which in turn suggested that it could be a rapid measure for the assessment of the prediction of high-risk atherosclerosis. Mainly, thinking of atherosclerosis to represent an important cause of ED raises the important of this developed model. As the developed model successes to predict high-risk atherosclerosis, it can be used to assist ED as well. Therefore, predicting the high-risk atherosclerosis at early stages could really improve the prevention of experiencing ED and improve the treatment methods. The analysis can be further extended to other cardiovascular risk factors such as hypertension, hyperlipidemia and smoking. These factors are not analyzed in this study due to limitation in the number of subjects with one of the particular above mentioned risk factors. However, there is no doubt that the assessment of arterial stiffness and the assessment of high-risk atherosclerosis will make a major contribution to the improved management of cardiovascular disease in clinical settings and to the process of diseases prevention.

4. References

[1] R Preston Mason. Optimal therapeutic strategy for treating patients with hypertension and atherosclerosis: focus on olmesartan medoxomil. Vascular Health and Risk Management 2011:7 405–416

[2] WHO. 2011. Cardiovascular diseases. World Health Organization. http://www.who.int/cardiovascular_diseases/en/ [22 Jan 2011]

[3] Blažeka, V., Hülsbusch, M., Herzog, M., Claudia, R., Blažek, H., Gunga, C., Kowoll, R & Waltraud, F. 2005. Behaviour of human hemodynamics under microgravity-a proposal for the 7th german parabolic flight campaign. *Advances in Electrical and Electronic Eng*: 107-111

[4] Galkina E, Ley K. Immune and inflammatory mechanisms of atherosclerosis. Annu Rev Immunol. 2009;27:165–197.

[5] Scott J. The pathogenesis of atherosclerosis and new opportunities for treatment and prevention. J Neural Transm Suppl. 2002;(63):1–17.

[6] Wasserman BA. Clinical carotid atherosclerosis. *Neuroimaging Clin N Am*. 2002;12(3):403–419.

[7] Li JJ, Chen JL. Inflammation may be a bridge connecting hypertension and atherosclerosis. *Med Hypotheses*. 2005;64(5):925–929.

[8] Matsushita M, Nishikimi N, Sakurai T, Nimura Y. Relationship between aortic calcification and atherosclerotic disease in patients with abdominal aortic aneurysm. *Int Angiol*. 2000;19(3):276–279.

[9] Simon A, Chironi G & Levenson J 2007. Comparative performance of subclinical atherosclerosis tests in predicting coronary heart disease in asymptomatic individual. European Heart Journal 28, 2967–2971 doi:10.1093/eurheartj/ehm48.

[10] Simon A, Levenson J 2005. May subclinical arterial disease help to better detect and treat high-risk asymptomatic individuals? J Hypertens; 23:1939–194

[11] MedicineNet. 2010. Definition of Arteriosclerosis. http://www.medterms.com/script/main/art.asp?articlekey=2336 [24 Nov 2010]

[12] Brunner H, Cockcroft JR, Deanfield J, et al. Endothelial function and dysfunction. Part II: association with cardiovascular risk factors and diseases. A statement by the Working Group on Endothelins and Endothelial Factors of the European Society of Hypertension. *J Hypertens*. 2005;23(2):233–246.

[13] Piero, M., Paolo, R., Stefano, G., Sarah, A., Alberto, B., Andrea, S. & Francesco, M. 2009. The Triad of Endothelial Dysfunction, Cardiovascular Disease, and Erectile Dysfunction: Clinical Implications. *European Urology supplements* 8: 58 - 66

[14] Vita, A., Treasure, B., Nabel, G., McLenachan, M., Fish, D., Yeung, C., Vekshtein, I., Selwyn, P. & Ganz, P. 1990. Coronary Vasomotor Response to Acetylcholine Relates to Risk Factors for Coronary Artery Disease. *Circulation* 81: 491-497.

[15] Black, R. 1992. *Cardiovascular Risk Factors In Heart Book* Edited by G.S. Genell, M.S. Subak-Sharpe, B.L. Zaret, M. Moser & L.S. Cohen. New York: Hearst Books.

[16] Celermajer, S., Sorensen, E., Gooch, M., Spiegelhalter, J., Miller, I., Sullivan, D., Lloyd, K. & Deanfield, E. 1992. Non-invasive detection of endothelial dysfunction in children and adults at risk of atherosclerosis. *Lancet* 340: 1111–1115

[17] Suwaidi, A., Hamasaki, S., Higano, T., Nishimura, A., Holmes, R. & Lerman, A. 2000. Long-term follow-up of patients with mild coronary artery disease and endothelial dysfunction. *Circulation* 101: 948–954

[18] Dierk, E. & Ernesto, S. 2004. Endothelial Dysfunction. *J Am Soc Nephrol* 15: 1983–1992

[19] Benetos, A., Safar, M., Rudnichi, A., Smulyan, H., Richard, JL., Ducimetieere, P. & Guize, L. 1997. Pulse pressure: a predictor of long-term cardiovascular mortality in a French male population. *Hypertension*. 30: 1410–1415.

[20] Hayashi, T., Nakayama, Y., Tsumura, K., Yoshimaru, K. & Ueda, H. 2002. Reflection in the arterial system and the risk of coronary heart disease. *Am J Hypertens*. 15: 405–409.

[21] Weber, T., Auer, J., O'Rourke, MF., Kvas, E., Lassnig, E., Berent, R. & Eber, B. 2004. Arterial stiffness, wave reflections, and the risk of coronary artery disease. *Circulation*. 20:109:184 –189.

[22] Van, LM., Duprez, D., Starmans-Kool, MJ., Safar, ME., Giannattasio, C., Cockcroft, J., Kaiser, DR. & Tuillez, C. 2002. Clinical applications of arterial stiffness, task force III: recommendations for user procedures. *Am J Hypertens* 15: 445– 452.

[23] Yan, Li., Ji-Guang, W. et al. 2006. Ambulatory Arterial Stiffness Index Derived From 24-Hour Ambulatory Blood Pressure Monitoring. DOI: 10.1161/01.HYP.0000200695.34024.4c

[24] Standridge JB. Hypertension and atherosclerosis: clinical implications from the ALLHAT trial. *Curr Atheroscler Rep*. 2005;7(2): 132–139.

[25] Munther, K. & Homoud, D. 2008. Coronary Artery Disease. http://ocw.tufts.edu/data/50/636849.pdf [20 Jan 2011]

[26] Kones R. Primary prevention of coronary heart disease: integration of new data, evolving views, revised goals, and role of rosuvastatin in management. A comprehensive survey. Drug Des Devel Ther. 2011;5:325-80

[27] Gul K, Ustun I, Aydin Y, Berker D, Erol K, Unal M, Barazi AO, Delibasi T, Guler S: Carotid intima-media thickness and its relations with the complications in patients with type 1 diabetes mellitus. *Anadolu Kardiyol Derg* 2010, 10(1):52-58

[28] Margeirsdottir HD, Stensaeth KH, Larsen JR, Brunborg C, Dahl-Jorgensen K: Early Signs of Atherosclerosis in Diabetic Children on Intensive Insulin Treatment: A Population-Based Study. *Diabetes Care* 2010.

[29] Singh TP, Groehn H, Kazmers A: Vascular function and carotid intimal-medial thickness in children with insulin-dependent diabetes mellitus. *J Am Coll Cardiol* 2003, 41(4):661-665

[30] Adam D. Gepner, BS, Claudia E. Korcarz, DVM, RDCS, Susan E. Aeschlimann, RDMS, RVT, Tamara J. LeCaire, MS, Mari Palta, PhD, Wendy S. Tzou, MD, and James H. Stein, MD, FASE, *Madison, Wisconsin*. Validation of a Carotid Intima-Media

Thickness Border Detection Program for Use in an Office Setting. *J Am Soc Echocardiogr 2006;19:223-228.*

[31] Mitchell JR, Schwartz CJ. Relationship between arterial disease in different sites: a study of the aorta and coronary, carotid, and iliac arteries. Br Med J 1962;5288:1293-301.

[32] Young W, Gofman J, Tandy R, Malamud N, Waters E. The quantitation of atherosclerosis III: the extent of correlation of degrees of atherosclerosis with and between the coronary and cerebral vascular beds. Am J Cardiol 1960;8:300-8.

[33] Hodis H, Mack W, LaBree L, Selzer R, Liu C, Liu C, et al. The role of carotid arterial intima-medial thickness in predicting clinical coronary events. Ann Intern Med 1998;128:262-9.

[34] Burke G, Evans G, Riley W, Sharrett A, Howard G, Barnes R, et al. Arterial wall thickness is associated with prevalent cardiovascular disease in middle-aged adults: the atherosclerosis risk in communities (ARIC) study. Stroke 1995;26:386-91.

[35] Chambless LE, Heiss G, Folsom AR, Rosamond W, Szklo M, Sharrett AR, et al. Association of coronary heart disease incidence with carotid arterial wall thickness and major risk factors: the atherosclerosis risk in communities (ARIC) study, 1987-1993. Am J Epidemiol 1997;146:483-94.

[36] Chambless LE, Folsom AR, Clegg LX, Sharrett AR, Shahar E, Nieto FJ, et al. Carotid wall thickness is predictive of incident clinical stroke: the atherosclerosis risk in communities (ARIC) study. Am J Epidemiol 2000;151:478-87.

[37] Greenland P, Abrams J, Aurigemma GP, Bond MG, Clark LT, Criqui MH, et al. Prevention conference V: beyond secondary prevention; identifying the high-risk patient for primary prevention–noninvasive tests of atherosclerotic burden, writing group III. Circulation 2000;101:E16-22.

[38] AHA. 2008. Risk Factors and Coronary Heart Disease. http://www.americanheart.org/presenter.jhtml?identifier=4726 [12 May 2010]

[39] Site Index. 2011. Carotid intima-media thickness (CIMT). http://www.drsobti.com/home/services/cimt/page3.html [19 Jan 2011]

[40] Hanna. P, Ari. P and Juha. H. Erectile dysfunction, physical activity and metabolic syndrome: differences in markers of atherosclerosis. *BMC Cardiovascular Disorders* 2011, 11:36

[41] Stocker R, Keaney JF Jr: Role of oxidative modifications in atherosclerosis. *Physiol Rev* 2004, 84:1381-1478.

[42] Kirby M, Jackson G, Simonsen U: Endothelial dysfunction links erectile dysfunction to heart Disease. *Int J Clin Pract* 2005, 59:225-229.

[43] Cohn J, Finkelstein S, McVeigh G, Morgan D, LeMay L, Robinson J, Mock J: Noninvasive Pulse Wave Analysis for the Early Detection of Vascular Disease. *Hypertension* 1995, 26:503-508.

[44] Boutouyrie P, Tropeano I, Asmar R, Gautier I, Benetos A, Lacolley P, Laurent S: Aortic stiffness is an independent predictor of primary coronary events in hypertensive patients. A longitudinal study. *Hypertension* 2002, 39:10-15.

[45] Van Popele N, Grobbee D, Bots M, Asmar R, Topouchian J, Reneman R, Hoeks A, Van der Kuip D, Hofman A, Witteman J: Association between arterial stiffness and atherosclerosis. The Rotterdam study. *Stroke* 2001, 32:454-460.

[46] Holvoet P, Mertens A, Verhamme P, Bogaerts K, Beyens G, Verhaeghe R, Collen D, Muls E, Van de Werf F: Circulating oxidized LDL is a useful marker for identifying patients with coronary artery disease. *Arterioscler Thromb Vasc Biol* 2001, 21:844-848.

[47] Fibrinogen Studies Collaboration: Plasma fibrinogen level and the risk of major cardiovascular diseases and nonvascular mortality: an individual participant metaanalysis. *JAMA* 2005, 294:1799-1809.

[48] Cooney M, Vartiainen E, Laatikainen T, Juolevi A, Dudina A, Graham I: Elevated resting heart rate is an independent risk factor for cardiovascular disease in healthy men and women. *Am Heart J* 2010, 159:612-619.

[49] Jackson G, Boon N, Eardley I, Kirby M, Dean J, Hackett G, Montorsi P, Montorsi F, Vlachopoulos C, Kloner R, Sharlip I, Miner M: Erectile dysfunction and coronary artery disease prediction: evidence-based guidance and consensus. *Int J Clin Pract* 2010, 64:848-857.

[50] Thompson I, Tangen C, Goodman P, Probstfield J, Moinpour C, Coltman C: Erectile dysfunction and subsequent cardiovascular disease. *JAMA* 2005, 294:2996-3002.

[51] Inman B, Sauver J, Jacobson D, McGree M, Nehra A, Lieber M, Roger V, Jacobsen S: A population-based, longitudinal study of erectile dysfunction and future coronary artery disease. *Mayo Clin Proc* 2009, 84:108-113.

[52] Araujo A, Hall S, Ganz P, Chiu G, Rosen R, Kupelian V, Travison T, McKinlay J: Does erectile dysfunction contribute to cardiovascular disease risk prediction beyond the Framingham risk score. *J Am Coll Cardiol* 2010, 55:350-356.

[53] Montorsi P, Ravagnani PM, Galli S, Rotatori F, Briganti A, Salonia A, Rigatti P, Montorsi F: The artery size hypothesis: a macrovascular link between erectile dysfunction and coronary artery disease. *Am J Cardiol* 2005, 96(Suppl):19M-23M.

[54] Michiaki Fukui, Muhei Tanaka, Hiroshi Okada, Hiroya Iwase, Yusuke Mineoka, Takafumi Senmaru, Masayoshi Ohnishi, Shin-ichi Mogami, Yoshihiro Kitagawa, Masahiro Yamazaki, Goji Hasegawa and Naoto Nakamura. Five-item version of the international index of erectile function correlated with albuminuria and subclinical atherosclerosis in men with type 2 diabetes. J Atheroscler Thromb, 2011; 18

[55] Jackson G, Rosen RC, Kloner RA, Kostis JB: The second Princeton consensus on sexual dysfunction and cardiac risk: new guidelines for sexual medicine. J Sex Med, 2006;3: 28-36

[56] Mass R, Schwedhelm E, Albsmeier J, Boger RH: The pathophysiology of erectile dysfunction related to endothelial dysfunction and mediators of vascular function. Vas Med 2002; 7: 213-215

[57] Newman AB, Sutton-Tyrell K, Vogt MT, Kuller LH; Morbidity and mortality in hypertensive adults with a low ankle/arm blood pressure index. JAMA, 1993;270: 487-489

[58] Davidson JM, Chen JJ, Crapo L, Gray GD, Greenleaf WJ, Catania JA. Hormonal changes and sexual function in aging men. J Clin Endocrinol Metab 1983;57:71-7.

[59] Harman SM, Metter EJ, Tobin JD, Pearson J, Blackman MR. Longitudinal effects of aging on serum total and free testosterone levels in healthy men. Baltimore Longitudinal Study of Aging. J Clin Endocrinol Metab 2001;86:724-31.

[60] Yassin AA, Saad F. Treatment of sexual dysfunction of hypogonadal patients with long-acting testosterone undecanoate (Nebido). World J Urol 2006;24:639-44.

[61] Yassin AA, Saad F. Improvement of sexual function in men with late-onset hypogonadism treated with testosterone only. J Sex Med 2007;4:497-501.

[62] Jae Il Kang, Byeong Kuk Ham, Mi Mi Oh, Je Jong Kim, Du Geon Moon. Correlation between Serum Total Testosterone and the AMS and IIEF Questionnaires in Patients with Erectile Dysfunction with Testosterone Deficiency Syndrome. Korean J Urol 2011;52:416-420

[63] Qawqzeh, Y., Mohd, A., Mamun, R. & Maskon, O. 2010. Photoplethysmogram Analysis of Artery Properties in Patients Presenting with Established Erectile Dysfunction. *2nd International Conference on Electronic Computer Technology (ICECT):* 165-168

[64] Fang J, Madhavan S, Cohen H, Alderman MH: Measures of blood pressure and myocardial infarction in treated hypertensive patients. J of Hypertens. 1995; 13:413–419.

[65] Amar, J. & Chamontin, B. 2007. Cardiovascular risk factors, atherosclerosis and pulse pressure. *Adv Cardiol* .44: 212-22.

[66] Patricia R. Hebert; Janet W. Rich-Edwards; JoAnn E. Manson; Paul M. Ridker; Nancy R. Cook; Gerald T. O'Connor; Julie E. Buring; Charles H. Hennekens. Height and Incidence of Cardiovascular Disease in Male Physicians. *Circulation 1993, 88:1437-1443*

[67] Palmer JR, Rosenberg L, Shapiro S. Stature and the risk of myocardial infarction in women. Am J Epidemiol. 1990;132:27-32.

[68] Walker M, Shaper AG, Phillips AN, Cook DG. Short stature, lung function and risk of a heart attack. Int J Epidemiol. 1989;18: 602-606.

[69] Bland, M. & Altman, G. 1999. Measuring agreement in method comparison studies. Statistical Methods in Medical Research 8: 135-160.

[70] Krouwer, S. 2008. Why Bland-Altman plots should use *X*, not (*Y*+*X*)/2 when *X* is a reference method. *Statistics in Medicine* 27: 778-780.

[71] Metz, E. 1978. Basic principles of ROC analysis. *Seminars in Nuclear Medicine* 8: 283-298.

[72] Zweig, H. & Campbell, G. 1993. Receiver-operating characteristic (ROC) plots: a fundamental evaluation tool in clinical medicine. *Clinical Chemistry* 39: 561-577.

[73] Griner, F., Mayewski, J., Mushlin, I. & Greenland, P. 1981. Selection and interpretation of diagnostic tests and procedures. *Annals of Internal Medicine* 94: 555-600

[74] Diamond, A. & Forrester, S. 1979. Analysis of probability as an aid in the clinical diagnosis of coronary artery disease. *N Engl J Med* 300: 1350-58 .

[75] Goldschlager, N. 1982. Use of the treadmill test in the diagnosis of coronary artery disease in patients with chest pain . *Ann InternMed* 97: 383-88.

[76] Rifkin, D. & Hood, B. 1977. Bayesian analysis of electrocardiographic exercise stress testing. *N Engl J Med* 297: 681-86

[77] David, S. & John, B. 1990. *Clinical Methods, 3rd edition. The History, Physical, and Laboratory Examinations.* Boston: Butterworths

[78] David, F. & Benjamin, R. 2002. Estimation of the area under the ROC curve. *Statist. Med*; 21: 3093–3106